Seasonal Affective Disorder

Practice and Research

Seasonal Affective Disorder
Practice and Research

Edited by

Timo Partonen
Department of Mental Health and Alcohol Research,
National Public Health Institute, Helsinki, Finland

Andres Magnusson
Research Forum and Department of Psychiatry, Ulleval Hospital,
Oslo, Norway

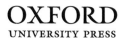
OXFORD
UNIVERSITY PRESS

OXFORD
UNIVERSITY PRESS

Great Clarendon Street, Oxford OX2 6DP

Oxford University Press is a department of the University of Oxford.
It furthers the University's objective of excellence in research, scholarship,
and education by publishing worldwide in

Oxford   New York

Athens Auckland Bangkok Bogotá Buenos Aires
Cape Town Chennai Dar es Salaam Delhi Florence Hong Kong Istanbul
Karachi Kolkata Kuala Lumpur Madrid Melbourne Mexico City Mumbai
Nairobi Paris São Paulo Shanghai Singapore Taipei Tokyo Toronto Warsaw
with associated companies in Berlin Ibadan

Oxford is a registered trade mark of Oxford University Press
in the UK and in certain other countries

Published in the United States
by Oxford University Press Inc., New York

Library of Congress Cataloging in Publication Data
Seasonal affective disorder: practice and research / edited by Timo Partonen and Andres Magnusson.
(Oxford medical publications)
Includes bibliographical references and index.
1. Seasonal affective disorder   I. Partonen, Timo. II. Magnusson, Andres. III. Series.
[DNLM: 1. Seasonal Affective Disorder. WM 171 S4388 2001]
RC545.S427 2001   616.85'27–dc21   2001021081

1 3 5 7 9 10 8 6 4 2

ISBN 0 19 263225 6 (Hbk)

Typeset by EXPO Holdings, Malaysia
Printed in Great Britain
on acid-free paper by T. J. International Ltd, Padstow, Cornwall

Preface

Man has been fascinated by the sun and the invariably changing seasons since the beginning of time. Ancient medical scripts include considerations on the variation of diseases through the seasons. Certain Greek and Roman physicians wrote on the effect of seasons and light on mental disorders such as mania and depression. Words and concepts for winter blues and depressions have also long existed in the languages spoken in the Nordic countries. However, systematic scientific enquiries into the season-bound changes in mood and behaviour are relatively recent.

A report from Dr N.E. Rosenthal and his co-authors published in the *Archives of General Psychiatry* in 1984 is considered to be the first systematic description of the syndrome called seasonal affective disorder (SAD) and its treatment with light therapy. Since this milestone, the field has been expanding rapidly. A recent literature search in eight major databases, including the MEDLINE, PSYCHLIT, and EXCERPTA MEDICA, identified over 1300 publications on SAD from 1988 to 2000. We would like to emphasize here that in this book the concept of SAD refers uniformly to the winter subtype of SAD, unless otherwise stated.

It is becoming increasingly difficult to be aware of everything that is happening in the field of winter SAD and to retain an overview of all the studies that range from epidemiology to molecular biology. This was one reason for us to embark on this project. The objective of this book is to summarize the knowledge that has been collected on winter SAD. We hope that the book will give the readers a clear overview of both research and practice and awareness of the many fascinating and relevant points of view linked to winter SAD. To aid our readers in this, the book is divided into two sections.

The first part is more clinically orientated and provides information for those involved in the care of patients. There are eleven chapters on the clinical picture, epidemiology, and treatment of winter SAD. Three 'key notes' elucidate in detail prevalence estimates from community-based studies, evidence-based data on treatment efficacy, and assessment instruments useful in everyday practice. This part of the book is aimed at a wide audience: psychiatrists, psychologists, primary care professionals, and others who work in health care settings. It may even be of value for patients who are willing to learn more about their condition, especially if they are familiar with reading scientific literature.

The second part is primarily targeted at academics and researchers working in this particular field of science. In eleven chapters on the pathogenesis of winter SAD, the authors discuss the hypotheses that have been put forward to explain the origin of the disorder and provide reviews on the experimental data both in favour of and against each theory. There are also three 'perspective notes' giving information about the key concepts and methods used in basic research on circadian clocks, with a particular reference to studies on winter SAD. The book begins with a retrospective historical glimpse and ends with a prospect on future research efforts.

Whenever a novel medical syndrome is described, it is reasonable to question its validity. Originally, we intended to include a chapter that would be critical towards the existence of

SAD and the efficacy of its treatment with light. However, since this particular field of science is becoming increasingly detailed and diverse, it would be difficult for one author to cover the topic. Therefore these items are touched upon by several contributors to the book. Readers who are especially interested in the more controversial issues of SAD are referred, for instance, to the discussions about the placebo effect in light-therapy studies (see Chapter 11), the efficacy of light visors (see Chapters 7 and 15), and the latitude gradient in the prevalence rates of SAD (see Chapter 13).

We would like to acknowledge and thank all the contributors. Our task as the editors was greatly facilitated by their swift and positive response to our initial enquiry, and thereafter by producing their manuscripts diligently and on time. We are most indebted to them as well as to all the others who have helped us with this interesting venture. Special thanks belong to Richard Marley who, on the behalf of the publisher, encouraged us throughout this project. Finally, we would like to thank our wives, Jarna and Aslaug, for bearing with us while we were immersed in the process of editing this volume.

T.P. and A.M., Helsinki and Oslo
2000

Contents

List of contributors

Janis L. Anderson
Department of Psychiatry,
Brigham and Women's Hospital,
Boston, MA,
USA.

Diane B. Boivin
Centre for Study and Treatment of Circadian
Rhythms,
Douglas Hospital,
Department of Psychiatry,
McGill University,
6875 LaSalle Boulevard,
Verdun, Quebec H4H 1R3,
Canada.
e-mail: boidia@douglas.mcgill.ca

Scott S. Campbell
Laboratory of Human Chronobiology,
Department of Psychiatry,
Cornell University Medical College,
White Plains,
New York, USA.

Nicolas Cermakian
Institut de Génétique et de Biologie Moléculaire et
Cellulaire,
CNRS–INSERM–Université Louis Pasteur,
1 rue Laurent Fries,
67404 Illkirch–Strasbourg,
France.
e-mail: paolosc@igbmc.u-strasbg.fr

Brian J. Cox
Mood Disorders Clinic,
Psychiatric Health Centre,
University of Manitoba,
PZ-430 771 Bannatyne Avenue,
Winnipeg, Manitoba,
Canada.

John M. Eagles
Mental Health Services,
Grampian Primary Care NHS Trust,
Royal Cornhill Hospital,
Aberdeen, UK.

Charmane I. Eastman
Biological Rhythms Research Laboratory,
Rush–Presbyterian St Luke's Medical Center,
Chicago, Illinois, USA.

Murray W. Enns
Mood Disorders Clinic,
Psychiatric Health Centre,
University of Manitoba,
PZ-430 771 Bannatyne Avenue,
Winnipeg, Manitoba,
Canada.
e-mail: menns@cc.umanitoba.ca

Mary–Anne Enoch
Laboratory of Neurogenetics,
National Institute on Alcohol Abuse and
Alcoholism,
National Institutes of Health,
12420 Parklawn Drive, Park 5 Building,
Room 451, MSC 8110,
Bethesda, MD 20892-8110,
USA.
e-mail: maenoch@dicbr.niaaa.nih.gov

David Goldman
Laboratory of Neurogenetics,
National Institute on Alcohol Abuse and
Alcoholism,
National Institutes of Health,
12420 Parklawn Drive, Park 5 Building,
Room 451, MSC 8110,
Bethesda, MD 20892-8110,
USA.

Christian Grimm
Department of Ophthalmology,
University Hospital Zürich,
8091 Zürich,
Switzerland.

Andreas Habeler
Department of General Psychiatry,
University of Vienna,
Währinger Gürtel 18–20,
A-1090 Vienna, Austria.

Farhad Hafezi
Department of Ophthalmology,
University Hospital Zürich,
8091 Zürich,
Switzerland.

Barbara Heßelmann
Department of General Psychiatry,
University of Vienna,
Währinger Gürtel 18–20,
A-1090 Vienna, Austria.

Eva Hilger
Department of General Psychiatry,
University of Vienna,
Währinger Gürtel 18–20,
A-1090 Vienna, Austria.

Siegfried Kasper
Department of General Psychiatry,
University of Vienna,
Währinger Gürtel 18–20,
A-1090 Vienna, Austria.
e-mail: SK@akh-wien.ac.at

Bengt F. Kjellman
Department of Psychiatry,
Institution for Clinical Neuroscience,
Karolinska Institute at St Göran's Hospital,
Stockholm, Sweden

Anastasios Konstantinidis
Department of General Psychiatry,
University of Vienna,
Währinger Gürtel 18–20,
A-1090 Vienna, Austria.

Kurt Kräuchi
Chronobiology and Sleep Laboratory,
Psychiatric University Clinic,
University of Basel,
Wilhelm–Klein–Strasse 27,
CH-4025 Basel,
Switzerland.

Megan R. Leahy
Department of Psychiatry,
VA CT Healthcare System and Yale University,
Mail Stop 116A,
950 Campbell Avenue,
West Haven, CT 06516,
USA.

Andres Magnusson
Research Forum and Department of Psychiatry,
Ullevål Hospital,
0407 Oslo, Norway.
e-mail: andres.magnusson@psykiatri.uio.no

Ybe Meesters
Department of Biological Psychiatry,
University Hospital Groningen,
P.O. Box 30001,
9700 RB Groningen,
The Netherlands.

Peter Paul A. Mersch
Department of Biological Psychiatry,
University Hospital Groningen,
P.O. Box 30001,
9700 RB Groningen,
The Netherlands.

Patricia J. Murphy
Laboratory of Human Chronobiology,
Department of Psychiatry,
Cornell University Medical College,
White Plains, New York,
USA.

Greg Murray
Department of Psychology,
University of Melbourne,
Parkville,
Victoria, Australia.

Alexander Neumeister
Department of General Psychiatry,
University of Vienna,
Währinger Gürtel 18–20,
A-1090 Vienna, Austria.
e-mail: alexander.neumeister@akh-wien.ac.at

Dan A. Oren
Department of Psychiatry,
VA CT Healthcare System and Yale University,
Mail Stop 116A, 950 Campbell Avenue,
West Haven, CT 06516,
USA.

Timo Partonen
Department of Mental Health and Alcohol
Research,
National Public Health Institute,
Mannerheimintie 166,
FIN-00300 Helsinki, Finland.
e-mail: timo.partonen@ktl.fi

Nicole Praschak–Rieder
Department of General Psychiatry,
University of Vienna,
Währinger Gürtel 1820,
A-1090 Vienna, Austria.

Martin R. Ralph
Departments of Psychology and Zoology,
University of Toronto,
100 St George Street,
Toronto, Ontario M5S 3GS,
Canada.

Ted Reichborn–Kjennerud
Psychiatric Institute,
University of Oslo,
Postbox 85,
Vinderen, N-0319 Oslo,
Norway.
e-mail: ted.reichborn-kjennerud@psykiatri.uio.no

Charlotte E. Remé
Department of Ophthalmology,
University Hospital Zürich,
8091 Zürich,
Switzerland.
e-mail: chreme@opht.unizh.ch

Norman E. Rosenthal
NIMH, National Institutes of Health,
Bethesda, MD,
USA.

Paolo SassoneCorsi
Institut de Génétique et de Biologie Moléculaire et
Cellulaire,
CNRS–INSERM–Université Louis Pasteur,
1 rue Laurent Fries,
67404 Illkirch–Strasbourg,
France.

David S. Schlager
Department of Psychiatry,
SUNY at Stony Brook,
Stony Brook, New York,
USA.

Colin M. Shapiro
Sleep and Alertness Clinic,
Department of Psychiatry,
The Toronto Hospital (Western Division),
Toronto, Ontario,
Canada.

Jianhua Shen
Sleep and Alertness Clinic,
Department of Psychiatry,
The Toronto Hospital (Western Division),
Toronto, Ontario,
Canada.

Jürgen Stastny
Department of General Psychiatry,
University of Vienna,
Währinger Gürtel 18–20,
A-1090 Vienna
Austria.

Michael Terman
Department of Psychiatry,
Columbia University,
New York State Psychiatric Institute,
New York, NY 10032,
USA.

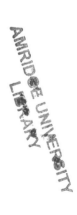

Chris Thompson
Department of Mental Health,
Royal South Hants Hospital,
Brinton's Terrace,
Southampton SO14 0YG, UK.

Russell G. Vasile
Department of Psychiatry,
Beth Israel Deaconess Medical Center,
Boston, MA, USA.

Andreas Wenzel
Department of Ophthalmology,
University Hospital Zürich,
8091 Zürich, Switzerland.

Matthäus Willeit
Department of General Psychiatry,
University of Vienna,
Währinger Gürtel 18–20,
A-1090 Vienna, Austria.

Janet B.W. Williams
Department of Psychiatry,
Columbia University,
New York State Psychiatric Institute,
New York, NY 10032,
USA.

Anna Wirz–Justice
Chronobiology and Sleep Laboratory,
Psychiatric University Clinic,
University of Basel,
Wilhelm–Klein–Strasse 27,
CH-4025 Basel,
Switzerland.

Michael A. Young
Institute of Psychology,
Illinois Institute of Technology,
Chicago, Illinois,
USA.

Part one

Chapter 1

Historical excerpts

Andres Magnusson

1.1 Ancient to modern times

Even some 4700 years ago, Wong Tai (cited by McCartney 1962) mentioned the variation of diseases with the seasons. Later, Hippocrates (quoted by Zilboorg 1941) wrote on the relationship between seasonal climatic conditions and manias and melancholias. Posidonius, in the fourth century AD, observed that mania is an intermittent disease that repeats itself once a year or more often, and he thought that melancholia occurred primarily in autumn and mania in summer (cited in Roccatagliata 1986). According to Eastwood (Eastwood and Peter 1988), Celsus thought that melancholia, madness, and epilepsy were at their peak in spring (Celsus 1838). Aretaeus, in the second century AD, recommended that 'lethargics are to be laid in the light and exposed to the rays of the sun' (reprinted 1856). In modern times, the seasonal variation in mental disorders has been studied by examining such parameters as suicide, prescription of antidepressive medication, administration of electroconvulsive therapy, and admission for mood disorders. Wehr and Rosenthal (1989), Eastwood (1988), Thompson (1989), Carney *et al.* (1989), and others have reviewed these studies.

1.2 Early cases of SAD

There are many early descriptions of psychiatric patients who, in retrospect, were probably suffering from SAD. In 1825, the French psychiatrist Esquirol, as quoted by Rosenthal (1989), described a patient from Belgium who for three successive winters had suffered a depressive episode which had lifted in spring. Esquirol advised the patient to spend the following winter in Italy, and his winter depression proved to be much milder there (Esquirol 1845).

In 1923, the British psychiatrist, J.G. Porter, wrote:

> ... it is obvious what a stimulating and beneficial influence artificial sunlight can exert on those whose fund of energy is seriously depleted by nervous or mental disorder, especially during the dull, sunless, and depressing months of our British winter ... several mental institutions have already installed apparatus for the production of artificial sunlight. (Quoted in Rosenthal 1993*a*)

In 1946, Dr G. Frumkes described a patient who today would seem to be suffering from typical SAD (cited by Rosenthal 1993*a*). In the same year, the German physician, Hellmut Marx, reported the use of bright artificial light to treat four men who had become depressed during an Arctic winter (Marx 1946). To quote Rosenthal (1993*a*):

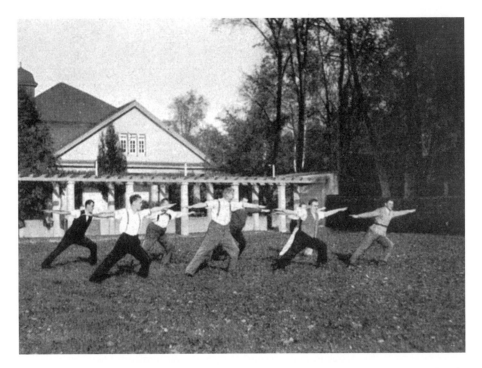

Fig. 1.1 Time-givers I; physical exercise. Patients doing gymnastics at the Psychiatric University Clinic in Basle, Switzerland in the 1930s. Source: Photo Archive, Psychiatric University Clinic Basel.

> Marx's work was impressive in that he recognised the recurrent nature of winter depression and even described the overeating that often accompanies the condition. Not only did he identify light deficiency as a trigger for this condition — and bright light as a treatment — but he also correctly suggested that light acted via the eyes to influence the hypothalamus.

However, Marx's report remained unknown to psychiatrists until very recently and had little influence on the course of events in psychiatric research and treatment.

1.3 **Scandinavia**

Throughout the ages the aborigines of North America, Greenland, Siberia, and northern Scandinavia have lived in closest encounter with the arctic winters. Unfortunately, we know little of how these people were affected mentally by the long winter, nor do we know if they applied any specific means to cope with it. Apart from these aborigines, the inhabitants of the Nordic countries are perhaps those who have wrestled hardest with the arctic winter. Professor Wetterberg has written that a thesis entitled 'On winter diseases' was published from the Uppsala University in Sweden in 1762 (see Rosenthal 1991). This thesis mentions that individuals with melancholia find it especially difficult to cope with the cold Swedish winter. Niels Finsen (1860–1904), who lived in Iceland, the Faeroe Islands, and Denmark, was awarded a Nobel Prize for his studies on the effect of light on various skin diseases. Finsen was said to have become interested in the therapeutic effect of light when he was a student in Reykjavik and noted that his concentration improved when he would read his books by the window. Finsen suffered from Pick's disease and wrote:

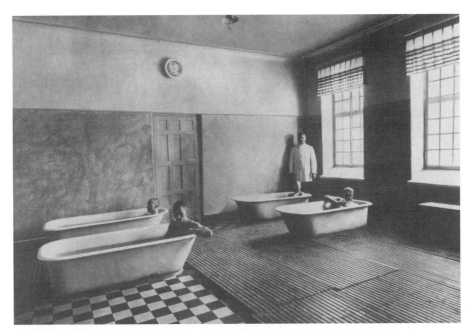

Fig. 1.2 Time-givers II: hot baths. Patients taking a bath at the Municipal Mental Hospital in Turku, Finland in 1912. Source: Department and Museum of Medical History, University of Helsinki.

I suffered from anaemia and tiredness, and since I lived in a house facing the north, I began to believe that I might be helped if I received more sun. (*http://www.nobel.se/laureates/medicine-1903-1-bi o.html*)

There are words for winter depression in both Icelandic and Swedish that are in common use. The Icelandic word is 'skammdegisthunglyndi' — 'Skamm' means short, 'degi' is day, 'thung' is heavy, and 'lyndi' means mood. Thus, 'skammdegisthunglyndi' means literally the heavy mood of the short days. The large heritage of literature in Icelandic includes the Icelandic sagas that were written some 800 years ago, which contain several descriptions of psychological phenomena (Høyersten 1998). There is for instance a description of treatment for depression consisting of regular interviews focusing on the traumatic event that triggered the depression (cited in Ivars thattur Ingimundarsonar 1999). In spite of this, the word 'skammdegisthunglyndi', or the related word 'skammdegisdrungi' (where 'drungi' means gloom), is not found in print until 1892 (Bjarnason 1892).

The Swedish word for winter depression is 'Lappsjuka'. 'Lapp' is the Scandinavian word for the aborigines of northern Scandinavia who live in Lapland and 'sjuka' means sickness. Interestingly, this word does not describe a condition of the Lapps but a state that those who come from the southern regions of Sweden experience when they travel north to Lapland in winter. The oldest citations of the word 'Lappsjuka', found in the University Library of Lund, Sweden, are from 1924. One of the two citations is by the well-known physicist Ångstrøm, who was a pioneer in the study of light and after whom the unit for wavelength of light (Å) is named. Ångstrøm wrote:

We are all dependent of light for our well being .... Many people are very sensitive to the lack of light while others are less so. The former will in arctic winters suffer from Lappsjuka. (Ångstrøm 1924)

Ångstrøm went on to ask:

> What quantity of light is necessary for an organism? Can the natural light emission be superseded by other means? In that case, how should the artificial irradiation be composed and how should it be administered? (op. cit.)

The Finns also have a word for winter depression — 'ruskavastavaikutus'. 'Ruskea' means brown (the derivation of that word is 'ruska' which denotes the colours of autumn) and 'vastavaikutus' means reaction. Thus 'ruskavastavaikutus' means the reaction that people experience in autumn. Väisänen *et al.* (1973) studied psychiatric reactions in northern and southern parts of Finland during spring and autumn 1970/71. They found higher prevalence of depression in autumn at the more northern location. They wrote:

> When the Ruska begins, the Lappish population seems to develop mental depression ... It is replaced with a slower pace of living during the long, dark winter. During the Ruska the persons are more sensitive because of the two or three months' light period already left behind, during which people are very active, stay awake a lot, as well as use up a great amount of energy. It is a slightly euphoric period. (Condensed from Väisänen *et al.* 1973)

Particularly interesting is the implication that depression in winter can be avoided by 'returning to a slower pace of living' or spending 'hämäränhyssyä', as commonly expressed in Finnish.

The English term 'cabin fever' is described in *Webster's Dictionary* (1966) as extreme irritability and restlessness resulting from living in isolation or within an confined indoor area for a prolonged time. Although cabin fever might have an element of SAD in it, it does not specifically refer to darkness, winter, nor depression.

1.4 **The present day history**

In the late 1970s and 1980s there was a growing interest in the relationship between biological rhythms and mood disorders. It was known that both circadian and annual rhythms in animals could be manipulated by light. Furthermore, the secretion in animals of the hormone melatonin, which is produced in the pineal gland, could be suppressed by light. However, it was not until 1980 that Lewy *et al.* showed that melatonin secretion could also be suppressed in humans, provided the light intensity was high enough (Lewy *et al.* 1980). Already in 1978, it was hypothesized that the seasonal pattern of mania and depression might be linked to seasonal behavioural rhythms, which in turn might be based on hours of daylight (Kripke *et al.* 1978). The first placebo controlled light treatment trial for depression was published in 1981 (Kripke 1981). However, the pieces did not start to fall into place until researchers realized that light treatment might not be helpful for all types of depression, but rather for a specific subtype of depression. But how did that occur?

An important step towards this end was the contribution of a patient named Herbert E. Kern. He had noted that every year he would become depressed in the autumn, and his depression would lift as the days lengthened again. Kern had kept a detailed diary of his seasonal mood swings (Rosenthal *et al.* 1983). He had suspected that they had something to do with light, and discussed this with his psychiatrist, Dr Peter S. Mueller. Later, Kern contacted a group at the National Institute of Mental Health (NIMH) after he had learned of their work with melatonin and light. Light therapy was administered when his depression recurred the following autumn, for three hours before dawn and three hours after dusk, thus simulating the long days of summer. It proved to be successful and the experiment was published in 1982 (Lewy *et al.* 1982). Subsequently, another patient with recurrent depression in winter and remissions in summer, was treated with bright lights, with favourable results.

These findings encouraged the NIMH group to search for more patients with this condition, which at that time was thought to be very rare. A short article describing the symptoms was published in the *Washington Post*, asking those with similar symptoms to contact the NIMH group. To the scientists' surprise, as many as two thousand people responded to the notice. The story of these individuals was strikingly similar, 'as if they had been cloned' (Rosenthal 1993*a*). Some of these patients were subsequently carefully studied. That led to a publication in the *Archives of General Psychiatry* in 1984, describing the characteristics of winter depression (SAD) and its treatment with light (Rosenthal *et al.* 1984). This article, by Rosenthal and colleagues, is generally considered to mark the birth of the modern era of SAD research; it has become a 'citation classic' (Rosenthal 1993*b*).

Many members of the NIMH group have moved to other parts of the USA and overseas to continue the research, and several other scientific groups have participated. However, the NIMH group, led by Dr Norman E. Rosenthal, has always played a leading role in SAD research. As of today, close to 1000 scientific articles have been published from all the corners of the world, describing different aspects of the disease and its treatment.

Acknowledgements

Several authors have written historical overviews on the history of SAD (Eastwood 1988; Wehr and Rosenthal 1989; Rosenthal 1989, 1997; Wetterberg 1993; Lam 1998). This overview has particularly borrowed from Rosenthal's book *Winter Blues* (1993a).

References

Ångstrøm, A. (1924) Studier over Sveriges straalingsklima. *Ymer* **44(1)**:1–23.

Anonymous (1999) Ivars thattur Ingimundarsonar. In: *Islendingasøgur, urval threttan thatta med inngangi, skyringum og skram* (ed. B. Halldorsson and K. Hafsteinsson). Mal og menning, Reykjavik.

Aretaeus (trans. 1856) *The extant works of Aretaeus, the Cappadocian.* Sydenham Society, London.

Bjarnason, B. (1892) Um husabaetur. *Bunadarritid* **42**.

Carney, P., Fitzgerald, C., and Monaghan, C. (1989) Seasonal variations in mania. In: Thompson C, Silverstone T, editors. *Seasonal affective disorder* (ed. C. Thompson and T. Silverstone) p. 278. CNS Publishers, London.

Celsus (trans. 1838) *Of medicine.* H. Renshaw Publishers, UK.

Eastwood, M.R. and Peter, A.M. (1988) Epidemiology and seasonal affective disorder. *Psychological Medicine* **18(4)**:799–806.

Esquirol, J. (1845) *Mental maladies: a treatise of insanity* pp. 31–3. Lea & Blanchard, Philadelphia.

Høyersten, J.G. (1998) *Personlighet og avvik: en studie i islendingesagaens menneskebilde, med særlig vekt på Njála.* University of Bergen.

http://www.nobel.se/laureates/medicine-19031-bio.html

Kripke, D.F., Mullaney D.J., Atkinson, M., and Wolf, S. (1978) Circadian rhythm disorders in manic-depressives. *Biological Psychiatry* **13(3)**:335–51.

Kripke, D. (1981) *Photoperiodic mechanisms for depression and its treatment.* Elsevier, Amsterdam.

Lam, R. (1998) *Seasonal affective disorder and beyond: light treatment for SAD and non-SAD conditions.* American Psychiatric Press, Washington DC.

Lewy, A.J., Wehr, T.A., Goodwin, F.K., Newsome, D.A., and Markey, S.P. (1980) Light suppresses melatonin secretion in humans. *Science* **210(4475)**:1267–9.

Lewy, A.J., Kern, H.A., Rosenthal, N.E., and Wehr, T.A. (1982) Bright artificial light treatment of a manic-depressive patient with a seasonal mood cycle. *American Journal of Psychiatry* **139**(11):1496–8.

Marx, H. (1946) 'Hypophysare Insuffizienz' bei Lichtmangel. *Klin Wochenschr* **24/25**:18–21.

McCartney, J. (1962) Seasonal variation in psychiatric illness. *Psychosomatics* **3**:312–16.

Roccatagliata, G. (1986) *History of ancient psychiatry.* Greenwood Press Inc., Westport.

Rosenthal, N. (1989) Letter. *Archives of General Psychiatry* **46**:194–5.

Rosenthal, N. (1991) *Ljus mot själens mörker: om orsakerna till årstidsbundna depressioner och hur de kan behandlas.* Bonniers, Stockholm.

Rosenthal, N. (1993*a*) *Winter blues: seasonal affective disorder, what it is and how to overcome it.* Guilford, New York.

Rosenthal, N. (1993*b*) This week's citational classic: a decade of SAD and light therapy. *Current Contents* **10**(8):March 8.

Rosenthal, N.E., Lewy, A.J., Wehr, T.A., Kern, H.E., and Goodwin, F.K. (1983) Seasonal cycling in a bipolar patient. *Psychiatry Research* **8**(1):25–31.

Rosenthal, N.E., Sack, D.A., Gillin, J.C., Lewy, A.J., Goodwin, F.K., Davenport, Y., *et al.* (1984) Seasonal affective disorder: a description of the syndrome and preliminary findings with light therapy. *Archives of General Psychiatry* **41**(1):72–80.

Thompson, C. (1989) Seasonality of depression. In: Thompson C, Silverstone T, editors. *Seasonal affective disorder* (ed. C. Thompson and T. Silverstone) pp. 1–18. CNS Publishers, London.

Väisänen, E., Lehtinen, V., and Rantanen, R. (1973) The 'Ruska' reaction: the effect of the seasonal alternation on the Lappish person. *Psychiatria Fennica* **4**:67–9.

Webster's Third New International Dictionary (1966). William Benton, Chicago.

Wehr, T.A. and Rosenthal, N.E. (1989) Seasonality and affective illness. *American Journal of Psychiatry* **146**(7):829–39.

Wetterberg, L. (1993) *Light and biological rhythms in man.* Pergamon Press, Oxford.

Zilboorg, G. (1941) *A history of medical psychology.* W.W. Norton & Co., New York.

Clinical picture

Chapter 2

Symptoms and course of illness

Timo Partonen and Norman E. Rosenthal

2.1 Introduction

SAD was originally defined as a syndrome in which depression developed during autumn or winter and remitted the following spring or summer for at least two successive years (Rosenthal *et al.* 1984). In addition, the SAD patient had to show a history of major depressive or bipolar disorder (see Table 2.1). Since then, two subtypes of SAD have been described in the literature: winter SAD and summer SAD, of which the former is far more frequent. Subsyndromal SAD is a condition with similar but milder symptoms that do not impair functioning to a major degree (Table 2.2). The tendency to experience seasonal changes in mood and behaviour (also known as seasonality) is manifested to a different degree in individuals, ranging from the extreme and

Table 2.1 Original criteria for SAD (Rosenthal *et al.* 1984)

- A history of major affective disorder, according to the Research Diagnostic Criteria (Spitzer *et al.* 1978).
- At least 2 consecutive years in which the depressive episodes had developed during the autumn or winter and remitted during the following spring or summer.
- Absence of any other Axis I mental disorder, according to the DSM-III (American Psychiatric Association 1980).
- Absence of any clear-cut, seasonally changing psychosocial factors that would account for the seasonal variation in mood and behaviour.

Table 2.2 Operational criteria for subsyndromal SAD (Kasper *et al.* 1989)

- A history of some difficulty during the winter months occurring on a regular basis (at least 2 consecutive winters) and lasting for a sustained period of time (at least 4 weeks). For example, decreased energy, decreased efficiency at work (concentration, completing tasks), decreased creativity or interest in socializing, and change in eating habit (eating more carbohydrates), weight (gaining weight), or sleep patterns (more sleep).
- Subjects have to regard themselves as normal — not suffering from an illness or a disorder.
- Subjects have not sought medical or psychological help specifically for the above difficulties, nor has anyone else suggested that they should do so.
- People who do not know them well do not recognize that they have a problem, or if they do, easily attribute it to circumstances such as 'flu' or 'overwork'.
- The symptoms experienced by the subjects have not disrupted their functioning to a major degree (for example, calling in sick several times per winter or severe marital discord).
- No history of major affective disorder in wintertime.
- No serious medical illness.

pathological end of the spectrum (namely patients with SAD), through the mildly pathological (as in subsyndromal SAD), to the normal.

2.2 Assessment of diagnosis

The original conceptualizations of SAD were eventually transformed into diagnostic criteria based on the *Diagnostic and Statistical Manual of Mental Disorders*. They were first published in 1987 (Table 2.3). In the latest version of this series of classifications, DSM-IV (American Psychiatric Association 1994), SAD is regarded as a specifier of either bipolar or recurrent major depressive disorder, with a seasonal pattern of major depressive episodes (codes 296.30 to 296.89; see Table 2.4).

The *ICD-10 Classification of Mental and Behavioural Disorders* gives only provisional diagnostic criteria for SAD on the grounds that its status is best regarded as uncertain (World Health Organization 1993). Subject to these reservations, SAD is recognized as a form of bipolar affective or recurrent depressive disorder, with episodes varying in degrees of severity (codes F31.0 to F31.9 or F33.0 to F33.9; see Table 2.5).

There are particular variations of these conditions with the seasonal pattern. They include recurrent affective disorders with a seasonal component that is not quite regular enough to

Table 2.3 Diagnostic criteria for the seasonal pattern specifier of mood disorders as defined by DSM-III-R (American Psychiatric Association 1987)

- There has been a regular temporal relationship between the onset of an episode of bipolar disorder (including bipolar disorder NOS) or recurrent major depression (including depressive disorder NOS) and a particular 60-day period of the year (for example, regular appearance of depression between the beginning of October and the end of November). **Note**: do not include cases in which there is an obvious effect of seasonally related psychosocial stressors (for example, regularly being unemployed every winter).
- Full remissions (or a change from depression to mania or hypomania) also occurred with a particular 60-day period of the year (for example, depression disappears from mid-February to mid-April).
- There have been at least 3 episodes of mood disturbance in 3 separate years that demonstrated the temporal seasonal relationship defined in the two criteria above; at least 2 of the years were consecutive.
- Seasonal episodes of mood disturbance, as described above, outnumbered any non-seasonal episodes of such disturbance that may have occurred by more than 3 to 1.

Table 2.4 Diagnostic criteria for the seasonal pattern specifier of mood disorders as defined by DSM-IV (American Psychiatric Association 1994)

- There has been a regular temporal relationship between the onset of major depressive episodes in bipolar I or bipolar II disorder or major depressive disorder, recurrent, and a particular time of the year (for example, regular appearance of the major depressive episode in the autumn or winter). **Note**: do not include cases in which there is an obvious effect of seasonal-related psychosocial stressors (for example, regularly being unemployed every winter).
- Full remissions (or a change from depression to mania or hypomania) also occur at a characteristic time of the year (for example, depression disappears in the spring).
- In the last 2 years, 2 major depressive episodes have occurred that demonstrate the temporal seasonal relationships defined in the two criteria above, and no non-seasonal major depressive episodes have occurred during that same period.
- Seasonal major depressive episodes (as described above) substantially outnumber the non-seasonal major depressive episodes that may have occurred over the individual's lifetime.

Table 2.5 Diagnostic criteria for research on SAD as defined by ICD-10 (World Health Organization 1993)

- Three or more episodes of mood (affective) disorder must occur, with onset within the same 90-day period of the year, for 3 or more consecutive years.
- Remissions also occur within a particular 90-day period of the year.
- Seasonal episodes substantially outnumber any non-seasonal episodes that may occur.

meet the criteria for SAD, subsyndromal SAD that is not quite severe enough to meet the criteria for SAD, and dysthymia with seasonal symptom exacerbation. These conditions may respond to some of the same modes of treatment, light therapy in specific, that benefit patients with winter SAD.

2.3 **Symptoms**

Clinical features associated with winter SAD are rather consistent across diverse series of patients from industrialised cultures (see Table 2.6). A characteristic of cardinal importance is the response to light exposure in the patient's history. This might manifest as mood

Table 2.6 Symptoms and signs in patients with winter SAD[a]

Frequent	%
• Sadness	96
• Decreased activity	96
• Social misfortune[b]	92
• Anxiety	86
• Irritability[b]	86
• Occupational misfortune	84
• Daytime tiredness[b]	81
Fairly frequent	%
• Increased sleep	76
• Poor quality of sleep[b]	75
• Increased weight	74
• Carbohydrate craving	70
• Decreased libido	68
• Increased appetite	65
Fairly infrequent	%
• Suicidal thoughts[c]	35
• Decreased sleep[c]	31
Infrequent	%
• Mixed or no change in appetite[b]	17
• Mixed or no change in weight[b]	17
• Decreased appetite	15
• Decreased weight	7
• Mixed or no change in sleep[c]	5
• No change in activity[c]	2

[a] Data are derived from the NIMH Seasonal Studies Program (N = 662)
[b] As [a] except for N = 366
[c] N = 46 from the Seasonal Mood Clinic at the University Hospital-UBC Site (Lam *et al.* 1989)

improvement when travelling to different regions during the winter, when living at different latitudes, when living or working in homes or offices with different levels of ambient lighting, or as reactions to spells of poor weather conditions even during the summertime. For example, most patients (94 per cent) have reported that travel to latitudes nearer the equator resulted in remission or at least a marked diminution of their symptoms.

A majority of patients develop, in addition to depressed mood, so-called atypical depressive symptoms (increased duration of sleep, increased appetite, weight gain, and carbohydrate craving) that are in fact common in winter SAD (Tam *et al.* 1997). These symptoms may frequently precede impaired functioning (Young *et al.* 1991). A minority of patients report the more typical symptoms of eating less, sleeping less, and losing weight. In addition to these vegetative symptoms, patients may suffer from more general symptoms of depression including diminished interest or pleasure, psychomotor agitation or retardation, fatigue or loss of energy, feelings of worthlessness or excessive or inappropriate guilt, diminished ability to think or concentrate, indecisiveness, and recurrent thoughts of death. A somatic symptom such as pain is often the presenting complaint at visits to general practice.

Despite the presence of physical symptoms, medical examination and laboratory studies are routinely normal in winter SAD, and the diagnosis therefore rests on the patient's history. Patients with winter SAD have less frequently suicidal ideation and morning worsening of mood than those with non-seasonal affective disorder. A family history of affective disorders, alcohol-related disorders, and SAD itself is common in the patient's first-degree relatives (Allen *et al.* 1993). Winter SAD is also seen in children who usually present with fatigue, irritability, sleep inertia, and school problems. Such children tend to attribute the cause of their problems to the external world (of family and school) rather than having insight into their symptoms (Swedo *et al.* 1995).

The impairment of functioning associated with winter SAD is often worse than that related to most chronic medical conditions (Schlager *et al.* 1995). Despite the depressive episodes seldom being severe enough to require absence from work, most patients with winter SAD do experience disability at work and in their social relations. Frequent symptoms, such as daytime tiredness and fatigue, are of concern not only for work performance but also for public safety, as they may adversely affect, for example, driving ability. Hence, the effort put into the detection and treatment of winter SAD seems justified in primary and occupational health care settings.

Depressive episodes typically begin during autumn, usually in September to November, depending on the latitude of residence. Untreated, these episodes generally resolve by the following spring, in most cases by February to April, although some individuals do not fully recover before the early summer (Lingjærde and Foreland 1999). Some patients have also reported short periods of depressed mood recurring during the summer if levels of ambient light are reduced for any reason such as poor weather conditions. In summer, some individuals may, in addition, experience a reversal of their symptoms, including affective periods with elation, increased libido, improved social activity and energy, and decreased need for sleep, reduced appetite, and loss of weight; manic episodes of bipolar disorder occur relatively seldom (5 per cent of cases) (Lingjærde and Reichborn–Kjennerud 1993). However, less severe hypomanic episodes are not infrequent in patients with winter SAD (34 per cent of cases). There is also a fair amount of hyperthymia that, although not sufficiently severe to qualify as hypomania, may nevertheless be clinically relevant.

The prolonged duration of the depressive episodes (5 to 6 months on average) distinguishes SAD from the so-called 'holiday blues', a short-lived reaction to psychosocial stresses that typically occur around the holiday season. The recurrent depressive episodes are not primarily attributable to a regularly recurring psychosocial stress, such as winter unemployment, though such distress may certainly exacerbate symptoms.

Depressive episodes are usually mild to moderate in severity, but about 10 per cent of patients have needed hospitalization and 2 per cent have been given electroconvulsive treatment due to severe depressive episodes. Judging from the statistics, patients with winter SAD seldom have psychotic symptoms or are at risk of suicide. However, this fact should not give too much reassurance to clinicians; patients suffering from a depressive episode, regardless of the primary diagnosis, need to be monitored carefully for emerging suicidal thoughts.

2.4 **Course of illness**

The onset of winter SAD typically occurs between 20 and 30 years of age, but the affected subject does not usually seek psychiatric attention for some years (Thompson and Isaacs 1988). Many subjects may in fact be more distressed by the decreased activity and fatigue than by the mood changes, and therefore will often initially seek the help of a physician rather than a psychiatrist. Many patients suffer from either more severe or longer episodes with time (Wirz–Justice *et al.* 1986). The course of illness is however variable, with some patients retaining their fundamentally seasonal pattern, others developing a more complicated course characterized by non-seasonal as well as seasonal episodes, and yet others appearing to remit.

After periods of 5 to 11 years since the initial diagnosis, less than half (22 to 42 per cent) of patients were still routinely suffering from winter SAD, as assessed by structured clinical interviews and collateral records, while over a third (33 to 44 per cent) had developed a non-seasonal pattern to subsequent episodes. Of the remaining patients, about 6 per cent had subsyndromal SAD or the disorder resolved completely (14 to 18 per cent). Since these data are derived from follow-up after treatment rather than from studying the natural course of the syndrome, it is unclear to what degree they reflect instability in the illness itself as opposed to the influence of treatment and awareness of the nature of the condition.

Data collected from case records and research diagnostic interviews suggest that the appearance of non-seasonal depressive episodes is associated with greater severity of the illness and poorer response to light, and bright-light therapy, while remaining as the treatment of choice for many, may be insufficient for more severely ill patients (Schwartz *et al.* 1996). A short duration of the index episode and a high frequency of episodes are linked to a continuing seasonal course of illness (Thompson *et al.* 1995), and the occurrence of atypical depressive symptoms is the best predictor of season-bound recurrence (Sakamoto *et al.* 1993, 1995). The age at onset of winter SAD or length of the disease history could not be identified as predictors of the subsequent course of illness in follow-up of 2 to 8 years (Leonhardt *et al.* 1994; Graw *et al.* 1997). According to these studies, there is a marked proportion of patients who recover completely with time, and winter SAD cannot be regarded as a prodromal or premature form of a more chronic or more severe affective disorder.

After all, SAD is a condition that is strongly influenced by behaviour, for example, how much time the individual chooses to spend outdoors or actively seeks light exposure. Therefore, awareness of the condition and the individual's behavioural response to it would be expected to affect its course and a favourable outcome can be due to either true recovery or simply good symptom control.

2.5 **Comorbid conditions**

Mixed conditions often compromise the search and recognition of winter SAD, and each may require specific intervention (see the chapter by Reichborn–Kjennerud). A number of bulimic patients suffer from seasonal depressive symptoms (Lam *et al.* 1991). Some data indicate that patients with winter SAD and those with bulimia nervosa have similar attitudes towards eating, reflected as distorted perceptions of body size and shape, but opposite styles of eating (low versus high scores of restraint eating behaviours respectively) (Berman *et al.* 1993; Kräuchi *et al.* 1997). Interestingly, whereas healthy subjects report sedation after ingestion of carbohydrates, depressed winter SAD patients experience activation and are less sensitive to the sweet taste (Rosenthal *et al.* 1989; Arbisi *et al.* 1996). Resting metabolic rates may also be increased in depressed winter SAD patients secondary to changes in appetite and caloric intake (Gaist *et al.* 1990).

The lifetime prevalence of anxiety disorders in patients with winter SAD is also high, though not different from the rate seen in non-seasonal recurrent major depression, and generalized anxiety disorder, simple phobias, and social phobia are among the most prevalent comorbid disorders (Levitt *et al.* 1993). It may well be that none of the key symptoms of winter SAD is the presenting complaint nor of principal concern in those patients with comorbid conditions. In such cases, the clinical picture needs to be assessed with taking a detailed history and monitoring the patient during short-interval visits before tailoring a specific intervention.

2.6 **Conclusion**

Winter SAD constitutes a group of patients with more atypical than classical symptoms of depression. The course of illness is characterized by recurrent depressive episodes that coincide with reduced hours of daylight during the winter season and disappear in summer. Since special investigations at present are uninformative, the diagnosis of winter SAD is based on the patient's history. Comorbid conditions influence the clinical picture of winter SAD by modulating the course of illness and make the diagnosis of winter SAD more difficult, particularly in patients presenting with non-specific complaints such as lack of energy, pain, and fatigue during the winter months.

References

Allen, J.M., Lam, R.W., Remick, R.A., and Sadovnick, A.D. (1993) Depressive symptoms and family history in seasonal and nonseasonal mood disorders. *Am J Psychiatry* **150**:443–8.

American Psychiatric Association (1980) *Diagnostic and statistical manual of mental disorders: DSM-III* (3rd edn). American Psychiatric Press, Washington DC.

American Psychiatric Association (1987) *Diagnostic and statistical manual of mental disorders: DSM-III-R* (3rd edn revised). American Psychiatric Press, Washington DC.

American Psychiatric Association (1994) *Diagnostic and statistical manual of mental disorders: DSM-IV* (4th edn). American Psychiatric Press, Washington DC.

Arbisi, P.A., Levine, A.S., Nerenberg, J., and Wolf, J. (1996) Seasonal alteration in taste detection and recognition threshold in seasonal affective disorder: the proximate source of carbohydrate craving. *Psychiatry Res* **59**:171–82.

Berman, K., Lam, R.W., and Goldner, E.M. (1993) Eating attitudes in seasonal affective disorder and bulimia nervosa. *J Affect Disord* **29**:219–25.

Gaist, P.A., Obarzanek, E., Skwerer, R.G., Duncan, C.C., Shultz, P.M., and Rosenthal, N.E. (1990) Effects of bright light on resting metabolic rate in patients with seasonal affective disorder and control subjects. *Biol Psychiatry* **28**:989–96.

Graw, P., Gisin, B., Wirz–Justice, A. (1997) Follow-up study of seasonal affective disorder in Switzerland. *Psychopathology* **30**:208–14.

Kasper, S., Rogers, S.L.B., Yancey, A., Schulz, P.M., Skwerer, R.G., and Rosenthal, N.E. (1989) Phototherapy in individuals with and without subsyndromal seasonal affective disorder. *Arch Gen Psychiatry* **46**:837–44.

Kräuchi, K., Reich, S., and Wirz–Justice, A. (1997) Eating style in seasonal affective disorder: who will gain weight in winter? *Compr Psychiatry* **38**:80–7.

Lam, R.W., Buchanan, A., and Remick, R.A. (1989) Seasonal affective disorder — a Canadian sample. *Ann Clin Psychiatry* **1**:241–5.

Lam, R.W., Solyom, L., and Tompkins, A. (1991) Seasonal mood symptoms in bulimia nervosa and seasonal affective disorder. *Compr Psychiatry* **32**:552–8.

Leonhardt, G., Wirz–Justice, A., Kräuchi, K., Graw, P., Wunder, D., and Haug H-J. (1994) Long-term follow-up of depression in seasonal affective disorder. *Compr Psychiatry* **35**:457–64.

Levitt, A.J., Joffe, R.T., Brecher, D., and MacDonald, C. (1993) Anxiety disorders and anxiety symptoms in a clinic sample of seasonal and non-seasonal depressives. *J Affect Disord* **28**:51–6.

Lingjærde, O. and Føreland, A.R. (1999) Characteristics of patients with otherwise typical winter depression, but with incomplete summer remission. *J Affect Disord* **53**:91–4.

Lingjærde, O. and Reichborn–Kjennerud, T. (1993) Characteristics of winter depression in the Oslo area (60° N). *Acta Psychiatr Scand* **88**:111–20.

Rosenthal, N.E., Sack, D.A., Gillin, J.C., Lewy, A.J., Goodwin, F.K., Davenport, Y., *et al.* (1984) Seasonal affective disorder: a description of the syndrome and preliminary findings with light therapy. *Arch Gen Psychiatry* **41**:72–80.

Rosenthal, N.E., Genhart, M.J., Caballero, B., Jacobsen, F.M., Skwerer, R.G., Coursey, R.D., *et al.* (1989) Psychobiological effects of carbohydrate- and protein-rich meals in patients with seasonal affective disorder and normal controls. *Biol Psychiatry* **25**:1029–40.

Sakamoto, K., Kamo, T., Nakadaira, S., Tamura, A., and Takahashi, K. (1993) A nationwide survey of seasonal affective disorder at 53 outpatient university clinics in Japan. *Acta Psychiatr Scand* **87**:258–65.

Sakamoto, K., Nakadaira, S., Kamo, K., Kamo, T., and Takahashi, K. (1995) A longitudinal follow-up study of seasonal affective disorder. *Am J Psychiatry* **152**:862–8.

Schlager, D., Froom, J., and Jaffe, A. (1995) Winter depression and functional impairment among ambulatory primary care patients. *Compr Psychiatry* **36**:18–24.

Schwartz, P.J., Brown, C., Wehr, T.A., and Rosenthal, N.E. (1996) Winter seasonal affective disorder: a follow-up study of the first 59 patients of the National Institute of Mental Health seasonal studies program. *Am J Psychiatry* **153**:1028–36.

Spitzer, R.L., Endicott, J., and Robins, E. (1978) Research diagnostic criteria: rationale and reliability. *Arch Gen Psychiatry* **35**:773–82.

Swedo, S.E., Pleeter, J.D., Richter, D.M., Hoffman, C.L., Allen, A.J., Hamburger, S.D., *et al.* (1995) Rates of seasonal affective disorder in children and adolescents. *Am J Psychiatry* **152**:1016–9.

Tam, E.M., Lam, R.W., Robertson, H.A., Stewart, J.N., Yatham, L.N., and Zis, A.P. (1997) Atypical depressive symptoms in seasonal and non-seasonal mood disorders. *J Affect Disord* **44**:39–44.

Thompson, C. and Isaacs, G. (1988) Seasonal affective disorder — a British sample: symptomatology in relation to mode of referral and diagnostic subtype. *J Affect Disord* **14**:1–11.

Thompson, C., Raheja, S.K., and King, E.A. (1995) A follow-up study of seasonal affective disorder. *Br J Psychiatry* **167**:380–4.

Wirz–Justice, A., Bucheli, C., Graw, P., Kielholz, P., Fisch, H-U., and Woggon, B. (1986) Light treatment of seasonal affective disorder in Switzerland. *Acta Psychiatr Scand* **74**:193–204.

World Health Organization (1993) *The ICD-10 classification of mental and behavioural disorders: diagnostic criteria for research.* World Health Organization, Geneva.

Young, M.A., Watel, L.G., Lahmeyer, H.W., and Eastman, C.I. (1991) The temporal onset of individual symptoms in winter depression: differentiating underlying mechanisms. *J Affect Disord* **22**:191–7.

Further reading

Blacker, C.V.R., Thomas, J.M., and Thompson, C. (1997) Seasonality prevalence and incidence of depressive disorder in a general practice sample: identifying differences in timing by caseness. *J Affect Disord* **43**:41–52.

Eagles, J.M., McLeod, I.H., and Douglas, A.S. (1997) Seasonal changes in psychological well-being in an elderly population. *Br J Psychiatry* **171**:53–5.

Eagles, J.M., Naji, S.A., Gray, D.A., Christie, J., and Beattie, J.A.G. (1998) Seasonal affective disorder among primary care consulters in January: prevalence and month by month consultation patterns. *J Affect Disord* **49**:1–8.

Eagles, J.M., Wileman, S.M., Cameron, I.M., Howie, F.L., Lawton, K., Gray, D.A., *et al.* (1999) Seasonal affective disorder among primary care attenders and a community sample in Aberdeen. *Br J Psychiatry* **175**:472–5.

Faedda, G.L., Tondo, L., Teicher, M.H., Baldessarini, R.J., Gelbard, H.A., and Floris, G.F. (1993) Seasonal mood disorders: patterns of seasonal recurrence in mania and depression. *Arch Gen Psychiatry* **50**:17–23.

Ghadirian, A-M., Marini, N., Jabalpurwala, S., and Steiger, H. (1999) Seasonal mood patterns in eating disorders. *Gen Hospital Psychiatry* **21**:354–9.

Gruber, N.P. and Dilsaver, S.C. (1996) Bulimia and anorexia nervosa in winter depression: lifetime rates in a clinical sample. *J Psychiatry Neurosci* **21**:9–12.

Halle, M.T. and Dilsaver, S.C. (1993) Comorbid panic disorder in patients with winter depression. *Am J Psychiatry* **150**:1108–10.

Levitan, R.D., Rector, N.A., and Bagby, R.M. (1998) Negative attributional style in seasonal and nonseasonal depression. *Am J Psychiatry* **155**:428–30.

Schlager, D., Schwartz, J.E., and Bromet, E.J. (1993) Seasonal variations of current symptoms in a healthy population. *Br J Psychiatry* **163**:322–6.

Terman, M., Levine, S.M., Terman, J.S., and Doherty, S. (1998) Chronic fatigue syndrome and seasonal affective disorder: comorbidity, diagnostic overlap, and implications for treatment. *Am J Med* **105(3A)**:115S–24S.

Wehr, T.A., Giesen, H.A., Schulz, P.M., Anderson, J.L., Joseph-Vanderpool, J.R., Kelly, K., *et al.* (1991) Contrasts between symptoms of summer depression and winter depression. *J Affect Disord* **23**:173–83.

Chapter 3

Comorbid disorders

Ted Reichborn–Kjennerud

3.1 Introduction

Comorbidity — that is, the co-occurrence of two or more mental disorder diagnoses within one individual — has been shown to affect the severity, course, prognosis, and outcome of individual disorders in several studies (Wittchen *et al.* 1999; Clark *et al.* 1995). Studies of comorbidity could also contribute to a deeper understanding of underlying aetiological mechanisms involved in psychopathology and thereby suggest new strategies for classification and treatment of mental disorders.

In this chapter, I shall review empirical studies of comorbidity in SAD, winter depression type (Rosenthal *et al.* 1984). I shall, however, first discuss some general aspects of comorbidity and comorbidity in non-seasonal depression as a background for interpreting the results for SAD.

3.2 Co-occurrence of mental disorders

Descriptive or phenomenological methods are most commonly used in studies of comorbidity. The best estimates of the co-occurrence of disorders in the general population are obtained from *epidemiological studies* using large representative samples. Studies using *clinical samples* give estimates of the comorbidity in help-seeking populations. These tend to be higher than those found in epidemiological studies because patients with comorbid disorders are more likely to seek treatment than those with single disorders (Galbaud du Fort *et al.* 1993; Kessler *et al.* 1994). The generalizability of such studies are therefore more limited.

Comorbidity is a direct consequence of the structure of our diagnostic systems. When most of the hierarchical exclusionary rules were dropped in DSM-III-R (Boyd *et al.* 1984), research on both community and clinical samples showed substantial rates of comorbidity (Clark *et al.* 1995). Two large epidemiological surveys in USA indicate that more than half of all individuals with a DSM disorder have at least one additional axis I diagnosis. In the Epidemiological Catchment Area (ECA) study, 60 per cent of the respondents with DSM-III-R axis I disorders had at least one comorbid disorder (Robins *et al.* 1991), and in the National Comorbidity Survey (NCS), 56 per cent of the respondents who were given lifetime diagnoses had at least two disorders (Kessler *et al.* 1994). In the NCS study, individuals with comorbid conditions accounted for 79 per cent of all lifetime diagnoses and 82 per cent of all 12-month diagnoses.

For axis II disorders, the comorbidity rates are usually even higher. Fabrega *et al.* (1992) found that 79 per cent of patients with a personality disorder (PD) also satisfied criteria for at least one axis I disorder, and Oldham *et al.* (1992) found that 80 per cent of patients with a PD had at least one comorbid axis II disorder, and that the mean number of personality disorder diagnoses were 3,4.

'Pure' conditions, as described by the DSM system, thus appear to be atypical in both clinical and community samples and are not likely to be representative of the overall population of people with the disorder.

Other approaches to comorbidity rely less on the descriptive aspects of disorders and focus instead on common aetiological mechanisms (Clark *et al.* 1995). *Genetic epidemiological* methods use twin or adoption designs or molecular genetic methods such as linkage or association studies to evaluate possible common genetic liability for different disorders. Kendler and co-workers (1992), for example, found that major depressive disorder (MDD) and generalized anxiety disorder (GAD) share a genetic liability, but that the environmental risk factors appear to be different for the two disorders. A finding of common underlying biological dysregulation or common treatment response in different disorders can also be an indication of common aetiological mechanisms and therefore of comorbidity. I shall return to these alternative approaches in the discussion.

3.3 **Comorbidity in non-seasonal depressive disorders**

Comorbidity is a well-established phenomenon in depressive disorders. Data from the ECA study show that 75 per cent of individuals with a lifetime diagnosis of depressive disorder had at least one comorbid disorder (Robins *et al.* 1991). In an international collaborative study, organized by the World Health Organization (Sartorius *et al.* 1996), 62 per cent of all depressive cases were found also to suffer from at least one other current mental disorder. In the NCS, 74 per cent of the respondents with a lifetime diagnosis of MDD had at least one lifetime disorder and 58.9 per cent had at least one 12-montn diagnosis. Nearly a third (31.9 per cent) had three or more lifetime diagnoses (Kessler *et al.* 1996). Lifetime diagnoses of anxiety disorders occurred in 58 per cent of the MDD group (social phobia, 27.1 per cent; GAD, 17.2 per cent; panic disorder, 9.9 per cent). A lifetime diagnosis of substance use disorders was found in 38.6 per cent of the respondents with MDD. The 12-month prevalences were 51.2 per cent for any anxiety disorder, 20 per cent for social phobia, and 18.5 per cent for any substance use disorder.

Estimates of frequencies of PD in non-seasonal MDD vary considerably due to methodological differences. For out-patients during a depressive episode, prevalences from 50 per cent to 86 per cent have been reported, dominated by disorders in cluster B and cluster C (Corruble *et al.* 1996). Numerous studies using dimensional approaches have reported significantly elevated scores for traits related to DSM-III-R cluster C, such as neuroticism (Bagby *et al.* 1995; Widiger *et al.* 1992), and harm avoidance (Joffe *et al.* 1993), in patients with non-seasonal MDD.

Several studies have shown that comorbidity influences the course and outcome in patients with MDD. Subjects with a lifetime comorbidity of anxiety and depression have been found to have lower psychosocial functioning scores, lower remission scores, and less favourable long-term course and outcome compared to those with pure depressive disorders (Wittchen *et al.* 1999). Kessler *et al.* (1994) found that non-remission of depression was significantly more likely in patients with a prior history of anxiety disorders. Furthermore, comorbid depression was more likely to result in hospitalization as well as an increased risk of suicide attempts. Johnson *et al.* (1990) reported a suicide rate of 8 per cent for pure cases of MDD, but 20 per cent for depressives with comorbid disorders. Comorbid axis II disorders have also been found to be a negative prognostic sign (Farmer and Nelson–Gray 1990; Shea 1996).

The majority of studies on response to antidepressant medication in patients with non-seasonal MDD, have found the presence of a DSM-III-R axis II disorder to be associated with less favourable outcome, and cluster C disorders were associated with poor treatment response in the majority of studies of out-patients. The presence of avoidant and dependent PD has been identified as a predictor of poor antidepressant treatment response in several studies (Ilardi and Craighead 1995). This has also been found for high pre-treatment scores of the personality trait, neuroticism and the temperament trait, harm avoidance (Ilardi and Craighead 1995; Joffe *et al.* 1993).

3.4 SAD — diagnostic issues

The way mental disorders are classified will determine the patterns of co-occurrence. In the original diagnostic criteria for SAD (Rosenthal *et al.* 1984), subjects with other axis I disorders were excluded. According to Rosenthal (personal communication, June 1992), this was considered useful to secure homogenous material for research purposes in an early stage when the entity of SAD was being identified. Samples selected by the use of these criteria will, for reasons already mentioned, probably not be representative for subjects with SAD in the general population or in clinical settings, and the generalizability of results from such studies will be limited. The same criteria do, however, permit axis II comorbidity.

In 1987, the validity of SAD was not found sufficient to justify the introduction of a new separate diagnostic category in DSM-III-R (Spitzer and Williams 1989). It was decided that seasonality should be incorporated as a 'pattern' of mood disturbances. Six years later it still appeared to be unclear whether what is identified as SAD represented a distinct affective syndrome, a subtype of recurrent affective disorder, or the most severe form of a widely distributed population trait (Bauer and Dunner 1993). It was therefore decided to retain seasonal pattern as a modifier for mood disorders in DSM-IV (American Psychiatric Association 1994). In both DSM-III-R and DSM-IV versions, multiple diagnoses are permitted, and both axis I and II comorbidity becomes relevant objects of study.

To diagnose SAD in epidemiological studies, a self-report screening instrument called the Seasonal Pattern Assessment Questionnaire (SPAQ) (Rosenthal *et al.* 1987) has been used. SPAQ includes a section measuring seasonal variation in six areas: mood, appetite, weight, sleep length, energy, and social functioning. Each item is scored from 0 to 4. The sum of these ratings is called the Global Seasonality Score (GSS), and has a range from 0 to 24. In addition, the questionnaire asks subjects to rate the degree to which the seasonal changes are experienced as a problem, and to identify the months of the year in which they feel worst and best. In epidemiological studies, the following criteria are commonly used for a diagnosis of SAD (Kasper *et al.* 1989):

1. GSS score of 10 or higher;

2. experiencing seasonal change as a problem at least to a moderate degree;

3. subjects feel worst during one of the winter months (January or February).

The SPAQ criteria has been used frequently in studies of comorbidity (see the chapter by Mersch). Magnusson (1996) found that 5 of 19 patients (26 per cent) with SPAQ-SAD also satisfied DSM-III-R criteria for major depression with a seasonal pattern. In a study of bulimic patients (n = 35) that satisfied SPAQ criteria for SAD (Levitan *et al.* 1994), it was found that only five of these patients (14 per cent) met full DSM-III-R criteria for fall/winter SAD according to interview data. Similar results have been found in other studies, and show that there is a limited overlap between the two diagnoses. Results with regard to comorbidity will therefore be different for the two classification systems, and thus not comparable.

3.5 Empirical studies of comorbidity in SAD

3.5.1 Anxiety disorders

As we have seen, there is a strong association between anxiety disorders and non-seasonal depression. In a study comparing seasonal (n = 18) and non-seasonal (n = 13) depressives (DSM-III), Garvey *et al.* (1988) found that 89 per cent of patients with SAD reported symptoms of anxiety during depression, compared to 77 per cent in the non-seasonal group. Thompson and Isaacs (1988) reported that 86 per cent of a sample of patients with SAD (n = 51) had symptoms of anxiety. In another study comparing seasonal and non-seasonal depressives, Levitt and collaborators (1993) found that in a sample of 38 patients with DSM-III-R major depression, seasonal pattern, 45 per cent had a lifetime diagnosis of an anxiety disorder (26 per cent, GAD; 10 per cent, social phobia; 5 per cent, panic disorder). There were no significant differences between seasonal and non-seasonal depressives in the prevalence of any anxiety disorder. Magnusson (1996) also found a very high prevalence (39 per cent) of GAD in a small sample (n=18) of patients with SPAQ diagnoses of SAD.

In a sample (n = 38) of patients with DSM-III-R major depression with a seasonal pattern, Halle and Dilsaver (1993) found that 23.7 per cent also fulfilled criteria for panic disorder. Panic attacks occurred exclusively in the context of a depressive syndrome; they were restricted to the months of the year during which the patients were depressed. Partonen and Lönnqvist (1995) found that 40 per cent of a sample of 20 females with SAD (DSM-III-R, seasonal pattern) had social phobia. Marriott *et al.* (1994) found significantly higher GSS scores in a sample (n = 133) of patients with panic disorder (DSM-III-R) compared to samples from the general population. They also found seasonal changes in anxiety and panic attacks. Using the SPAQ criteria with a cut-off point of 9 on the GSS scale, 30.1 per cent of the panic patients could be defined as suffering from SAD.

3.5.2 Eating disorders

Disturbances in eating behaviour, namely increased appetite and eating, occur frequently in patients with SAD. It is therefore not surprising that eating disorders and especially bulimia nervosa (BN) have been associated with SAD. In a mixed sample (n = 259) of patients with eating disorders (53.7 per cent with BN), 27 per cent were found to meet SPAQ criteria for SAD (Ghadirian *et al.* 1999). Hardin and co-workers (1991) studied seasonality in six clinical populations (winter SAD, summer SAD, subsyndromal SAD (Kasper *et al.* 1989), eating disorders, major affective disorder, bipolar disorder) and two normal control groups. They found that patients with eating disorders (10 with a history of anorexia nervosa (AN), 31 with a history of BN) had GSS scores significantly higher than patients with non-seasonal disorders, but not significantly different from patients with winter SAD. GSS scores for the eating disorder group were higher than for both the summer SAD and the subsyndromal group, but this difference was not significant.

To clarify the relationship of the specific eating disorders diagnoses, the same group (Brewerton *et al.* 1994) later evaluated SPAQ scores for patients with BN (n = 109), AN (n = 30), and BN + AN (n = 20). They found that all subgroups of eating disorders had significantly higher GSS scores than normal controls. Thirteen per cent of the sample of patients with eating disorders met SPAQ criteria for SAD. Patients with both AN and BN had significantly higher scores than the two other patient groups. Patients with BN showed a significantly higher prevalence of all seasonal syndromes as defined by SPAQ.

Lam *et al.* (1996*a*), comparing patients with BN (n = 60) and AN (n = 31) with normal controls (n = 50), found that the BN group had higher GSS scores and more presumptive diagnoses of SAD than the other two groups. The AN patients did not differ from the normal controls. Fornari *et al.* (1994) reported that patients with AN (n = 60) had significantly lower GSS scores than patients with BN, and less seasonal change in mood, weight, and energy. Lam *et al.* (1991) found that 42 per cent of BN patients met SPAQ criteria for SAD. As a group their mean GSS scores were 11,7 (+ 5,8). Levitan and co-workers (1994) found that 69 per cent of a sample of patients with BN (n = 103) also satisfied the SPAQ criteria for SAD. The majority of these patients also had a marked seasonal fluctuation in BN symptoms such as binge eating This was also reported by Blouin *et al.* (1992) after assessing 197 patients with BN several times over a 4-year period.

A clinical overlap between SAD and BN was found by Berman *et al.* (1993), comparing 30 female SAD patients with 30 matched patients with BN. In a treatment study of phototherapy for BN (Lam *et al.* 1994), 17 female patients with DSM-III-R BN were found to have a mean GSS of 13,7 (+ 5,3), and 6 patients (35 per cent) also met DSM-III-R criteria for major depression with a seasonal pattern. In a similar study by Braun *et al.* (1999), 44.1 per cent of patients with BN met SPAQ criteria for SAD, but did not meet DSM-IV criteria for current major depression with a seasonal pattern specifier.

3.5.3 **Personality disorders**

Estimates of personality disorders are influenced by several methodological factors (for example, depressive state, self-report questionnaires vs. structured interviews), and results therefore vary considerably (Zimmerman 1994). Schultz *et al.* (1988), using structured interviews, found that 34 per cent of patients with SAD (n = 28) in the depressive state satisfied DSM-III-R criteria for at least one PD. In an interview study, we found that 23 per cent of a group of SAD patients (n = 57) fulfilling DSM-III-R criteria for MDD, recurrent, seasonal pattern, met DSM-III-R criteria for one or more axis II diagnosis (Reichborn–Kjennerud *et al.* 1994). Disorders in cluster C occurred in 18 per cent of the sample, disorders in cluster B in 12 per cent, and disorders in cluster A in 5 per cent.

Using a self-report questionnaire for the assessment of PD (ReichbornKjennerud *et al.* 1997), we found that 58 per cent of the 45 patients with SAD fulfilled the criteria for one or more DSM-III-R PD, in the depressed state; cluster C disorders were most prevalent (49 per cent). Avoidant PD was the most frequent single disorder, diagnosed in 31 per cent of the sample. In a non-depressed state the prevalence of any PD fell to 47 per cent. Again, cluster C diagnoses were most prevalent, occurring in 38 per cent of the sample, and avoidant PD was the most prevalent individual PD (24 per cent). Twenty-seven per cent of the patients had a cluster A disorder and 22 per cent had a cluster B diagnosis. Although the number of categorical diagnoses were lower in the euthymic state, the differences were not significant for any cluster or individual PD.

Partonen and Lönnqvist (1995), using interview data, reported that 50 per cent of a sample of female patients with SAD (n = 20) satisfied criteria for avoidant PD. The severity of symptoms of comorbid avoidant PD was reduced simultaneously with an improvement in the severity of the depressive episode by bright light treatment.

3.5.4 Personality traits

After having found elevated levels of neuroticism in non-seasonal depression (Bagby *et al.* 1995), the same group later reported no significant differences in neuroticism between seasonal and non-seasonal depressives (Bagby *et al.* 1996), but both scores were significantly higher than normative scores from the general population. The scores on the dimension of openness was significantly higher in the SAD patients. Jain *et al.* (1999) reported consistent findings in a later study, and found that scores on the openness domain remained elevated also after treatment. The finding of elevated scores on the neuroticism scale has been replicated in several studies. Murray *et al.* (1995), in a twin study, found a correlation of 0.38 between seasonality and neuroticism, and Jang *et al.* (1997) found a correlation of 0.35 between GSS and neuroticism in a media-recruited sample (n = 297) from the general population. Gordon *et al.* (1999), in a group of SAD patients (n = 45), found elevated scores for neuroticism relative to the normal population, but no significant correlation with GSS.

3.5.5 Late luteal phase dysphoric disorder

Late luteal phase dysphoric disorder (LLPDD) was found to occur in 70 per cent of a small sample (n = 20) of females with DSM-III-R MDD, seasonal pattern (Partonen and Lönnqvist 1995). In a sample of 100 women with LLPDD, significantly elevated seasonality scores, compared to a non-clinical control group, was found (Maskall *et al.* 1997). The estimated rate of SPAQ-SAD was 38 per cent.

3.5.6 Chronic fatigue syndrome

Several symptoms involved in chronic fatigue syndrome (CFS) such as fatigue, hypersomnia, hyperphagia weight gain and mood, show seasonal variation in the general population. Garcia–Borreguero *et al.* (1998), however, found significantly lower scores on multiple SPAQ-derived measures in a group (n = 41) of patients with CFS compared to controls. In a sample of 110 patients with CFS, Terman *et al.* (1998) found that 73 subjects reported seasonal fluctuations in symptoms. Of these, 37 per cent had a GSS of 10 or more. They concluded that a subgroup of patients with CFS show seasonal symptom variation resembling SAD with winter exacerbation, and might benefit from light treatment.

3.5.7 Comorbidity and treatment outcome

In a sample of patients with SAD, Lilie *et al.* (1990) found that subjects without axis II psychopathology were more likely than patients with PDs to be bright light responders and to fully remit in summer. Partonen and Lönnqvist (1995) found that SAD patients with comorbid avoidant PD chose to use light therapy significantly longer than patients without avoidant PD indicating that these patients respond less well to phototherapy. In a study of PDs and temperament as predictors of response to light therapy in patients with SAD (Reichborn–Kjennerud *et al.* 1997), we found that subjects with a diagnosis of any DSM-III-R, axis II PD were significantly less likely to respond to phototherapy than patients without axis II pathology. Poor treatment outcome was also significantly associated with one or more PDs in cluster C, avoidant PD, and high score on the harm avoidance scale of the Tridimensional Personality Questionnaire (TPQ). Levitt *et al.* (1993), however, found that the presence of any anxiety disorder was associated with a better response rate to light therapy in SAD patients.

3.6 **Discussion**

In clinical samples and unrepresentative samples of volunteers from the general population, high rates of comorbidity between SAD and other axis I disorders, PDs, and personality traits have been reported. There are no data on the comorbidity of SAD from epidemiological studies using representative samples from the general population. In the NCS in USA (the only epidemiologic study of SAD using interviews), the prevalence of DSM-III-R major depression with a seasonal pattern was found to be 0.4 per cent (Blazer *et al.* 1998). This is very low compared to studies using SPAQ-criteria (Kasper *et al.* 1989; Rosen *et al.* 1990), indicating that the two methods identify different diagnostic entities (see Partonen and Lönnqvist 1998). Furthermore, findings from clinical samples or samples recruited among volunteers through advertisement are biased in several different ways and therefore cannot be directly compared with each other. Studies using seasonality (GSS) assessed by a questionnaire (SPAQ) with limited psychometric qualities (Raheja *et al.* 1996) represent a weak foundation for generalization. We must therefore conclude that there are few valid data on the comorbidity of SAD as diagnosed by the DSM system.

With these limitations taken into consideration, the results of the studies on co-occurrence show the overall pattern of comorbidity between seasonal and non-seasonal MDD to be similar with regard to anxiety disorders, eating disorders, PDs, and personality traits. Social phobia, GAD, and panic disorder are prevalent in both kinds of depression. High prevalences of cluster B and cluster C PDs (especially avoidant PD) and neuroticism have been found in both seasonal and non-seasonal depression. The prevalence of substance use disorder has been found to be high in non-seasonal MDD (Kessler *et al.* 1996), but so far we have little information on these disorders for SAD.

Scores on the openness domain seem to be elevated in patients with SAD compared to non-seasonal affective disorders (Bagby *et al.* 1996; Jain *et al.* 1999). This indicates a unique personality profile in patients with SAD, also suggested by Schuller *et al.* (1993) and Pendse *et al.* (1999), and should be further explored. It does not, however, alter the general impression that seasonal and non-seasonal MDD co-occur with similar disorders. In longitudinal follow-up studies of patients with SAD, it has been found that more than a third of the patients develop non-seasonal MDD (Partonen and Lönnqvist 1998). If lifetime prevalence was used as a criterion, high rates of comorbidity would thus be found between seasonal and non-seasonal depression.

The co-occurrence of two or more distinct disorders in the same individual can have different causes:

1. One disorder causes or increases the liability for another disorder.

2. Both disorders are caused by the same underlying factor(s).

3. Two disorders are aetiologically distinct, but when they occur together one influences the clinical manifestation, course. and outcome of the other.

4. The two disorders are causally unrelated. The co-occurrence is a chance result due to high prevalence of both disorders in a specific population or overlapping diagnostic criteria.

The quality of the studies on comorbidity in SAD do not permit firm conclusions to be drawn regarding these hypotheses. Longitudinal studies would be required to test the first hypothesis. We have, however, several lines of evidence that point to common aetiological factors through indications of common pathophysiological mechanisms, common treatment response, and common genetic liability in many of the disorders found to co-occur in the descriptive studies.

Given the characteristic symptom pattern of SAD (with hypersomnia, hyperphagia, and carbohydrate craving) and the fact that serotonergic systems have been shown to play an important role in the regulation of appetite and sleep, it is not surprising that evidence suggests a dysregulation of the serotonergic (5-HT) systems in SAD (see Partonen and Lönnqvist 1998). Serotonergic dysregulation have also been found in non-seasonal depression (Mann 1999), anxiety disorders (Ninan 1999), eating disorders (Jimerson *et al.* 1997; Brewerton and Jimerson 1996), and personality (Knutson *et al.* 1998; Lesch *et al.* 1996).

Response to serotonergic agents like selective serotonin reuptake inhibitors (SSRIs), previously found in non-seasonal depression, anxiety disorders, eating disorders, LLPDD, and personality (Masand and Gupta 1999; Knutson *et al.* 1998), have also been found in SAD (Partonen and Lönnqvist 1998; Ruhrmann *et al.* 1998). Several studies have showed that tryptophan depletion produced a rapid and robust, but transient, reversal of antidepressant effects of light therapy (Lam *et al.* 1996*b*; Neumeister *et al.* 1997), thus giving support to the theory that serotonergic mechanisms may be involved in the mechanisms of action of light therapy.

Three studies of the effect of phototherapy for the treatment of BN have been published (Lam *et al.* 1994; Blouin *et al.* 1996; Braun *et al.* 1999). Two of these found significant effect on binge frequency in women with BN. Light treatment has also been found to have an effect on non-seasonal depression (Kripke 1998) and LLPDD (Lam *et al.* 1999). These findings are all consistent with the hypothesis that the disorders have pathophysiological mechanisms in common.

Genetic studies suggest a common aetiological mechanism between SAD and comorbid disorders. In a twin study (n = 297) of volunteers from the general population, Jang and collaborators (1998) found a genetic correlation of .52 between GSS and neuroticism, implying that approximately 27 per cent of the genetic influences affecting seasonality and neuroticism are the same. The proportion of environmental influence was nearly zero. Neuroticism has been found to be associated with a polymorphism in the regulatory region of the serotonin (5-HT) transporter gene (5-HTTLPR) (Lesch *et al.* 1996). This same genetic polymorphism has also been found to be associated with seasonality (GSS) in patients with SAD (Rosenthal *et al.* 1998) and with GSS in a sample drawn from the general population (Sher *et al.* 1999).

Taken together, these studies strongly indicate that serotonergic dysregulation is a common causal factor in SAD and the disorders that have been found to co-occur with it.

With regard to the third hypothesis, we have seen that comorbid disorders influence treatment outcome in patients with SAD. Further studies are required to explore the relationship between comorbidity and severity, course, and outcome in patients with SAD and to test whether comorbidity could be a chance result due to sampling bias.

Future research must include epidemiological studies with representative samples from the general population, using reliable structured interviews and validated diagnostic criteria. Genetic epidemiological methods are needed to explore causal mechanisms. Longitudinal designs are important to determine the diagnostic stability of SAD and thereby the relationship between seasonal and non-seasonal depression and the influence of comorbid disorders on course and outcome. Studies of comorbidity are important for the development of more valid classification systems and will contribute to determining the future diagnostic status of SAD. The understanding of the effect of comorbid disorders on treatment outcome could help us design more sophisticated treatment strategies.

References

American Psychiatric Association (1994) *Diagnostic and Statistical Manual of Mental Disorders* (4th edn). American Psychiatric Association, Washington DC.

Bagby, R.M., Joffe, R.T., Parker, J.D.A., Kalemba,V., and Harkness, K.L. (1995) Major depression and the five factor model of personality. *Journal of Personality Disorders,* 9:224–34.

Bagby, R.M., Schuller, D.R., Levitt, A.J., Joffe, R.T., and Harkness, K.L. (1996) Seasonal and non-seasonal depression and the five factor model of personality. *Journal of Affective Disorders,* 38:89–95.

Bauer, M.S. and Dunner, D.L. (1993) Validity of seasonal pattern as a modifier for recurrent mood disorders for DSM-IV. *Comprehensive Psychiatry,* 34:159–70.

Berman, K., Lam, R.W., and Goldner, E.M. (1993) Eating attitudes in seasonal affective disorder and bulimia nervosa. *Journal of Affective Disorders,* 29:219–25.

Blazer, D.G., Kessler, R.C., and Swartz, M.S. (1998) Epidemiology of recurrent major depression with a seasonal pattern: the National Comorbidity Survery. *British Journal of Psychiatry,* 172:164–7.

Blouin, A.G., Blouin, J.H., Aubin, P., Carter, J. Goldstein, C., Boyer, H., *et al.* (1992) Seasonal pattern of bulimia nervosa. *American Journal of Psychiatry,* 149:73–81.

Blouin, A.G., Blouin, J.H., Iversen, H. Carter, J. Goldstein, C., Goldfield, G., *et al.* (1996) Light therapy in bulimia nervosa: a double-blind, placebo-controlled study. *Psychiatry Research,* 60:1–9.

Boyd, J.H., Bruke, J.D., Gruenberg, E., Holzer, C.E., and Rae, D.S. (1984) Exclusion criteria of DSM-III: a study of hierarchy-free syndromes. *Archives of General Psychiatry,* 41:983–9.

Braun, D.L., Sunday, S.R., Fornari, V.M., and Halmi, K.A. (1999) Bright light therapy decreases binge frequency in women with bulimia nervosa: a double blind, placebo-controlled study. *Comprehensive Psychiatry,* 40:442–8.

Brewerton, T.D., Krahn, D.D. Hardin, T.A., Wehr, T.A., and Rosenthal, N.E. (1994) Findings from the Seasonal Pattern Assessment Questionnaire in patients with eating disorders and control subjects: effects of diagnoseis and location. *Psychiatry Research,* 52:71–84.

Brewerton, T.D. and Jimerson, D.C. (1996) Studies of serotonin function in anorexia nervosa. *Psychiatry Research,* 62:31–42.

Clark, L.A., Watson, D., and Reynolds, S. (1995) Diagnosis and classification of psychopathology: challenges to the current system and future directions. *Annual Review of Psychology,* 46: 121–53.

Corruble, E., Ginestet, D., and Guelfi, J.D. (1996) Comorbidity of personality disorders and unipolar major depression: a review. *Journal of Affective Disorders,* 37:157–70.

Fabrega, H., Ulrich, R., Pilkonis, P., and Mezzich, J.E. (1992) Pure personality disorders in an intake psychiatric setting. *Journal of Personality Disorders,* 6:153–61.

Farmer, R. and Nelson–Gray, R.O. (1990) Personality disorders and depression: hypothetical relations and methodological considerations. *Clinical Psychology Review,* 10:453–76.

Fornari, V.M., Braun, D.L., Sunday, S.R., Sandberg, D.E., Matthews, M., Chen, I., *et al.* (1994) Seasonal pattern in eating disorder subgroups. *Comprehensive Psychiatry,* 35:450–6.

Galbaud du Fort, G., Newman, S.C., and Bland, R.C. (1993) Psychiatric comorbidity and treatment seeking: sources of selection bias in the study of clinical populations. *Journal of Nervous and Mental Disorders,* 181:467–74.

Garcia–Borreguero, D., Dale, J.K., Rosenthal, N.E., Chiara, A., O'Fallon, A., Bartko, J.J., *et al.* (1998) Lack of seasonal variation of symptoms in patients with chronic fatigue syndrome. *Psychiatry Research,* 77:71–7.

Garvey, M.J., Wesner, R., and Godes, M. (1988) Comparison of seasonal and nonseasonal affective disorders. *American Journal of Psychiatry,* 145:100–2.

Ghadirian, A.M., Marini, N., Jabalpurwala, S., and Steiger, H. (1999) Seasonal mood patterns in eating disorder. *General Hospital Psychiatry*, **21**:35–49.

Gordon, T., Keel, J., Hardin, T.A., and Rosenthal, N.E. (1999) Seasonal mood change and neuroticism: the same construct? *Comprehensive Psychiatry*, **40**:415–17.

Halle, M.T. And Dilsaver, S.C. (1993) Comorbid panic disorder in patients with winter depression. *American Journal of Psychiatry*, **150**:1108–10.

Hardin, T.A., Wehr, T.A., Brewerton, T.D., Kasper, S., Berrettini, W., Rabkin, J., *et al.* (1991) Evaluation of seasonality in six clinical populations and two normal populations. *Journal of Psychiatry Research*, **25**:75–87.

Ilardi, S.S. and Craighead W.E. (1995) Personality pathology and response to somatic treatments for major depression: a critical review. *Depression*, **2**:200–17.

Jain, U., Blais, M.A., Otto, M.W., Hirshfeld, D.R., and Sachs, G.S. (1999) Five-factor personality traits in patients with seasonal depression: treatment effects and comparison with bipolar patients. *Journal of Affective Disorders*, **55**:51–4.

Jang, K.L., Lam, R.W., Harris, J.A., Livesley, W.J., and Vernon, P.A. (1997) The relationship between seasonal mood change and personality: more apparent than real? *Acta Psychiatrica Scandinavica*, **95**:539–43.

Jang, K.L., Lam, R.W., Harris, J.A., Vernon, P.A., and Livesley, W.J. (1998) Seasonal mood change and personality: an investigation of genetic co-morbidity. *Psychiatry Research*, **78**:1–7.

Jimerson, D.C., Wolfe, B.E., Metzger, E.D., Finkelstein, D.M., Cooper, T.B., and Levine, J.M. (1997) Decreased serotonin function in bulimia nervosa. *Archives of General Psychiatry*, **54**:529–34.

Joffe, R.T., Bagby, R.M., Levitt, A.J., Regan J.J., and Parker, J.D.A. (1993) The Tridimensional Personality Questionnaire in major depression. *American Journal of Psychiatry*, **150**:959–60.

Johnson, J., Weissman, M.M., and Klerman, G.L. (1990) Panic disorder, comorbidity and suicide attempts. *Archives of General Psychiatry*, **47**:805–8.

Kasper, S., Wehr, T.A., Bartko, J.J., Gaist, P.A., and Rosenthal, N.E. (1989) Epidemiological findings of seasonal changes in mood and behavior. A telephone survey of Montgomery County, Maryland. *Archives of General Psychiatry*, **46**:823–33.

Kendler, K.S., Neale, M. C., Kessler, R. C., Heath, A. C., Eaves, L. J. (1992) Major depression and generalized anxiety disorder: same genes, (partly) different environments? *Archives of General Psychiatry*, **49**, 716–22.

Kessler, R.C., McGongale, K.A., Zhao, S., Nelson, C.B., Hughes, M., *et al.* (1994) Lifetime and 12-month prevalence of DSM-III-R psychiatric disorders in the United States: results from the National Comorbidity Survey. *Archives of General Psychiatry*, **51**:8–19.

Kessler, R.C., Nelson, C.B., McGonagle, K.A., Liu, J., Schwartz, M., and Blazer, D.G. (1996) Comorbidity of DSM-III-R major depressive disorder in the general population: results from the National Comorbidity Survey. *British Journal of Psychiatry*, **168** (suppl. 30):17–30.

Knutson, B., Wolkowitz, O.M., Cole, S.W., Chan, T., Moore, E.A., Johnson, R.C., *et al.* (1998) Selective alteration of personality and social behavior by serotonergic intervention. *American Journal of Psychiatry*, **155**:373–9.

Kripke, D.F. (1988) Light treatment for nonseasonal depression: speed, efficacy, and combined treatment. *Journal of Affective Disorders*, **49**:109–17.

Lam, R.W., Solyom, L., and Tompkins, A. (1991) Seasonal mood symptoms in bulimia nervosa and seasonal affective disorder. *Comprehensive Psychiatry*, **32**:552–8.

Lam, R.W., Goldner, E.M., Solyom, L., and Remick, R.A. (1994) A controlled study of light therapy for bulimia nervosa. *American Journal of Psychiatry*, **151**:744–50.

Lam, R.W., Goldner, E.M., and Grewal, A. (1996a) Seasonality of symptoms in anorexia and bulimia nervosa. *International Journal of Eating Disorders*, **1**:35–44.

Lam, R.W., Zis, A.P., Grewal, A.K., Delgado, P.L., Charney, D.S., and Krystal, J.H. (1996b) Effects of tryptophan depletion in light-remitted patients with seasonal affective disorder. *Archives of General Psychiatry*, **53**:41–4.

Lam, R.W., Carter, D., Misri, S., Kuan, A.J., Yatham, L.N., and Zis, A.P. (1999) A controlled study of light therapy in women with late luteal phase dysphoric disorder. *Psychiatry Research*, **86**:185–92.

Lesch, K.P., Bengel, D., Heils, A., Sabol, S.Z., Greenberg, B.D., Petri, S., *et al.* (1996) Association of anxiety-related traits with a polymorphism in the serotonin transporter gene regulatory region. *Science*, **274**:1527–31.

Levitan, R.D., Kaplan, A.S., Levitt, A.J., and Joffe, R.T. (1994) Seasonal fluctuation in mood and eating behavior in bulimia and eating disorders. *International Journal of Eating Disorders*, **16**:295–9.

Levitt, A.J., Joffe, R.T., Brecher, D., and McDonald, C. (1993) Anxiety disorders and anxiety symptoms in a clinical sample of seasonal and non-seasonal depressives. *Journal of Affective Disorders*, **28**:51–6.

Lilie, J.K., Lahmeyer, H.W., Watel, L.G., and Eastman, C.I. (1990) The relation of personality to clinical outcome in SAD. *Society for Light Treatment and Biological Rhythms Abstract* 2:213.

Magnússon, A. (1996) Validation of the Seasonal Pattern Assessment Questionnaire (SPAQ). *Journal of Affective Disorders*, **40**:121–9.

Mann, J.J. (1999) Role of the serotonergic system in the pathogenesis of major depression and suicidal behavior. *Neuropsychopharmacology*, **2(suppl.)**:99S–105S.

Marriott, P.F., Greenwood, K.M., and Armstrong, S.M. (1994) Seasonality in panic disorder. *Journal of Affective Disorders*, **31**:75–80.

Masand, P.S. and Gupta, S. (1999) Selective serotonin reuptake inhibitors: an update. *Harvard Review of Psychiatry*, **7**:69–84.

Maskall, D.D., Lam, R.W., Misri, S., Carter, D. Kuan, A.J., Yatham, L.N., *et al.* (1997) Seasonality symptoms in women with late luteal phase dysphoric disorder. *American Journal of Psychiatry*, **154**:1436–41.

Murray, G.W., Hay, D.W., and Armstrong, S.M. (1995) Personality factors in seasonal affective disorder: is seasonality an aspect of neuroticism? *Personality and Individual Differences*, **19**:613–18.

Neumeister, A., Praschak–Rieder, N., Heßelmann, B., Rao, M.L., Gluck, J., and Kasper, S. (1997) Effects of tryptophan depletion on drug-free patients with seasonal affective disorder during a stable response to bright light therapy. *Archives of General Psychiatry*, **54**:133–8.

Ninan, P.T. (1999) The functional anatomy, neurochemistry and pharmacology of anxiety. *Journal of Clinical Psychiatry*, **60(suppl. 22)**:18–22.

Oldham, J.M., Skodol, A.E., Kellman, H.D., Hyler, S.E., Rosnick, L., and Davies, M. (1992) Diagnosis of DSM-III-R personality disorders by two structured interviews: patterns of comorbidity. *American Journal of Psychiatry*, **149**:213–20.

Partonen, T. and Lönnqvist, J. (1995) The influence of comorbid disorders and of continuation light treatment on remission and recurrence in winter depression. *Psychopathology*, **28**:256–62.

Partonen, T. and Lönnqvist, J. (1998) Seasonal affective disorder. *Lancet*, **352**:1369–74.

Pendse, B., Westrin, Å., and Engström, G. (1999) Temperament traits in seasonal affective disorder, suicide attempters with non-seasonal major depression and healthy controls. *Journal of Affective Disorders*, **54**:55–65.

Raheja, S.K., King, E.A., and Thompson, C. (1996) The Seasonal Pattern Assessment Questionnaire for identifying seasonal affective disorders. *Journal of Affective Disorders*, **41**:193–9.

Reichborn–Kjennerud, T., Lingjærde, O., and Dahl, A.A. (1994) Personality disorders in patients with winter depression. *Acta Psychiatrica Scandinavica*, **90**:413–19.

Reichborn–Kjennerud, T. and Lingjærde, O. (1996) Response to light therapy in seasonal affective disorder: personality disorders and temperament as predictors of outcome. *Journal of Affective Disorders*, **41**:101–10.

Reichborn–Kjennerud, T., Lingjærde, O., and Dahl, A.A. (1997) DSM-III Personality disorders in seasonal affective disorder: change associated with depression. *Comprehensive Psychiatry*, **38**:43–8.

Robins, L.N., Locke, B.Z., and Regier, D.A. (1991) An overview of psychiatric disorders in America. In *Psychiatric Disorders in America* (ed. L.N. Robins and L.B.Z. Locke), pp. 328–66. Free Press, New York.

Rosen, L.N., Targum, S.D. Terman, M., Bryant, M.J., Hoffman, H., Kasper, S., *et al.* (1990) Prevalence of seasonal affective disorder at four lattitudes. *Psychiatry Research*, **31**:131–44.

Rosenthal, N.E., Sack, D.A., Gillin, C., Lewy, A.J., Goodwin, F.K., Davenport Y., *et al.* (1984) Seasonal affective disorder. A description of the syndrome and preliminary findings with light therapy. *Archives of General Psychiatry*, **41**:72–80.

Rosenthal, N.E., Genhardt, M., Sack, D.A., Skwerer, R., and Wehr, T.A. (1987). Seasonal affective disorder: relevance for treatment and research of bulimia. In *Psychobiology of bulimia* (ed. J.I. Hudson and H.G. Pope), pp. 205–28. American Psychiatric Press, Washington DC.

Rosenthal, N.E., Mazzani, C.M., Barnett, R.L., Hardin, T.A., Turner, E.H., Lam, G.K., *et al.* (1998) Role of serotonin transporter promoter repeat length polymorphism (5-HTTLPR) in seasonality and seasonal affective disorder. *Molecular Psychiarty*, **3**:175–7.

Ruhrmann, S., Kasper, S., Hawellek, B., Martinez, B., Höflich, G., Nickelsen, T., *et al.* (1998) Effects of fluoxetine versus bright light in the treatment of seasonal affective disorder. *Psychological Medicine*, **28**:923–33.

Sartorius, N., Üstün, T.B., Lecrubier, Y., and Wittchen, H-U. (1996) Depression comorbid with anxiety: results from the WHO study on psychological disorders in primary health care. *British Journal of Psychiatry*, **168(suppl. 30)**:38–43.

Schuller, D.R., Bagby, R.M., Levitt, A.J., and Joffe, R.T. (1993) A comparison of personality characteristics of seasonal and nonseasonal major depression. *Compre hensive Psychiatry*, **34**:360–2.

Schultz, P.M., Goldberg, S., Wehr, T.A., Sack, D.A., Kasper, S., and Rosenthal, N.E. (1988) Personality as a dimension of summer and winter depression. *Psychopharmacological Bulletin*, **24**:476–83.

Shea, M.T. (1996) The role of personality in recurrent and chronic depression. *Current Opinion in Psychiatry*, **9**:117–20.

Sher, L., Hardin, T.A., Greenberg, B.D., Murphy, D.L., Qian, L., and Rosenthal, N.E. (1999) Seasonality associated with the serotonin transporter promotor repeat length polymorphism. *American Journal of Psychiatry*, **156**:1837.

Spitzer, R.L. and Williams, J.B.W. (1989) The validity of SAD. In *Seasonal affective disorder and phototherapy* (ed. N.E. Rosenthal and M. Blehar), pp. 79–84. Guilford Press, New York.

Terman, M., Levine, S.M., Terman, J.S., and Doherty, S. (1998) Chronic fatigue syndrome and seasonal affective disorder: comorbidity, diagnostic overlap, and implications for treatment. *American Journal of Medicine*, **105**:115S–124S.

Thompson, C. and Isaacs, G. (1988) Seasonal affective disorder — a British sample: symptomatology in relation to mode of referral and diagnostic sub-type. *Journal of Affective Disorders*, **14**:1–11.

Widiger, T. and Trull, T. (1992) Personality and psychopathology: an application of the five factor model. *Journal of Personality*, **60**:363–92.

Wittchen, H-U., Lieb, R., Wunderlich, U., and Schuster, P. (1999) Comorbidity in primary care: presentation and consequences. *Journal of Clinical Psychiatry*, **60(suppl. 7)**:29–36.

Zimmerman, M. (1994) Diagnosing personality disorders. A review of issues and research methods. *Archives of General Psychiatry*, **51**:225–45.

Epidemiology

Chapter 4

Sociodemographic aspects

John M. Eagles

4.1 Introductory comments

In this chapter, the sociodemographic characteristics of people who suffer from SAD are described. To avoid having to repeat certain caveats, a few points are made here at the beginning which should be borne in mind while reading the chapter.

It is much easier to describe accurately the sociodemographics of a condition, such as breast cancer or tuberculosis, which has a recognized set of readily identifiable diagnostic criteria that can be externally validated, than to do the same for SAD. When the diagnosis of SAD relies so heavily on self-reporting of retrospective symptoms, one's conclusions about the sociodemographics of SAD may say as much about the sociodemographics of self-reporting as they do about SAD itself. For example, in completing the Seasonal Pattern Assessment Questionnaire (SPAQ), it is not implausible that younger women might be more likely to recognize, report, and describe as a problem a level of symptoms which would be less recognized, reported, and complained about by older men. As a related point, Nayyar and Cochrane (1996) have shown that people can be quite fallible in their retrospective evaluation of seasonal changes, as required when completing the SPAQ. Since much of what we think we know about the sociodemography of SAD derives from SPAQ data, it would be appropriate to remember that recall of seasonal fluctuations in well-being may be influenced by these very sociodemographic variables.

In reaching sociodemographic conclusions from population screening studies, it is necessary not only to have clear information about the characteristics of the surveyed population but also to consider the possible effects of response rates from that population. Kasper *et al.* (1989), in their telephone survey in Maryland, found that if respondents had heard of SAD then they were more likely to suffer from it. Since it seems highly probable that people will be more likely to complete and to return a questionnaire when they recognize symptoms therein to which they can relate personally, it is thus likely that respondents to SPAQ surveys have higher levels of seasonal pathology than do non-respondents. Especially since there is a wide reported range of response rates in SPAQ screening studies — for example, 82 per cent among a study by Magnusson and Axelsson (1993) in Manitoba against 14 per cent in a study by Muscettola *et al.* (1995) in Italy, possible response bias should lead to considerable caution in comparing population rates from such studies.

Furthermore, responders to surveys may differ sociodemographically from non-responders, and middle-aged, well-educated females have been characterized as likely to be the most conscientious respondents. As already mentioned, if response is linked to a higher likelihood of SAD, then this factor will serve to lower comparatively the apparent prevalence of SAD among higher responding subgroups. As it happens, well-educated, middle-aged females are generally found to be at increased risk of SAD (see p. 00), which may indicate that response bias would, if anything, *under*estimate the magnitude of these sociodemographic differences. That does not, however, significantly undermine the principle that response bias might limit how definitive one can be in drawing conclusions about the epidemiology of SAD.

Finally, it is necessary to avoid drawing simplistic aetiological conclusions from the sociodemographic data about SAD. It is probably justified to infer that it is a fairly pure effect of gender through which females suffer much more often from breast cancer than do men. With SAD, the preponderance of female sufferers may indeed reflect a biological predisposition, but it may also relate to differences in gender role, not only in a psychosocial context but also with regard to gender differences in such things as diet, taking exercise, and levels of daylight exposure. Such possibilities will be touched on later but merit background consideration while reading the presented data.

4.2 **Age**

It is a little difficult to disentangle age and gender in the epidemiology of SAD, and some points relating to sex differences will be raised in this section. Age and gender effects are shown together in Table 4.1 and Figs. 4.1 and 4.2. The relationship between age and SAD is subdivided into childhood, adulthood, and old age.

4.2.1 **Childhood**

Rosenthal *et al.* (1986) first described childhood SAD in a group of seven children. Irritability and seasonal work difficulties were more prominent than in adult cohorts, but affected children improved with light therapy, as they did in the study by Sonis *et al.* (1987). Since then, there have been only a few large epidemiological studies of SAD in children and adolescents.

Sonis (1989) described a sample of 779 high-school children (an 87 per cent response rate). His group had developed their own self-report screening questionnaire and the five symptoms of fatigue, headache, craving for sweets, crying, and worrying accounted for differences in total scores. The children's ages ranged from 14 to 18 years and 6.4 per cent were classified as 'highly seasonal'. Girls aged 16 years scored significantly higher than other age and sex combinations.

Carskadon and Acebo (1993) contacted children aged 9 to 12 years, and their parents, at 78 schools across the USA. Responses were received from 892 girls and 788 boys. As well as questions directed specifically at the parents, children received a 6-page questionnaire and parents were asked to complete a 2-page survey about their child. This large amount of material may have partly accounted for the fairly low response rate (46 per cent from girls and their parents, 39 per cent from boys and their parents). The parents' questionnaires were 'taken roughly from the SPAQ' and required 'Yes/No' responses. When children were identified as 'cases' on the basis that they 'seemed sad' in the winter and had at least two other seasonal symptoms, then 2.9 per cent, 4.2 per cent, 4.7 per cent, and 4.0 per cent of 9, 10, 11, and 12 year olds respectively were deemed to be affected. These figures suggest an increase in prevalence after age 9 but may relate to the fact that parents had to have noted seasonal changes for at least 2 years. This study relied heavily on parental judgements, and it is possible that, especially in households where parents suffered from SAD, children might have been erroneously identified as sufferers through family interaction, projection, and projective identification.

Swedo *et al.* (1995) modified the SPAQ to include the areas of school performance, irritability, and conduct problems and obtained usable responses from 1835 out of 2269 (81 per cent) school students, aged 9 to 19 years, in Washington DC. The results are reported by school grade, from grade 6 up to grade 12, rather than by the ages of the children, and researchers found that rates of SAD increased significantly from grade 10 onwards (that is, from around the age of 15 years). This increase seemed to coincide with puberty, a proxy measure of this being menstruation in girls and axillary hair growth in boys. However, while the rate in pre- and post-pubertal boys was very similar, at around 3 per cent, girls had a pre-pubertal rate of 1.7 per cent and a post-pubertal rate of 4.5 per cent. Given the alterations made to the SPAQ, it would be invalid to make direct comparisons with rates of SAD in adults, but Swedo *et al.* (1995) concluded that it was a real problem for some children and estimated that over a million children aged 10 to 18 years in the USA suffer from SAD.

Sourander *et al.* (1999) also deployed the SPAQ as modified by Swedo *et al.* (1995) in their study of school attendees at two latitudes in Finland. They received evaluable responses from 1458 adolescents from two school grades, with age ranges of 13 to 14 and 15 to 17 respectively. In this study, no differences in seasonal well-being were established between these age groups, but girls, especially in the sample at higher latitude, had more problems than boys in February and March. These authors concluded that symptoms of seasonal mood changes among adolescents living at higher latitudes were so common that they should be considered to be 'almost normative concerns'.

4.2.2 Adulthood

As for other sociodemographic variables, much of what we know about the relationship between age and SAD derives from SPAQ screening studies, and these will be described after findings from other publications.

From an early clinical sample of 220 patients, Rosenthal and Wehr (1987) reported that 'onset of illness typically occurs in the third decade', and while the mean age at presentation was 37 years, the onset had been on average 15 years earlier. Lingjærde and Reichborn–Kjennerud (1993) recruited sufferers through the Norwegian media and these were most commonly aged 40 to 49 with a mean age of onset of 26 years. Hansen *et al.* (1998), conducting a study of air pollution at a latitude of 70° in northern Norway, embedded issues relating to seasonal changes in their questionnaires, thus hopefully avoiding some of the suggestion and sensitization which may arise in completing the SPAQ. Depression perceived as evoked by the polar night peaked in men aged 40 to 49 and in women aged 50 to 59 years. In the National Comorbidity Survey in the USA, Blazer *et al.* (1998) found that older respondents among over 8000 surveyed were more likely to have DSM-IIIR diagnosis of both major and minor recurrent depression with a seasonal pattern. They noted that the definition of recurrence was more likely to be satisfied by older subjects.

Among SPAQ studies, there is more agreement that SAD is common among younger adults (see Magnusson 2000). Table 4.1 shows rates of winter problems (the categories of SAD and subsyndromal – SAD [s-SAD] combined) in our own study (Eagles *et al.* 1999) of 4557 people in Aberdeen, grouped by age and sex, who were waiting to see a doctor in primary care. In both sexes, rates peak in the 35 to 44 years age group and decline thereafter. Broken into SAD and S-SAD, the rates are shown graphically by age and sex in Figs. 4.1 and

Table 4.1 Winter problems (combined SAD and S-SAD) by age and sex. Aberdeen primary care study (Eagles *et al.* 1999)

Age group (years)	Males	Females
16–24	30 / 224 (13.4%)	137 / 545 (25.1%)
25–34	51 / 331 (15.4%)	193 / 774 (24.9%)
35–44	78 / 369 (21.1%)	195 / 683 (28.6%)
45–54	65 / 366 (17.8%)	104 / 559 (18.6%)
55–64	50 / 304 (16.4%)	70 / 402 (17.4%)
ALL	274 / 1594 (17.2%)	709 / 2963 (23.9%)

4.2. As we found in a previous study (Eagles *et al.* 1996), there is a suggestion, especially among females, of a peak in S-SAD at age 25 to 34, with women then 'graduating' to full SAD, with a peak at age 35 to 44 years.

The relationship between age and SAD is variously reported in different SPAQ studies, and a brief synopsis of findings follows. In Alaska, Booker and Hellekson (1992) compared under 40s with over 40s, and found the younger group to have a 2.8-fold and a 3.9-fold increased rate of SAD and S-SAD respectively. Hegde and Woodson (1996), screening staff and students at a Texas University, found that respondents over the age of 50 experienced significantly fewer seasonal changes. In Iceland, Magnusson and Stefansson (1993) found the highest prevalence of SAD and S-SAD in the under 25 age group. Mersch *et al.* (1999a), in a large study in the Netherlands, found that respondents without SAD had a mean age of 39.7 while those with SAD had a mean age of 36.5 and with S-SAD, a mean age of 35.6 years. Rosen *et al.* (1990) reported low rates of SAD in their four-centre study of subjects aged over 54. Two large SPAQ studies — Okawa *et al.* (1996) in Japan and Saarijärvi *et al.* (1999) in northern Finland — have not found a significant relationship between age and SAD.

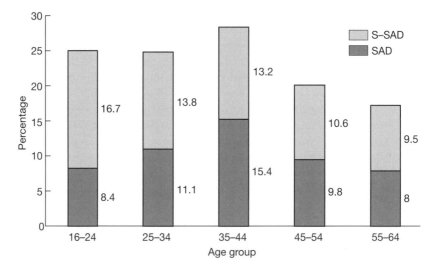

Fig. 4.1 SPAQ prevalence of females with SAD and S-SAD, by age group. Aberdeen primary care study (Eagles *et al.* 1999).

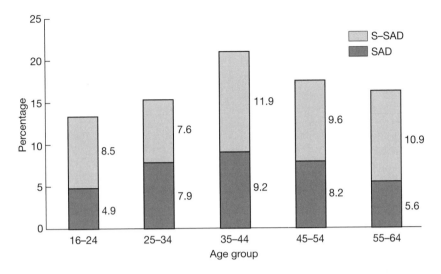

Fig. 4.2 SPAQ prevalence of males with SAD and S-SAD, by age group. Aberdeen primary care study (Eagles *et al.* 1999).

The relationship between age and the global seasonality score (GSS) within the SPAQ has also been investigated. In general, there are statistically significantly negative correlations between GSS and age — –0.25 (Kasper *et al.* 1989), –0.11 (Eagles *et al.* 1996), –0.29 for women and –0.14 for men (Muscettola *et al.* 1995). Magnusson and Axelsson (1993), in their sample from Manitoba, estimated that GSS decreased by a mean of 0.05 with each increasing year of age. Taking an age cut-off of 41/42 years, Dam *et al.* (1998) in Copenhagen found that the younger age group were significantly more seasonal within the GSS and perceived themselves as being more profoundly affected by weather conditions. Mersch *et al.* (1999*a*) noted that highest GSS scores occurred in younger respondents, but only in later years were seasonal fluctuations in well-being perceived as significant problems, giving rise to subjects constituting a 'case' on the SPAQ.

Certainly in SPAQ studies, therefore, younger adults predominate among SAD sufferers. It is worth noting that this contrasts with non-seasonal depression, for which both sexes tend to exhibit an age peak in their early 60s (Lehtinen and Joukamaa 1994).

Old age

Literature on SAD among older adults is much more sparse, but confirms the decline in prevalence among older age groups that has been described earlier. Harris and Dawson–Hughes (1993) interviewed 250 post-menopausal women aged 43 to 72 years (mean age 62) for a trial of vitamin D in bone loss at four points during a year. These women exhibited a small peak of psychological morbidity in autumn rather than in winter. In Maryland, Genhart *et al.* (1993) recruited 140 people out of 265 available residents (53 per cent) in age-segregated housing units, with a mean age of 79 years. They had a very low mean global seasonality score of 2.0. A trial of light therapy tended to exacerbate, rather than to improve, symptomatology on the Hamilton Depression Rating Scale.

Within a large urban/rural primary care practice in north-east Scotland, Eagles *et al.* (1997) looked at self-ratings of psychopathology made by an elderly population (mean age 73 years) during the course of a study which spanned a 21-month period. There was a 98 per cent completion rate. The ratings of the 387 subjects surveyed during winter (December, January, and February) were compared with the 1079 subjects responding during other months. Five different rating scales were deployed, and while winter levels of psychopathology were significantly higher on each scale, in terms of rates of actual cases there was only a slight (and statistically non-significant) difference. For example, 13.2 per cent and 10.4 per cent were cases on the General Health Questionnaire in winter and during the rest of the year respectively.

4.2.4 Summary

Rates of SAD in children increase at puberty (in females if not in males), prevalence reaches a peak in the middle of the reproductive years, and then falls off in old age.

4.3 Gender

Some gender differences in the epidemiology of SAD have been alluded to earlier, since the effects of age differ between the sexes. Pre-pubertally, boys and girls seem to be fairly equally affected (Swedo *et al.* 1995), and in the only study which has looked at possible gender differences in old age (Eagles *et al.* 1997) there was no evidence that elderly females experienced any more seasonal fluctuations in well-being than did their male counterparts. At the extremes of lifespan, therefore, there is no evidence of a gender difference in prevalence, but the situation is different during the middle years (roughly age 14 to 50), and in the following I focus on that age group. Again, studies which have not involved the SPAQ will be covered first.

Among clinical cohorts of patients with SAD, females have predominated since the first description by Rosenthal *et al.* (1984), of whose first 29 patients, 25 were female. As the patient group in the Washington DC area was enlarged, a female preponderance persisted — 182 out of 220 (Rosenthal and Wehr 1987). Among a study by Lingjærde and Reichborn–Kjennerud (1993), 81 per cent were women among a media recruited sample. Indeed, it is instructive to note the predominance of female subjects in trials of light therapy. Lee and Chan (1998) reviewed 40 such studies and found that among 1129 subjects, females outnumbered males by nearly 3.5 to 1. In three more recently conducted trials of light therapy, there was an even higher proportion of females (83 per cent) among the 307 subjects (Eastman *et al.* 1998; Lewy *et al.* 1998; Terman *et al.* 1998). These figures are likely to reflect, in part, a greater willingness among females to seek treatment and to engage in research studies.

Nevertheless, females predominate, albeit to a lesser extent, in studies of non-clinical samples. Schlager *et al.* (1993) screened 1870 employees of a large company in Pennsylvania from October through to the following August. Comparing winter scores (December, January, and February) with those during other months, women experienced significant winter increases in rates of psychopathology (low mood, anxiety, and somatization) but men did not. Two studies in the far north (Hansen *et al.* 1998; Nilssen *et al.* 1999) have reported that polar nights are more likely to evoke depression in women than in men. Blazer *et al.*'s (1998) study gave rise to atypical findings when deploying DSM-III-R diagnostic criteria. In comparison to people with non-seasonal depression, males were more likely to have seasonally recurrent *major* depression while females were more likely to suffer from seasonally recurrent *minor* depression. Another study which utilized tight diagnostic criteria, including DSM-IV, conducted at a higher latitude in Scotland (Eagles *et al.* 1999) estimated the community prevalence of SAD at 4.8 per cent in females and 2.1 per cent in males. Interestingly, among subjects who were cases of SAD on the SPAQ, a higher proportion of females (45 per cent) than of males (28 per cent) satisfied more stringent diagnostic criteria.

Among SPAQ studies, there is a wealth of evidence that females endure more seasonally mediated pathology, certainly in populations distant from the equator (Magnusson 2000). Studies often compare rates between the sexes for both SAD and S-SAD, but for brevity I shall mention only comparisons of SAD. Female to male ratios of SPAQ cases of SAD can often be calculated and these include 3.5 in a telephone study in Maryland (Kasper *et al.* 1989), 3.0 in Alaska (Booker and Hellekson 1992), 1.5 among Icelanders (Magnusson and Stefansson 1993), 4.0 among psychiatric nurses in Aberdeen (Eagles *et al.* 1996), 1.6 in Copenhagen (Dam *et al.* 1998), 1.5 among primary care attendees in north-east Scotland (Eagles *et al.* 1998), 3.1 in the Netherlands (Mersch *et al.* 1999*a*), 2.0 in northern Finland (Saarijärvi *et al.* 1998), and 3.3 among college students in Maine, USA (Rohan and Sigmon 2000). Most of these studies also reported that females had significantly higher scores than males on the GSS.

Interestingly, studies which have found lesser or no female preponderance among sufferers on the SPAQ have been conducted at lower latitudes, for example, in employees of a large company in the Philippines (Ito *et al.* 1992), in staff and students at a Texas university (Hegde and Woodson 1996), in two Japanese samples (Ozaki *et al.* 1995; Okawa *et al.* 1996), and among students in China (Han et al. 2000*a*, 2000*b*). Two of these studies (Ito *et al.* 1992; Hegde and Woodson 1996) did find greater female pathology on the GSS. Findings suggest, however, that higher latitudes of residence may be more likely to invoke seasonal changes in females than in males.

Other methods of investigation suggest increased rates of seasonal problems in females. In Birmingham, Suhail and Cochrane (1998) found that females but not males had a winter peak of admissions with depression. Spring peaks in suicide in Europe seem to be higher among men, with autumn peaks more evident among females (Näyhä 1982; Preti 1997).

Finally, it is worth remembering that disorders of mood and anxiety are generally significantly more prevalent among females and, certainly for depression, this seems to be a transcultural phenomenon (Gater *et al.* 1998). That is to say, while this increased morbidity may well in part reflect a variety of psychosocial factors (Jenkins 1985), females are likely to have an increased biological propensity to develop affective disorders in general. Their increased rates of SAD should be viewed in this context.

4.4 Socio-economic and educational status

Since socio-economic and educational levels are highly correlated variables, they will be dealt with together.

Socio-economic disadvantage and lower levels of education are both risk factors for the development of non-seasonal depression. Socially disadvantaged children are more likely to become depressed adults (Sadowski *et al.* 1999) and current low income and poor social environment also predispose to non-seasonal depression (Lynch *et al.* 1997; Mathiesen *et al.* 1999). Lower levels of education are consistently found to be associated with depression during adult and late life (Blazer *et al.* 1994; van Os *et al.* 1997; Kubzansky *et al.* 1998).

It is thus somewhat surprising that a different situation seems to prevail for SAD. Blazer *et al.* (1998) found that people in households with annual incomes of more than $70 000 were significantly more likely to satisfy DSM-IIIR criteria for SAD (odds ratio 3.7) than those in poorer families. In northern Finland, Saarijärvi *et al.* (1999) looked at the risk of suffering from winter seasonality on the SPAQ compared against subjects with no vocational education, and found educational groupings to have the following significantly elevated odds ratios: vocational education 1.6, college degree 1.6, university degree 2.2. Mersch *et al.* (1999*a*) did not detect any relationship between educational attainment and the likelihood of having SAD in the Netherlands, and neither educational level nor income were related to the risk of depressive symptoms among people over-wintering in Antarctica (Palinkas *et al.* 1995).

While most studies of SAD have not included investigation of these particular sociodemographic variables, it is intriguing that on the available evidence, SAD does seem to differ from non-seasonal depression. Saarijärvi *et al.* (1999) suggested that higher educational achievers would be more likely to work indoors and thus to suffer from SAD through light deprivation, but this idea lacks supporting evidence (see the next section 'Employment'), and wondered if better educated people might simply be more aware of seasonal fluctuations in well-being. It is worth noting that in families of patients with bipolar affective disorder (but not with major depression), there is an over-representation of higher occupational class (Verdoux and Bourgeois 1995). This may well indicate that the genetics of bipolar affective disorder link to those of high achievement, and perhaps a similar situation pertains with SAD, with SAD sufferers (being less seriously affected than those with bipolar disorder) remaining able to achieve their genetic potential rather than it being observed through the achievement of their relatives.

4.5 **Employment**

Perhaps the most obvious way in which employment might relate to SAD is that a dimly lit workplace and/or a job which allows little time for daylight exposure during the darker months of the year might give rise to winter depression through light deprivation. There are anecdotal reports to this effect (Eagles 1994; Rosenthal 1998). Few studies, however, have systematically investigated the relationship between employment and SAD.

Magnusson and Stefansson (1993) found no differences in rates of SAD in their Icelandic subjects with regard to whether they worked indoors or outdoors. They did not give figures in their paper however, and one suspects that the proportion of outdoor workers was relatively small and that a larger cohort would be required to generate adequate statistical power in this type of comparison. It has been said, anecdotally, that SAD was rediscovered in the twentieth century since at the beginning of the nineteenth century 90 per cent of people in developed countries worked outdoors compared with 90 per cent who now work indoors. Especially since people with SAD may 'self-select' to work outdoors, this very imbalance of indoor/outdoor workers makes the relationship difficult to research.

Shift work desynchronizes sleepwake cycles, not infrequently having deleterious psychological effects (Regestein and Monk 1991), and the chronobiology of such effects can be likened to the presumed aetiology of SAD. While I suspect that shift workers may be over-represented among referrals to my SAD clinics, when psychiatric nurses in Aberdeen completed SPAQs there was no indication of an elevated risk of SAD among those working night shifts (Eagles *et al.* 1996). Again, self-selection may have played a part in this negative finding in that nurses who found that their psychological well-being was not affected by working at night may have gravitated towards this shift.

Booker and Hellekson (1992) found no differences in rates of SAD in Alaska between employed and unemployed people in their sample. In their larger study in the Netherlands, Mersch *et al.* (1999*a*) found that 41 per cent of people with SAD were employed. This was significantly less than respondents with subsyndromal SAD (59 per cent) or without significant seasonal pathology (57 per cent). Self-evidently, it is not possible to extricate cause from effect in this relationship, especially since people with SAD in this study were more likely to take time off work due to seasonally mediated ill health.

Suicide statistics can yield data which give rise to hypotheses about employment and seasonal changes in mood. Chew and McCleary (1995) investigated seasonality of suicides in 28 countries between the 1960s to 1980s, and found that the size of the spring peak was correlated with the size of a country's agricultural workforce. Only for women in temperate countries was there evidence of an autumn peak. Näyhä (1982), writing before the rediscovery of SAD, noted that the autumn peak in suicides in Finland was most obvious in women and those in 'modern' (that is, indoor) occupations, while a spring peak was evident in agricultural workers. Noting the autumn peak as characteristic of people working in 'man-made environments', she related her findings to variations in ambient daylight levels.

In summary, we have little data on the relationship between SAD and employment. As data accrue, it will be important to note the likely interrelationship between type of employment and other sociodemographic variables, notably educational level, age, and gender.

4.6 **Marital status and fertility**

While the effect may be stronger for men than for women, marriage is usually found to be associated with lower levels of psychiatric morbidity (for example, Hope *et al.* 1999). The available evidence suggests that this effect also prevails in SAD, although the relationship of seasonal symptoms to marital status has not been frequently investigated. Saarijärvi *et al.* (1999) found no relationship between marital status and seasonality in Finland, and in Alaska, Booker and Hellekson (1992) found a slightly, but statistically non-significantly, lower rate of SAD among married people. Mersch *et al.* (1999*a*) found that among subjects with SAD, 53 per cent were married, and among S-SAD subjects, 54 per cent were married. This compared with 61 per cent of unaffected subjects. They analysed these data in a 3 by 2 chi-squared and concluded that marriage and seasonality were not related. However, if one compares a 'winter problems' group (SAD and S-SAD combined) against unaffected subjects in a 2 by 2 chi-squared then this gives a figure of $\chi^2 = 5.27$, d.f. $= 1$, p $= 0.02$, and an odds ratio of 0.76 (95% CI 0.60 to 0.97). In our own group's study of psychiatric nurses, logistic regression analysis of risk factors for SAD found that marriage conferred a significantly lower risk (odds ratio of 0.19, 95% CI 0.06 to 0.59). Among 119 people over-wintering in Antarctica, being married was an independent predictor of *greater* likelihood of suffering from winter depression (Palinkas *et al.* 1995). The authors attributed this to the prolonged separation of married people from spouses and families.

If married people are indeed less likely to suffer from winter depression, what is likely to be the direction of causality? That is to say, does marriage protect against SAD, or are people who suffer from SAD less likely to be married? In that married/cohabiting people living with a partner seem to be less likely to have SAD and married people separated from spouses seem more likely to experience SAD, it seems very likely that marriage is a protective factor. As a corollary, the data would not support the contention that SAD might confer a social disadvantage with regard to the likelihood of marrying.

However, the studies finding low rates of SAD among Icelanders both in Iceland and in Manitoba (Magnusson and Stefansson 1993; Magnusson and Axelsson 1993) concluded that the findings represented a genetic adaptation to living at high latitudes, given that winter depression was biologically disadvantageous to reproduction. It was acknowledged that this was 'an assumption that as yet has no independent support' (Magnusson and Axelsson 1993).

Schlager's (1998) review discusses the evolution of biological rhythms and concludes that it is difficult to see SAD conferring evolutionary advantages. Wehr and Rosenthal (1989), however, hypothesized that seasonality might maximize efficiency of energy use. Lester (1997), adopting month by month suicide rates in the USA as a proxy measure of depression in the population, found a significant negative correlation (Spearman's $r = -0.54$) with birth rates nine months later. Given the human gestation period of nine months, in earlier centuries SAD may have conferred an advantage if it increased the likelihood of spring/summer conception and thus of late winter/spring births, following which babies born away from the equator would anticipate warmer weather and more plentiful food supplies in the early months of life, thus presumably enhancing their chances of survival.

If SAD and fertility are linked then reproductive patterns of people with SAD should differ from people without seasonal pathology. In Aberdeen, we matched subjects who had been quite tightly diagnosed with SAD (see Eagles *et al.* 1999) each with two age- and sex-matched controls who had exhibited little or no seasonal pathology on the SPAQ. Out of 73 respondents with SAD, 49 were married or cohabiting (67 per cent) as against 97 out of 128 controls (76 per cent) — this difference not being statistically significant. The fertility of the SAD subjects was actually slightly greater than that of controls with an average of 1.62 and 1.46 children respectively. Furthermore, there was no apparent difference with regard to the months in which the two groups' children were born. Taking January to July as the optimal months to be born, in line with the aforementioned hypothesis, 58 per cent of the 118 children of SAD subjects and 54 per cent of the 187 children of controls were born during this period of the year. On the basis of this relatively small study, therefore, there is no evidence of reduced fertility or of a change in seasonal birth patterns among people with SAD.

In larger samples, the seasons clearly influence human fertility — see Bronson (1995) for a full review. In most European countries there is a spring peak in births, and most industrialized countries show a reduction in birth seasonality over the past hundred years (Lam and Miron 1991). Moving north from the southern states of the USA to Canada, a spring trough of births is replaced by a spring peak (Bronson 1995). These findings suggest, at higher latitudes, a pattern of evolutionary advantage of spring birth which has been flattened out by industrialization, and might be taken as indirect evidence that SAD conferred a reproductive advantage rather than the disadvantage hypothesized by Magnusson and Axelsson (1993).

4.7 Societal factors

Social influences are difficult to extricate from effects of ethnicity (see the chapter by Magnusson) and will be touched on only briefly here.

As noted at the start of this chapter, self-reporting of symptoms of SAD may be influenced by several demographic and social factors. Noting that rates of SAD on the SPAQ in North America are generally about twice as high as those reported in Europe, Mersch *et al.* (1999*b*) suggested that this may reflect a difference in the cultural acceptability of acknowledging and admitting to psychological problems. Murase *et al.* (1995) administered the Beck Depression

Inventory to 242 Japanese subjects who had moved to Stockholm. The authors had anticipated that recent arrivals would show more winter exacerbation of depressive symptoms, but in fact this was significantly more marked among respondents who had been in Stockholm for more than 10 years. The authors thought that this finding may have related to progressive acceptance of Swedish culture and lifestyle the longer the period of immigration continued. When people move to societies in the far north, however, then there is a trend for seasonal morbidity to *decline* with longer duration of residence (Booker and Hellekson 1992; Saarijärvi *et al.* 1999) — although this finding may relate to reducing seasonal morbidity with advancing age.

What the findings from these four studies may indicate is that immigrants may adopt a level of stoicism/openness to acknowledge psychological difficulties which they deem appropriate to the level which prevails in the society to which they have moved. This underlines the vagaries of inferring biological differences between populations with regard to SAD, especially when differences are based on self-report measures such as the SPAQ.

4.8 Conclusions

It seems justified to conclude that, certainly at more northerly latitudes, females are significantly more at risk than males of suffering from SAD. This gender difference is apparently confined to the female reproductive years, and seasonally mediated changes in psychological well-being decline after the middle years of life. Marriage may be a protective factor against SAD but, contrary to non-seasonal depression, the disorder may be more prevalent among the socially and educationally advantaged.

These sociodemographic differences are likely to reflect both biological and psychological factors. The pattern of age and gender effects lends strong support to a link with female reproductive hormones (Kasper *et al.* 1989; Partonen 1995). Other intervening variables, which may relate to the aetiology of SAD, could account in part for sociodemographic variations in prevalence. People with SAD have a greater seasonal change in light exposure than non-sufferers, while men have consistently more light exposure than women across the seasons of the year (Mersch *et al.* 1999*a*). In temperate climates, exercise is taken more frequently in summer than in winter (Dannenberg *et al.* 1989), and women exercise less than men, although the gradient of greater levels of exercise with increasing socio-economic prosperity (Eyler *et al.* 1997) argues against the importance of exercise as a protective intervening variable. Age, gender, and educational level all influence diet (Haines *et al.* 1992) and, given that winter seasonality is positively correlated with body mass index (Saarijärvi 1999), which may in turn correlate with exercise levels and light exposure (Graw *et al.* 1999), any possible relationship between diet and the sociodemographics of SAD is likely to be complex.

Research into SAD is, relatively speaking, in its infancy. Despite the complexities of sociodemographic research, we should persist with studies in this area, which can ultimately yield much evidence about the aetiology of SAD.

Acknowledgements

I am grateful to statistician Jane Andrew who provided data and statistical analyses for this chapter. Additional data were presented from our local studies, which were conducted in collaboration with Simon Naji, Samantha Wileman, Isobel Cameron, Fiona Howie, Ken Lawton,

Carol Robertson, Douglas Gray, Mysore Dharmendra, and Kirsty Webb. The secretarial work was done by Lana Hadden.

References

Blazer, D.G., Kessler, R.C., McGonagle, K.A., and Swartz, M.S. (1994). The prevalence and distribution of major depression in a national community sample: the National Comorbidity Survey. *American Journal of Psychiatry*, **151**:979–86.

Blazer, D.G., Kessler, R.C., and Swartz, M.S. (1998). Epidemiology of recurrent major and minor depression with a seasonal pattern. *British Journal of Psychiatry*, **172**:164–7.

Booker, J.M. and Hellekson, C.J. (1992). Prevalence of seasonal affective disorder in Alaska. *American Journal of Psychiatry*, **149**:1176–82.

Bronson, F.H. (1995). Seasonal variation in human reproduction: environmental factors. *Quarterly Review of Biology*, **70**:141–64.

Carskadon, M.A. and Acebo, C. (1993). Parental reports of seasonal mood and behavior changes in children. *Journal of the American Academy of Child and Adolescent Psychiatry*, **32**:264–9.

Chew, K.S.Y. and McCleary, R. (1995). The spring peak in suicides: a cross-national analysis. *Social Science and Medicine*, **2**:223–30.

Dam, H., Jakobsen, K., and Mellerup, E. (1998). Prevalence of winter depression in Denmark. *Acta Psychiatrica Scandinavica*, **97**:1–4.

Dannenberg, A.O., Keller, J.B., Wilson, P.W., and Castelli, W.P. (1989). Leisure time physical activity in the Framingham offspring study. Description, seasonal variation, and risk factor correlates. *American Journal of Epidemiology*, **129**:76–88.

Eagles, J.M. (1994). The relationship between mood and daily hours of sunlight in rapid cycling bipolar illness. *Biological Psychiatry*, **36**:422–4.

Eagles, J.M., Mercer, G., Boshier, A.J., and Jamieson, F. (1996). Seasonal affective disorder among psychiatric nurses in Aberdeen. *Journal of Affective Disorders*, **37**:129–35.

Eagles, J.M., McLeod, I.H., and Douglas, A.S. (1997). Seasonal changes in psychological well-being in an elderly population. *British Journal of Psychiatry*, **171**:53–5.

Eagles, J.M., Naji, S.A., Gray, D.A., Christie, J., and Beattie, J.A.G. (1998). Seasonal affective disorder among primary care consulters in January: prevalence and month by month consultation patterns. *Journal of Affective Disorders*, **49**:1–8.

Eagles, J.M., Wileman, S.M., Cameron, I.M., Howie, F.L., Lawton, K., Gray, D.A., *et al.* (1999). Seasonal affective disorder among primary care attenders and a community sample in Aberdeen. *British Journal of Psychiatry*, **175**:472–5.

Eastman, C.I., Young, M.A., Fogg, L.F., Liu, L., and Meaden, P.M. (1998). Bright light treatment of winter depression. *Archives of General Psychiatry*, **55**:883–9.

Eyler, A.A., Brownson, R.C., King, A.C., Brown, D., Donatelle, R.J., and Heath, G. (1997). Physical activity and women in the United States: an overview of health benefits, prevalence, and intervention opportunities. *Women & Health*, **26**:27–49.

Gater, R., Tansella, M., Korten, A., Tiemens, B.G., Mavreas, V.G., and Olatawura, M.O. (1998). Sex differences in the prevalence and detection of depressive and anxiety disorders in general health care settings. *Archives of General Psychiatry*, **55**:405–13.

Genhart, M.J., Kelly, K.A., Coursey, R.D., Datiles, M., and Rosenthal, N.E. (1993). Effects of bright light on mood in normal elderly women. *Psychiatry Research*, **47**:87–97.

Graw, P., Recker, S., Sand, L., Krauchi, K., and Wirz–Justice, A. (1999). Winter and summer outdoor light exposure in women with and without seasonal affective disorder. *Journal of Affective Disorder*, **56**:163–9.

Haines, P.S., Hungerford, D.W., Popkin, B.M., and Guilkey, D.K. (1992). Eating patterns and energy and nutrient intakes of US women. *Journal of the American Dietetic Association*, **92**:698–704.

Han, L., Wang, K., Du, Z., Cheng, Y., Simons, J.S., and Rosenthal, N.E. (2000a). Seasonal variations in mood and behavior among Chinese medical students. *American Journal of Psychiatry*, **157**:133–5.

Han, L., Wang, K., Cheng, Y., Du, Z., Rosenthal, N.E., and Primeau, F. (2000b). Summer and winter patterns of seasonality in Chinese college students: a replication. *Comprehensive Psychiatry*, **41**:57–62.

Hansen, V., Lund, E., and Smith–Sivertsen, T. (1998). Self-reported mental distress under the shifting daylight in the high north. *Psychological Medicine*, **28**:447–52.

Harris, S. and Dawson–Hughes, B. (1993). Seasonal mood changes in 250 normal women. *Psychiatry Research*, **49**:77–87.

Hegde, A.L. and Woodson, H. (1996). Prevalence of seasonal changes in mood and behavior during the winter months in central Texas. *Psychiatry Research*, **62**:265–71.

Hope, S., Rodgers, B., and Power, C. (1999). Marital status transitions and psychological distress: longitudinal evidence from a national population sample. *Psychological Medicine*, **29**:381–9.

Ito, A., Ichihara, M., Hisanaga, N., Ono, Y., Kajukawa, Y., Ohta, T., *et al.* (1992). Prevalence of seasonal mood changes in low latitude area. *Japanese Journal of Psychiatry*, **46**:249.

Jenkins, R. (1985). Sex differences in minor psychiatric morbidity. *Psychological Medicine*, **Monograph Supplement 7**:1–53.

Kasper, S., Wehr, T.A., Bartko, J.J., Gaist, P.A., and Rosenthal, N.E. (1989). Epidemiological findings of seasonal changes in mood and behavior. A telephone survey of Montgomery Country, Maryland. *Archives of General Psychiatry*, **46**:823–33.

Kubzansky, L.D., Berkman, L.F., Glass, T.A., and Seeman, T.E. (1998). Is educational attainment associated with shared determinants of health in the elderly? *Psychosomatic Medicine*, **60**:578–85.

Lam, D.A. and Miron J.A. (1991). Seasonality of births in human populations. *Social Biology*, **38**:51–78.

Lee, T.M. and Chan, C.C.H. (1998). Vulnerability by sex to seasonal affective disorder. *Perceptual and Motor Skills*, **87**:1120–2.

Lehtinen, V. and Joukamaa, M. (1994). Epidemiology of depression: prevalence, risk factors and treatment situation. *Acta Psychiatrica Scandinavica*, **377**:7–10.

Lester, D. (1997). Seasonal depression and conception. *Perceptual and Motor Skills*, **85**:256.

Lewy, A.J., Bauer, V.K., Cutler, N.L., Sack, R.L., Ahmed, S., Thomas, K.H., *et al.* (1998). Morning vs evening light treatment of patients with winter depression. *Archives of General Psychiatry*, **55**:890–6.

Lingjærde, O. and Reichborn–Kjennerud, T. (1993). Characteristics of winter depression in the Oslo area (60N). *Acta Psychiatrica Scandinavica*, **88**:111–20.

Lynch, J.W., Kaplan, G.A., and Shema, S.J. (1997). Cumulative impact of sustained economic hardship on physical, cognitive, psychological and social functioning. *New England Journal of Medicine*, **337**:1889–95.

Magnusson, A. (2000). An overview of epidemiological studies on seasonal affective disorder. *Acta Psychiatrica Scandinavica*, **101**:176–84.

Magnusson, A. and Axelsson, J. (1993). The prevalence of seasonal affective disorder is low among descendants of Icelandic emigrants in Canada. *Archives of General Psychiatry*, **50**:947–51.

Magnusson, A and Stefansson, J.G. (1993). Prevalence of seasonal affective disorder in Iceland. *Archives of General Psychiatry*, **50**:941–6.

Mathiesen, K.S., Tambs, K., and Dalgard, O.S. (1999). The influence of social class, strain and social support on symptoms of anxiety and depression in mothers of toddlers. *Social Psychiatry and Psychiatric Epidemiology*, **34**:61–72.

Mersch, P.P.A., Middendorp, H.M., Bouhuys, A.L., Beersma, D.G.M., and van den Hoofdakker, R.H. (1999a). The prevalence of seasonal affective disorder in the Netherlands: a prospective and retrospective study of seasonal mood variation in the general population. *Biological Psychiatry*, **45**:1013–22.

Mersch, P.P.A., Middendorp, H.M., Bouhuys, A.L., Beersma, D.G.M., and van den Hoofdakker, R.H. (1999b). Seasonal affective disorder and latitude: a review of the literature. *Journal of Affective Disorders*, **53**:35–48.

Murase, S., Murase, S., Kitabatake, M., Yamauchi, T., and Mathé, A.A. (1995). Seasonal mood variation among Japanese residents of Stockholm. *Acta Psychiatrica Scandinavica*, **92**:51–5.

Muscettola, G., Barbato, G., Ficca, G., Beatrice, M., Puca, M., Aguglia, E., *et al.* (1995). Seasonality of mood in Italy: role of latitude and sociocultural factors. *Journal of Affective Disorders*, **33**:135–9.

Näyhä, S. (1982). Autumn incidence of suicides re-examined: data from Finland by sex, age and occupation. *British Journal of Psychiatry*, **141**:512–17.

Nayyar, S. and Cochrane, R. (1996). Seasonal changes in affective state measured prospectively and retrospectively. *British Journal of Psychiatry*, **168**:627–32.

Nilssen, O., Brenn, T., Høyer, G., Lipton, R., Boiko, J., and Tkatchev, A. (1999). Self-reported seasonal variation in depression at 78 degree north. *Original Research*, **58**:14–23.

Okawa, M., Shirakawa, S., Uchiyama, M., Oguri, M., Kohsaka, M., Mishima, K., *et al.* (1996). Seasonal variation of mood and behaviour in a healthy middle-aged population in Japan. *Acta Psychiatrica Scandinavica*, **94**:211–16.

Ozaki, N., Ono, Y., Ito, A., and Rosenthal, N.E. (1995). Prevalence of seasonal difficulties in mood and behavior among Japanese civil servants. *American Journal of Psychiatry*, **152**:1225–7.

Palinkas, L.A., Cravalho, M., and Browner, D. (1995). Seasonal variation of depressive symptoms in Antarctica. *Acta Psychiatrica Scandinavica*, **91**:423–9.

Partonen T. (1995). Estrogen could control photoperiodic adjustment in seasonal affective disorder. *Medical Hypotheses*, **45**:35–6.

Preti, A. (1997). The influence of seasonal change on suicidal behaviour in Italy. *Journal of Affective Disorders*, **44**:123–30.

Regestein, Q.R. and Monk, T.H. (1991). Is the poor sleep of shift workers a disorder? *American Journal of Psychiatry*, **148**:1487–93.

Rohan, K.J. and Sigmon, S.T. (2000). Seasonal mood patterns in a northeastern college sample. *Journal of Affective Disorders*, **59**:85–96.

Rosen, L.N., Targum, S.D., Terman, M., Bryant, M.J., Hoffman, H., Kasper, S.F., *et al.* (1990). Prevalence of seasonal affective disorder at four latitudes. *Psychiatry Research*, **31**:131–44.

Rosenthal, N.E. (1998). *Winter blues*, p. 51. Guilford Press, New York.

Rosenthal, N.E., Sack, D.A., Gillin, J.C., Lewy, A.J., Goodwin, F.K., Davenport, Y., *et al.* (1984). Seasonal affective disorder. *Archives of General Psychiatry*, **41**:72–80.

Rosenthal, N.E., Carpenter, C.J., James, S.P., Parry, B.L., Rogers, S.L.B., and Wehr, T.A. (1986). Seasonal affective disorder in children and adolescents. *American Journal of Psychiatry*, **143**:356–8.

Rosenthal, N.E. and Wehr, T.A. (1987). Seasonal affective disorders. *Psychiatric Annals*, **17**:670–4.

Saarijärvi, S., Lauerma, H., Helenius, H., and Saarilehto, S. (1999). Seasonal affective disorders among rural Finns and Lapps. *Acta Psychiatrica Scandinavica*, **99**:95–101.

Sadowski, H., Ugarte, B., Kolvin, I., Kaplan, C., and Barnes, J. (1999). Early life family disadvantages and major depression in adulthood. *British Journal of Psychiatry*, **174**:112–20.

Schlager, D. (1998). Evolution of biological rhythms. *Light Treatment and Biological Rhythms*, **10(2)**:1–5, 17.

Schlager, D., Schwartz, J.E., and Bromet, E.J. (1993). Seasonal variations of current symptoms in a healthy population. *British Journal of Psychiatry*, **163**:322–6.

Sonis, W.A. (1989). Seasonal affective disorder of childhood and adolescents: a review. In *Seasonal affective disorders and phototherapy* (ed. N.E. Rosenthal and M.C. Blehar), pp. 55–63. Guilford Press, New York.

Sonis, W.A., Yellin, A.M., Garfinkel, B.D., and Hoberman, H.H. (1987). The antidepressant effect of light in seasonal affective disorder of childhood and adolescence. *Psychopharmacology Bulletin*, **23**:360–3.

Sourander, A., Koskelainen, M., and Helenius, H. (1999). Mood, latitude and seasonality among adolescents. *Journal of the American Academy of Child and Adolescent Psychiatry*, **38**:1271–6.

Suhail, K. and Cochrane, R. (1998). Seasonal variations in hospital admissions for affective disorders by gender and ethnicity. *Social Psychiatry and Psychiatric Epidemiology*, **33**:211–17.

Swedo, S.E., Pleeter, J.D., Richter, D.M., Hoffman, C.L., Allen, A.J., Hamburger, S.D., *et al.* (1995). Rates of seasonal affective disorder in children and adolescents. *American Journal of Psychiatry*, **152**:1016–19.

Terman, M., Terman, J.S., and Ross, D.C. (1998). A controlled trial of timed bright light and negative air ionization for treatment of winter depression. *Archives of General Psychiatry*, **55**:875–82.

van Os, J., Jones, P., Lewis, G., Wadsworth, M., and Murray, R. (1997). Development precursors of affective illness in a general population birth cohort. *Archives of General Psychiatry*, **54**:625–31.

Verdoux, H. and Bourgeois, M. (1995). Social class in unipolar and bipolar probands and relatives. *Journal of Affective Disorders*, **33**:181–7.

Wehr, T.A. and Rosenthal, N.E. (1989). Seasonality and affective illness. *American Journal of Psychiatry*, **146**:829–39.

Chapter 5

Acclimatization

Andres Magnusson

5.1 **Ethnicity**

Twin studies have revealed that genes may influence the tendency to experience seasonal changes in mood and behaviour (Madden *et al.* 1996; Jang *et al.* 1997) and hence it is theoretically possible that the prevalence of SAD may differ among ethnic groups.

The issue of ethnicity and SAD has been addressed in at least 13 studies. The first studies came from Alaska. In a community survey employing the SPAQ in Alaska (65° N), Booker and Hellekson examined whether rates of SAD and S-SAD differed among whites, blacks, and native Alaskans (Booker and Hellekson 1992). No statistically significant differences were found. Native Alaskans have been exposed to arctic winters for hundreds of generations, while there is hardly any winter at all in large parts of Africa. Still, the rates for winter problems (SAD and S-SAD) were remarkably similar in blacks (a ratio of 8 to 23) and native Alaskans (a ratio of 6 to 19). The same authors also collaborated on a SPAQ study in the former Soviet Union. The details of that study have not yet been published, but preliminary results have been presented (Booker *et al.* 1991). In that study, which was carried out at four different sites (38° N to 64° N), the prevalence of SAD proved to be fairly similar to surveys from other parts of the world (Magnusson 2000). An exception was the natives in Providenia in Siberia. No cases of SAD were found among the 92 natives examined (Booker *et al.* 1991).

Certain features of SAD seem to be unique to the Japanese population. For example, exceptionally low prevalence rates of SAD and S-SAD have been found in Japan (Takahashi *et al.* 1991; Ozaki *et al.* 1995). Furthermore, in contrast to findings from other countries, there is little or no preponderance of females among SAD sufferers in Japan (Takahashi *et al.* 1991; Ozaki *et al.* 1995; Okawa *et al.* 1996). In addition, while SAD and S-SAD is usually more common in the young, there has been little effect of age in Japanese surveys (Takahashi *et al.* 1991; Ozaki *et al.* 1995; Okawa *et al.* 1996). Genetic factors have been suggested as an explanation for these differences (Ozaki *et al.* 1995). However, a study of Japanese residing in Stockholm found that those who had lived there for several years suffered much more seasonal variation in mood than those who had lived there for less than two years (Murase *et al.* 1995). This indicates that the low prevalence of SAD among Japanese might be determined by environmental rather than genetic factors.

The aborigines of northern Scandinavia (called Lapps, Samer, or Kvener) have been studied by four groups. Näyhä *et al.* administered the Cornell Medical Index questionnaire to 1251 reindeer herders in northern Finland throughout a year. Ten per cent of the participants were Lapps. Näyhä and colleagues reported that seasonal variations in depressive symptoms and other psychiatric symptoms did not seem to differ between Lapps and Finns (Näyhä *et al.* 1994). Saarijärvi and co-workers administered the SPAQ to 598 Finns and 126 Lapps in northern Finland (68° N to 70° N) (Saarijärvi *et al.* 1999). The odds ratio for SAD was 2.2 for Finns against Lapps. Holte, Konradsen, and associates surveyed an area in northern Norway with the SPAQ. Twenty-five aborigines (Samer and Kvener) were included. The mean seasonality score (see the chapter by Mersch) did not differ between this group and other Norwegians in the same location (Konradsen 1995). Hansen and colleagues surveyed a group of 3736 individuals living in a small community in northern Norway (70° N). They reported that 4.8 per cent of the men and 11.1 per cent of the women suffered problems with depression in winter, while only 0.1 per cent had this problem in summer (Hansen *et al.* 1998). There was no statistically significant difference in the risk for winter depression between the aborigines (Samer) and the other Norwegians.

Nilssen and co-workers examined two populations in Svalbard (78° N), the northern-most regularly inhabited settlement in the world (Nilssen *et al.* 1999); 517 Norwegians and 450 Russians participated. The seasonality score scale of the SPAQ and other instruments were used. The one year prevalence of depression was 2–3 times higher among Russians compared to the Norwegians. In addition, 80 per cent of the Russians reported experiencing their depression in the dark period of the year, but only 40 to 50 per cent of the Norwegians did so. About half of the Norwegians were recruited from the northern part of Norway, whereas the Russians primarily came from southern Russia and the Ukraine. The Russians reported the transition from southern Russia to Svalbard to be extremely difficult, especially the polar night. The Norwegians on the other hand were more familiar with the climatic condition in Svalbard.

Suhail and Cochrane administered the Hospital Anxiety and Depression scale (HAD) monthly, for a year, to 25 white British women and 25 women of Asian origin born in Britain (Suhail and Cochrane 1997). The latter group proved to have more marked seasonal variation in mood. However, the authors were of the opinion that this difference was not caused by genetic factors. The same authors examined hospital admission rates for depression in Birmingham, UK. There was a three-fold higher number of admissions in winter than in summer in a group of patients of Asian origin, but only a 26 per cent winter increase among whites (Suhail and Cochrane 1998).

Iceland is an isolated island in the north Atlantic ocean, and the Icelandic population has lived in virtual isolation during the past thousand years since it was inhabited. In SPAQ surveys in Iceland and the USA, SAD and S-SAD were found to be less common in Iceland than on the east coast of the USA (Magnusson and Stefansson 1993). The authors speculated that Icelandic ancestors with a genetic predisposition towards SAD might have been at an disadvantage to survive and ensure the survival of their offspring. To test this hypothesis of a population selection towards increased tolerance of winter darkness, SAD was studied in a population of immigrants of wholly Icelandic descent in Canada (Magnusson and Axelsson 1993). The prevalence of SAD and S-SAD was several times lower among the immigrants than on the east coast of the USA (see Fig. 5.1). These findings have recently been replicated in a study comparing Canadians of Icelandic descent living in Winnipeg in Canada with other citizens of Winnipeg (Axelsson *et al.* 1998).

These studies of Icelanders have been based on the SPAQ, with the limitations that it imposes. However, seasonal variation in mood has also been examined by cross-sectional methods in Iceland (Magnusson *et al.* 2000). The HAD scale was administered in winter, spring, summer, and autumn. No seasonal variation in mood was detected. This is in contrast with cross-sectional surveys from several other countries (Magnusson 2000).

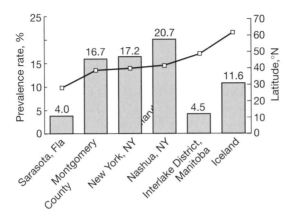

Fig. 5.1 Combined prevalence rates of SAD and S-SAD at different latitudes (line with squares) in three locations in the USA, in Iceland, and among people of wholly Icelandic descent in Canada. (Reproduced with permission from *Archives of General Psychiatry*.)

To conclude, it appears that the propensity to experience SAD differs between ethnic groups. The idea of a genetic adaptation to SAD in groups residing for several generations at high latitudes suggests that SAD has been a maladaptive rather than an adaptive response to the changing of the seasons. There is, however, no independent support for this yet.

5.2 Acclimatization

Do people acclimatize to the long, dark winter at high northern locations? In a SPAQ survey from Alaska, Booker and Hellekson found that the subjects with SAD had lived on average 14.8 years in Alaska; individuals with S-SAD, 11.9 years; and unaffected individuals, 17.6 years (Booker and Hellekson 1992). Thus it appears as if those who have lived for a shorter time in Alaska are more prone to winter problems. Williams and Schmidt (1993) examined records from an out-patient clinic in north Canada with a catchment area of 23 000 individuals living between 54° N and 60° N. Using relatively strict and objective criteria, they were only able to identify six patients with SAD. Of these six, all but one had immigrated from a more southern location. Eighty per cent is a striking proportion, but the low numbers involved make it difficult to draw definite conclusions.

Eagles and co-workers surveyed 443 psychiatric nurses in Aberdeen (north-east Scotland) with the SPAQ. They asked the respondents: 'Were you resident in north-east Scotland for 5 years prior to joining the services?' The prevalence of SAD and S-SAD amongst those who had moved into north-east Scotland was 17.0 per cent but only 10.6 per cent among the natives (p = 0.076) (Eagles *et al.* 1996). However, the mean seasonality score (see the chapter by Terman and Williams) was very similar in these two groups.

Suhail and Cochrane surveyed three groups of women in Birmingham, UK (52° N): white British women, Asian women who had recently moved to the UK, and women of Asian origin who were born in the UK. The Asian countries of origin were from 12° N to 28° N. Twenty-five women from each group were interviewed monthly, for a year, and the HAD scale was administered. The two Asian groups had similar mean HAD scores of 4.6 in summer, but the Asian-born group had a mean HAD score of 8.4 in winter while the Asian women born in Britain had a mean score of 6.2 (Suhail and Cochrane 1997) (see Fig. 5.2). This suggests that the women who had spent their whole life in Britain were in some ways better adapted to the long winter.

Saarijärvi and co-workers mailed out 3000 SPAQ questionnaires to two random samples in Finland: one on the south-west coast (below 61° N) and the other in northern Finland (68° N to 70° N) (Saarijärvi *et al.* 1999). On univariate analysis, there was a statistically significant association between seasonality (SAD/S-SAD/non-SAD) and the number of years the subjects had lived in the area: the longer they had resided in the area, the fewer seasonal symptoms were reported. This difference was not statistically significant on multivariate analysis.

Low and Feissner surveyed 76 students in a college in northern New England with the SPAQ and the Beck Depression Inventory (BDI) in October and February. They compared four groups of students categorized according to the location of their home town: students from the local area, from Western areas, from the mid-Atlantic area, and from the southern states of the USA. The difference in the BDI scores across seasons was most pronounced among the students that had come from the southern regions of the USA, and they also had a higher seasonality score on the SPAQ (Low and Fleissner 1998). Although the differences were statistically significant, the results need to be interpreted cautiously since there were only 12 students in the southern group.

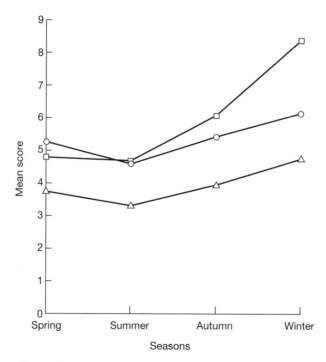

Fig. 5.2 Change in HAD depression score in groups across seasons: □ = Asian group; △ = white group; ○ = Asian–British group. (Reproduced with permission from Social Psychiatry and Psychiatric Epidemiology.)

The six studies previously cited suggest that people may acclimatize or adapt to the long winters at high latitudes. However, three studies have failed to find this effect, or even found contrary results. Partonen and colleagues surveyed a working population of 1000 Finns between 60° N and 70° N (Partonen *et al.* 1993). The structured interview guide for Hamilton Depression Rating Scale, seasonal affective disorder version, self-rating format (SIGH-SAD-SR) was administered in November. Fifty-four depressed individuals were identified; of the 41 of these who returned the questionnaire again the following May, 23 were judged to have SAD. Of these, 12 had migrated southward and only four northward.

In the Hansen *et al.* study (1998) from northern Norway (70° N), the respondents were classified according to whether they had stayed for less or more than half their life in the north (as described on p. 00). There was no statistically significant difference in the risk for winter depression between these two groups.

Murase *et al.* (1995) examined Japanese residing in Stockholm (around 59° N). They compared two groups of Japanese: those who had lived in Stockholm for less than 2 years against those who had lived there for more than 10 years. The BDI was administered to the two groups during summer and winter. There was no indication that the Japanese who had stayed longer in Stockholm had acclimatized to the long Scandinavian winter. In fact, that group had significantly more seasonal variation in mood than those who had only stayed for 2 years.

A lower rate of winter depression among natives compared to persons recently relocated to northern regions does not necessarily mean that they have acclimatized. Firstly, individuals who have recently relocated to new surroundings, often with a resulting poor social network, may be more sensitive to any adversities, including the stressors accompanying a long harsh winter. Second, selection factors may be at work. Nowadays there is much geographic mobility in populations at high northern locations (see following discussion). It is possible that those prone to SAD more frequently migrate away from high latitudes, and thus the natives with which the newcomers are compared are in fact a selected group with less propensity for SAD. Therefore, studies are needed that compare those who have moved southwards from high northern locations with the 'natives' of the new southern residence.

To conclude, the results of six studies indicate that those who migrate to higher latitudes are more prone to SAD, but three studies have not been able to find this effect.

5.3 Ethnicity, geographic mobility, and the latitude gradient

Most studies on SAD have been carried out in the USA and northern Europe where the geographic mobility is high. The studies on acclimatization clearly show that the inhabitants at high northern latitudes frequently relocate. In the Booker and Hellekson study from Alaska (1992), the mean age of the participants was around 40 years. However, they had on average only lived in Alaska for approximately 16 years. In the survey of psychiatric nurses in Aberdeen (Eagles *et al.* 1996), the respondents were asked: 'Were you resident in north-east Scotland for 5 years prior to joining the services?'. Only two-thirds responded affirmative to this question. In the Partonen *et al.* study (1993) already discussed, a total of 41 depressed individuals were identified. Of those, 28 (or more than two-thirds) had moved, most commonly southwards. At the extreme northern location, Svalbard (78° N), the Russians had lived there for 1.5 years while the median length of stay for the Norwegians was four years (Nilssen *et al.* 1999).

Within a given country, geographic mobility probably increases with higher northern latitudes. This is at least the case for Norway (*http://www.ssb.no/emner/02/02/20/flytting/tab-1999–08–25–03.html*). It is primarily young women who move southward in Norway (*http://www.ssb.no/emner/02/aktuell_befolkning/9807/9807t10 .shtml*), and that is indeed the group in which SAD is most prevalent (see the chapter by Eagles).

If the propensity to experience SAD does influence who decides to move southwards, it will affect population surveys conducted across several latitudes. It will be more difficult to detect latitude gradients (see the chapter by Mersch) in the prevalence rates of SAD if the most susceptible individuals have already removed themselves from the highest latitudes. In addition, if the aborigines, who usually reside at the northernmost locations, have adapted to the arctic winter, it will be even more difficult to uncover the effect of latitude on the prevalence of SAD.

5.4 **Future directions**

Hitherto, most epidemiological studies on SAD have been carried out either by the SPAQ (see the chapter by Mersch) or by successive cross-sectional surveys (Magnusson 2000). Diagnostic criteria have also been applied to large population samples (Blazer *et al.* 1998). Each study method has strengths and disadvantages. Today, prospective studies are needed. That is, one has to measure mood and other variables regularly, over years, in each individual. These types of studies are both resource- and time-consuming, and they need motivated participants. However, it is possible to accomplish this (see the chapter by Murray).

If these studies do validate that aborigines in northern America and Europe have adapted to the arctic winter, it might encourage the search for genes that predispose to SAD. Furthermore, if acclimatization proves to hold true in prospective studies, we might focus our attention towards identifying the coping mechanisms that protect against SAD. What are the active ingredients of the coping techniques of the natives and aborigines? If we can identify these, and the methods can be applied in modern societies, a great deal of unnecessary suffering might be relieved.

References

Axelsson, J., Karlsson, M., Stefansson, J.G., and Magnusson, A. (1998) Seasonal affective disorders: the relevance of Icelandic and Icelandic-Canadian evidence to aetiological hypotheses. In *10th Annual Meeting of the Society for Light Treatment and Biological Rhythms, 1998*. Florida, USA.

Blazer, D.G., Kessler, R.C., and Swartz, M.S. (1998) Epidemiology of recurrent major and minor depression with a seasonal pattern. The National Comorbidity Survey (see comments). *Br J Psychiatry* **172**:164–7.

Booker, J.M. and Hellekson, C.J. (1992) Prevalence of seasonal affective disorder in Alaska. *Am J Psychiatry* **149(9)**:1176–82.

Booker, J.M., Hellekson, C.J., Putilov, A.A., and Danilenko, K.V. (1991) Seasonal depression and sleep disturbances in Alaska and Siberia: a pilot study. *Arctic Med Res* **Suppl**:281–4.

Eagles, J.M., Mercer, G., Boshier, A.J., and Jamieson, F. (1996) Seasonal affective disorder among psychiatric nurses in Aberdeen. *J Affect Disord* **37(23)**:12935.

Hansen, V., Lund, E., and Smith, S.T. (1998) Self-reported mental distress under the shifting daylight in the high north. *Psychol Med* **28(2)**:447–52.

http://www.ssb.no/emner/02/02/20/flytting/tab-1999–08–25–03.html

http://www.ssb.no/emner/02/aktuell_befolkning/9807/9807t10.shtml

Jang, K.L., Lam, R.W., Livesley, W.J., and Vernon, P.A. (1997) Gender differences in the heritability of seasonal mood change. *Psychiatry Res* **70(3)**:145–54.

Konradsen, H. (1995) *Årstidsavhengig affektiv forstyrrelse: en emperisk undersøkelse av forekomst blant 6300 unge voksne fra 58 til 70° N.* University of Tromsø.

Low, K. and Fleissner, J. (1998) Seasonal affective disorder in college students: prevalence and latitude. *J Am Coll Health* **47**(3):135–7.

Madden, P.A., Heath, A.C., Rosenthal, N.E., and Martin, N.G. (1996) Seasonal changes in mood and behavior. The role of genetic factors. *Arch Gen Psychiatry* **53**(1):47–55.

Magnusson, A. (2000) An overview of epidemiological studies on seasonal affective disorder. *Acta Psychiatr Scand* **101**(3):176–84.

Magnusson, A. and Stefansson, J.G. (1993) Prevalence of seasonal affective disorder in Iceland. *Arch Gen Psychiatry* **50**(12):941–6.

Magnusson, A. and Axelsson, J. (1993) The prevalence of seasonal affective disorder is low among descendants of Icelandic emigrants in Canada. *Arch Gen Psychiatry* **50**(12):947–51.

Magnusson, A., Axelsson, J., Karlsson, M.M., and Oskarsson, H. (2000) Lack of seasonal mood change in the Icelandic population: results of a cross-sectional study. *Am J Psychiatry* **157**(2):234–8.

Murase, S., Murase, S., Kitabatake, M., Yamauchi, T., and Mathe, A.A. Seasonal mood variation among Japanese residents of Stockholm. *Acta Psychiatr Scand* **92**(1):51–5.

Näyhä, S., Väisänen, E., and Hassi, J. (1994) Season and mental illness in an Arctic area of northern Finland. *Acta Psychiatr Scand* **Suppl 377**:46–9.

Nilssen, O., Brenn, T., Hoyer, G., Lipton, R., Boiko, J., and Tkatchev, A. (1999) Self-reported seasonal variation in depression at 78 degree north. The Svalbard study. *Int J Circumpolar Health* **58**(1):14–23.

Okawa, M., Shirakawa, S., Uchiyama, M., Oguri, M., Kohsaka, M., Mishima, K., *et al.* (1996) Seasonal variation of mood and behaviour in a healthy middle-aged population in Japan. *Acta Psychiatr Scand* **94**(4):211–6.

Ozaki, N., Ono, Y., Ito, A., and Rosenthal, N.E. (1995) Prevalence of seasonal difficulties in mood and behavior among Japanese civil servants. *Am J Psychiatry* **152**(8):1225–7.

Partonen, T., Partinen, M., and Lönnqvist, J. (1993) Frequencies of seasonal major depressive symptoms at high latitudes. *Eur Arch Psychiatry Clin Neurosci* **243**(3–4):189–92.

Saarijärvi, S., Lauerma, H., Helenius, H., and Saarilehto, S. (1999) Seasonal affective disorders among rural Finns and Lapps. *Acta Psychiatr Scand* **99**:95–101.

Suhail, K. and Cochrane, R. (1997) Seasonal changes in affective state in samples of Asian and white women. *Soc Psychiatry Psychiatr Epidemiol* **32**(3):149–57.

Suhail, K. and Cochrane, R. (1998) Seasonal variations in hospital admissions for affective disorders by gender and ethnicity. *Soc Psychiatry Psychiatr Epidemiol* **33**(5):211–17.

Takahashi, K., Asano, Y., Kohsaka, M., Okawa, M., Sasaki, M., Honda, Y., *et al.* (1991) Multi-center study of seasonal affective disorders in Japan. A preliminary report. *J Affect Disord* **21**(1):57–65.

Williams, R.J. and Schmidt, G.G. (1993) Frequency of seasonal affective disorder among individuals seeking treatment at a northern Canadian mental health center. *Psychiatry Res* **46**(1):41–5.

Chapter 6

Longitudinal measurement

Greg Murray

6.1 Introduction

Although SAD (originally defined by Rosenthal *et al.* 1984) is described in DSM as a variant of categorical mood disorder, it is typically understood as the extreme end of a continuum of normative seasonal variation in mood and behaviour (Gordon et al. 1999; Hardin *et al.* 1991; Madden *et al.* 1996). It has in fact been suggested that the tendency towards seasonal variation in mood ('seasonality') may have more empirical support than categorical SAD (Bauer and Dunner 1993). The operationalization and measurement of seasonality is therefore an important aspect of the epidemiology of SAD. This chapter presents a brief review of insights into seasonality that have arisen using prospective methodologies.

6.2 Prospective versus retrospective designs

The majority of epidemiological research into SAD has measured seasonality on the Seasonal Pattern Assessment Questionnaire (SPAQ) (Rosenthal *et al.* 1987). The SPAQ is a retrospective self-report instrument, originally designed to screen for SAD. A major strength of the SPAQ is that it is a brief questionnaire with good face validity. It has therefore been used widely (for example, Blacker *et al.* 1997; Booker and Hellekson 1992; Kasper et al. 1989*b*; Magnusson and Axelsson 1993; Rosen *et al.* 1990; Terman 1988; Thompson *et al.* 1988) and provides an invaluable benchmark for seasonality research in different locales.

Studies using the SPAQ in various countries in the temperate zones have concluded that the most prominent form of mood seasonality is the 'winter pattern' — feeling worst in winter relative to other seasons, particularly summer and spring (Bauer and Dunner 1993; Rosen *et al.* 1990)[1]. SPAQ studies also suggest that seasonality might be more pronounced amongst females and decrease in later middle age (Lam and Levitt 1998; Levitt and Boyle 1997; Rosen *et al.* 1990).

The limitations of retrospective estimation of seasonality are commonly noted, especially by authors of prospective studies (for example, Harmatz *et al.* 2000; Harris and Dawson–Hughes 1993; Murray *et al.* 1999; Nayyar and Cochrane 1996; Schlager *et al.* 1993; Suhail and Cochrane 1997). Possible confounds in retrospective report include preconceptions

---

1 SAD is generally considered synonymous with winter SAD (see, for example, Bauer and Dunner 1993), but other patterns of seasonal difficulties have been recorded and must be accounted for in prospective research (Stiles *et al.* 1993; Terman *et al.* 1989), along with non-seasonal sources of mood variation.

(Eastwood and Peter 1988; Stiles *et al.* 1993) and restrictions on long-term recall (Wicki *et al.* 1992). There is in fact growing consensus that SPAQ-based studies may overestimate both the prevalence of SAD and the magnitude of the seasonal effect on mood (Blazer *et al.* 1998; Levitt and Boyle 1997; Murray *et al.* 2000; Nayyar and Cochrane 1996; Raheja *et al.* 1996).

6.3 Overview of prospective studies of seasonality

Some sixteen northern hemisphere projects have generated prospective data on seasonal mood variation in the general population (our recent Australian study will be discussed separately in this chapter). These studies form a heterogeneous set, using a variety of sampling procedures, mood measures, periods of reflection (ranging from one to four weeks), and definitions of seasonal pattern. The majority of studies have used transverse (repeated cross-sectional) designs, with only three studies tracking the same individuals across the seasonal year (true longitudinal designs; see Menard 1991 for a discussion of longitudinal methodologies).

Of the sixteen reviewed studies, ten found the expected seasonal pattern of mood, with winter and summer as its extreme poles (Eagles *et al.* 1997; Haggag *et al.* 1990; Harmatz *et al.* 2000; Mersch *et al.* 1999; Murase *et al.* 1995; Palinkas *et al.* 1995; Schlager *et al.* 1993 (amongst females but not males); Smith 1979; Suhail and Cochrane 1997; Terman *et al.* 1989). Included amongst these ten 'positive' studies is the large (n = 2819) and rigorous project of Mersch and colleagues (Mersch *et al.* 1999) and one of the few true longitudinal studies (Suhail and Cochrane 1997).

Three projects failed to find significant seasonal trends in mood (Hansen *et al.* 1991; Magnusson *et al.* 2000; Stiles *et al.* 1993). Both Hansen *et al.* and Magnusson *et al.* investigated large random samples, but the former project did not take measurements in summer, and the latter was conducted amongst the Icelandic population, which may be unusually aseasonal (Magnusson 1999; Magnusson and Axelsson 1993; Magnusson and Stefansson 1993). The research of Stiles and colleagues used only a small number of subjects (40 psychotherapy patients) and an indirect measure of mood (subjective reports of severity of identified life problems).

Finally, three studies found non-winter peaks in lowered mood. Consistent with the common epidemiological conclusion that there is a spring peak in the incidence of suicide and other traces of severe depression (Eastwood and Peacocke 1976; Eastwood and Peter 1988; Eastwood and Stiasny 1978), spring peaks in depressed mood were found in two studies (Lacoste and Wirz–Justice 1989; Näyhä *et al.* 1994). However, the findings of Näyhä and colleagues may not generalize beyond the somewhat unusual sample tested (reindeer herders in the north of Finland), and a relatively small sample (n = 285 in a transverse design) was used by Lacoste and Wirz–Justice. Harris and Dawson–Hughes (1993) found an autumn peak in lowered mood, but this finding is difficult to interpret: time sampling did not correspond to any common definition of the seasons, and the participants were post-menopausal women.

In prospective designs, season-linked effects on mood must compete with other potential sources of mood variation, and hence the magnitude of the seasonal effect can be meaningfully quantified. Terman *et al.* (1989) report effect sizes in the order of 2 per cent for a variety of mood variables. By applying standard formulae (Cohen 1988)[2], an estimate of effect size was calculated

---

2 Calculations were based on means and variances presented in the published papers, and must therefore be considered approximations.

from a further three of the published studies that identified winter worsening of mood. The maximum size of the winter pattern effect was found to be approximately 4 per cent (Mersch *et al.* 1999), 6 per cent (amongst females only, Schlager *et al.* 1993), and 1 per cent (in an elderly sample, Eagles *et al.* 1997). It is noteworthy that this simple effect size analysis is consistent with SPAQ data in suggesting that winter pattern seasonality might be positively associated with being female and negatively associated with being elderly.

Two conclusions can be drawn from the review of prospective investigations of mood seasonality. First, on balance, findings are consistent with retrospective studies in suggesting that winter pattern seasonality of mood is a discernible group-level phenomenon in the general population (Mersch *et al.* 1999). Second, the effect is of modest magnitude[3].

6.4 A theoretically-driven investigation of seasonality

We have recently published results of a longitudinal study conducted amongst a large, random, general population sample in Melbourne, Australia (Murray *et al.* 1999). Our research aimed to advance the science of seasonality in two ways. First, the study was designed to measure seasonality across time within the same individuals. A peak in cross-sectional incidence does not mean that the pattern exists longitudinally in any individual (Eastwood and Peter 1988). However, only a handful of true longitudinal studies have been conducted in non-clinical samples (viz. Harmatz *et al.* 2000; Harris and Dawson–Hughes 1993; Suhail and Cochrane 1997). None of these studies collected data across more than one annual cycle, and therefore trends in seasonality within an individual could not be investigated. Participants in our research gave mood reports in winter (July–August) and summer (January–February) across three years.

Second, mood constructs were drawn from recent research into the structure and dynamics of mood (Depue and Zald 1993; Kardum 1999; McConville and Cooper 1999; Watson and Clark 1997; Watson *et al.* 1999; Williams 1989, 1990). Positive affect (PA) and behavioural engagement (BE) were selected as the mood variables most likely to demonstrate seasonality in the general population (Depue *et al.* 1987, 1989; Watson and Clark 1997; Watson *et al.* 1999). Depue's BE and Watson *et al.*'s PA are closely related constructs, both being understood as the subjective component of a fundamental engagement motivation system. They stand in contrast to negative affect (NA) or anxiety, a transitory response to threat which should not vary with predictable cycles in the availability of resources (Clark *et al.* 1989; Watson *et al.* 1999). In our study, BE data were collected across three years, PA and NA data across two[4]. The SPAQ was also included as a retrospective measure of seasonality[5].

Amongst the 245 respondents with complete valid data across six seasons statistically significant winter lowering of BE was found. Consistent with research in the northern

---

3 Effect sizes of 1–2 per cent can be described as small (Cohen 1988). As a point of comparison, in our recent longitudinal study (Murray *et al.* 1999), the personality trait of neuroticism, measured in summer, explained 16.8 per cent of variance in Beck Depression Inventory scores in the subsequent winter.

4 PA and NA were measured on the positive and negative affect scales (PANAS) (Watson *et al.* 1988), while the BE construct was measured on a modified version of the inventory of seasonal variation (ISV) (Spoont *et al.* 1991). Joint factor analysis confirmed that the BE scale was predominantly a measure of the PA construct, as measured against the 'gold standard' of the PA scale.

5. The study's interest in seasonality of mood was obscured from participants, and the SPAQ was completed at T4 and T5.

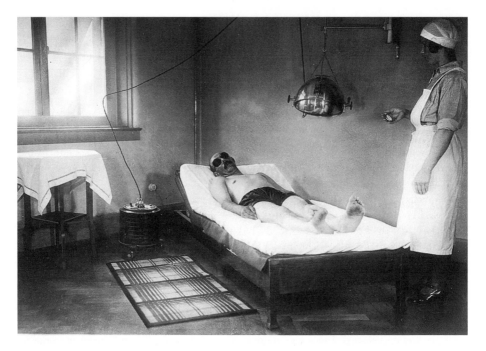

Figure 6.1 Time-givers III: artificial light. A patient having ultraviolet light treatment at the Psychiatric University Clinic in Basle, Switzerland in the 1930s.
Source: Photo Archive, Psychiatric University Clinic Basel

hemisphere, the effect was small in magnitude (2.1 per cent of the total variance on the BE scale was explained by the season effect), and more marked in females. Based on SPAQ response (self-report as winter pattern), a subgroup with more robust seasonality could be identified. This winter pattern subgroup (n = 84; 34.3 per cent of the final sample) exhibited a stronger seasonal effect (7.7 per cent of variance in BE scores). Significant winter pattern seasonal variation on the PA scale was not found in the group as a whole, but was measured amongst the winter pattern subgroup (7.7 per cent of variance in PA scores was explained by the season effect). As expected, NA showed no seasonal variation in either the entire sample or the robustly seasonal subgroup.

There was no evidence in the entire sample that the annual seasonality effect (calculated as summer minus winter levels of BE) remained stable within an individual during a number of years, and only ambiguous evidence amongst the winter pattern subgroup. The prospective data did not, therefore, offer evidence for the stable trait of seasonality assumed by many researchers (for example, Bauer and Dunner 1993; Depue *et al.* 1989; Kasper *et al.* 1989*a*; Madden *et al.* 1996; Raheja *et al.* 1996). However, the longitudinal demonstration of stability in personality characteristics demands aggregation over many years (Zuckerman 1991), and only 3 years were observed in our study.

It could be argued that retrospective self-report on the SPAQ involves a subjective aggregation of many situations, and hence the demonstrated congruence between retrospective report as winter pattern type and prospective estimation of winter pattern seasonality constitutes some evidence for stability in seasonality. Nonetheless, long-term SAD follow-up studies suggest that, even amongst individuals in whom the trait is presumably most pronounced, the course of depressions remains strictly seasonal in less than half (Leonhardt *et al.* 1994; Sakamoto *et al.* 1995; Schwartz *et al.* 1996; Thompson *et al.* 1995). Stability data, amongst both patients and non-patients, is therefore consistent with the effect size analysis described here in suggesting that seasonality of mood is a subtle tendency within individuals.

6.5 **Summary**

Much remains unknown about the extent, the quality, the pattern, and the potential correlates of season-linked mood changes. However, research over the past decade has substantially advanced our understanding of this theoretically and clinically important process. The majority of prospective studies (in accord with retrospective research) suggest that a seasonal rhythm in human mood can be discerned amongst the general population living in the temperate zones. The rhythm has summer and winter as its extreme poles, with winter being associated with greater depressed mood (which may be most directly measured in lowered PA or BE). The seasonal effect is small to medium in size, which may explain both negative conclusions in some studies and our finding that demonstration of the season effect depends on the measurement scale chosen. Equally, stability across time appears to be difficult to demonstrate in such a subtle tendency. The pattern may be more pronounced amongst females, especially younger females, and there is some evidence that self-report as winter pattern type identifies a subgroup of the population in which the tendency is qualitatively and quantitatively more marked.

When researchers measure seasonality longitudinally, attention must be paid to mood constructs and measurement instruments, time sampling options, and the potentially competing role of non-seasonal sources of mood variation and stability. In contrast, when seasonality of mood is measured by retrospective self-report, important aspects of the construct's operationalization are effectively left to the respondent. Therefore, while prospective designs are expensive and constrained by the restrictions on repeated measures over long periods, they will continue to prove efficient for illuminating the boundaries of the seasonality construct.

References

Bauer, M.S. and Dunner, D.L. (1993). Validity of seasonal pattern as a modifier for recurrent mood disorders for DSM-IV. *Comprehensive Psychiatry*, **34(3)**:159–70.

Blacker, C.V.R., Thomas, J.M., and Thompson, C. (1997). Seasonality prevalence and incidence of depressive disorder in a general practice sample: identifying differences in timing by caseness. *Journal of Affective Disorders*, **43**:41–52.

Blazer, D.G., Kessler, R.C., and Swartz, M.S. (1998). Epidemiology of recurrent major and minor depression with a seasonal pattern: the national comorbidity survey. *British Journal of Psychiatry*, **172**:164–7.

Booker, J.M. and Hellekson, C.J. (1992). Prevalence of seasonal affective disorder in Alaska. *American Journal of Psychiatry*, **149(9)**:1176–82.

Clark, L.A., Watson, D., and Leeka, J. (1989). Diurnal variation in the positive affects. *Motivation and Emotion*, **13(3)**:205–34.

Cohen, J. (1988). *Statistical power analysis for the behavioral sciences* (2nd edn). Lawrence Erlbaum, Hillsdale (NJ).

Depue, R.A., Krauss, S.P., and Spoont, M.R. (1987). A two-dimensional threshold model of seasonal bipolar affective disorder. In *Psychopathology: an interactional perspective* (ed. D. Magnusson and A. Ohman), pp. 95–123. Academic Press, Orlando.

Depue, R.A., Arbisi, P., Spoont, M.R., Leon, A., and Ainsworth, B. (1989). Dopamine functioning in the behavioral facilitation system and seasonal variation in behavior: normal population and clinical studies. In *Seasonal affective disorders and phototherapy*) ed. N.E. Rosenthal and M.C. Blehar). Guilford Press, New York.

Depue, R.A. and Zald, D.H. (1993). Biological and environmental processes in nonpsychotic psychopathology: a neurobehavioral perspective. In *Basic issues in psychopathology* (ed. N.E. Rosenthal and M.C. Blehar). The Guilford Press, New York.

Eagles, J.M., McLeod, I.H., and Douglas, A.S. (1997). Seasonal changes in psychological well-being in an elderly population. *British Journal of Psychiatry*, **171**:53–5.

Eastwood, M.R. and Peacocke, J. (1976). Seasonal patterns of suicide, depression and electroconvulsive therapy. *British Journal of Psychiatry*, **129**:472–5.

Eastwood, M.R. and Stiasny, S. (1978). Psychiatric disorder, hospital admission and season. *Archives of General Psychiatry*, **35**:76971.

Eastwood, M.R. and Peter, A.M. (1988). Epidemiology and seasonal affective disorder. *Psychological Medicine*, **18**:799–806.

Gordon, T., Keel, J., Hardin, T.A., and Rosenthal, N.E. (1999). Seasonal mood change and neuroticism: the same construct? *Comprehensive Psychiatry*, **40**:415–17.

Haggag, A., Eklund, B., Linaker, O., and Götestam, K.G. (1990). Seasonal mood variation: an epidemiological study in northern Norway. *Acta Psychiatrica Scandinavica*, **81**:141–5.

Hansen, V., Jacobsen, B.K., and Husby, R. (1991). Mental distress during winter: an epidemiologic study of 7759 adults north of Arctic Circle. *Acta Psychiatrica Scandinavica*, **84**:137–41.

Hardin, T.A., Wehr, T.A., Brewerton, T., Kasper, S., Berrettini, W., Rabkin, J., *et al.* (1991). Evaluation of seasonality in six clinical populations and two normal populations. *Journal of Psychiatric Research*, **25**(3):75–87.

Harmatz, M.G., Well, A.D., Overtree, C.E., Kawamura, K.Y., Rosal, M., and Ockene, I.S. (2000). Seasonal variation of depression and other moods: a longitudinal approach. *Journal of Biological Rhythms*, **15**(4):344–50.

Harris, S. and Dawson-Hughes, B. (1993). Seasonal mood changes in 250 normal women. *Psychiatry Research*, **49**(1):77–87.

Kardum, I. (1999). Affect intensity and frequency — their relation to mean level and variability of positive and negative affect and Eysenck's personality traits. *Personality and Individual Differences*, **26**(1):33–47.

Kasper, S., Rogers, S.L.B., Yancey, A., Skwerer, R.G., Schulz, P.M., and Rosenthal, N.E. (1989*a*). Psychological effects of light therapy in normals. In *Seasonal affective disorders and phototherapy* (ed. N.E. Rosenthal and M.C. Blehar). Guilford Press, New York.

Kasper, S., Wehr, T.A., Bartko, J.J., Gaist, P.A., and Rosenthal, N.E. (1989*b*). Epidemiological findings of seasonal changes in mood and behavior: a telephone survey of Montgomery County, Maryland. *Archives of General Psychiatry*, **46**:823–33.

Lacoste, V. and Wirz-Justice, A. (1989). Seasonal variation in normal subjects: an update of variables current in depression research. In *Seasonal Affective Disorders and Phototherapy* (ed. N.E. Rosenthal and M.C.). Guilford Press, New York.

Lam, R.W. and Levitt, A.J. (1998). Canadian consensus guidelines for the treatment of Seasonal Affective Disorder. *The Canadian Journal of Diagnosis*, **Suppl. (October)**:3–15.

Leonhardt, G., Wirz-Justice, A., Kräuchi, K., Graw, P., Wunder, D., and Haug, H.J. (1994). Long-term follow-up of depression in Seasonal Affective Disorder. *Comprehensive Psychiatry*, **35**(6):457–64.

Levitt, A.J. and Boyle, M.H. (1997). *Latitude and the variation in seasonal depression and seasonality of depressive symptoms*. Paper presented at the Ninth annual meeting of the Society for Light Treatment and Biological Rhythms, Vancouver, BC.

Madden, P.A.F., Heath, A.C., Rosenthal, N.E., and Martin, N.G. (1996). Seasonal changes in mood and behavior: the role of genetic factors. *Archives of General Psychiatry*, **53**:47–55.

Magnusson, A. (1999). *Do populations at far northern locations adapt to the long winter?* Paper presented at the International Congress on Chronobiology, Washington DC.

Magnusson, A. and Axelsson, J. (1993). The prevalence of seasonal affective disorder is low among descendants of Icelandic emigrants in Canada. *Archives of General Psychiatry,* **50***:947–51.*

Magnusson, A. and Stefansson, J.G. (1993). Prevalence of seasonal affective disorder in Iceland. *Archives of General Psychiatry,* **50**:941–6.

Magnusson, A., Axelsson, J., Karlsson, M.M., and Oskarsson, H. (2000). Lack of seasonal mood change in the Icelandic population: results of a cross-sectional study. *American Journal of Psychiatry,* **157**:234–8.

McConville, C. and Cooper, C. (1999). Personality correlates of variable moods. *Personality and Individual Differences,* **26**:65–78.

Menard, S. (1991). *Longitudinal research* (Vol. 76). Sage, London.

Mersch, P.P.A., Middendorp, H.M., Bouhuys, A.L., Beersma, D.G.M., and van den Hoofdakker, R.H. (1999). The prevalence of seasonal affective disorder in the Netherlands: a prospective and retrospective study of seasonal mood variation in the general population. *Biological Psychiatry,* **45**:1013–22.

Murase, S., Murase, S., Kitabatake, M., Yamauchi, T., and Mathe, A.A. (1995). Seasonal mood variation among Japanese residents of Stockholm. *Acta Psychiatrica Scandinavica,* **92**:5–15.

Murray, G.W., Allen, N.B., and Trinder, J. (1999). Construct validation of seasonality in Australia [abstract]. International Congress on Chronobiology Abstracts, 27.

Murray, G.W., Lam, R.W., Magnusson, A., Mersch, P-P.A., and Levitt, A.J. (2000). Contemporary issues in the epidemiology of SAD and seasonality. *Bulletin of the Society for Light Treatment and Biological Rhythms,* **11**:5–11.

Näyhä, S., Väisänen, E., and Hassi, J. (1994). Season and mental illness in an arctic area of northern Finland. *Acta Psychiatrica Scandinavica,* **Suppl.** 377:46–9.

Nayyar, K. and Cochrane, R. (1996). Seasonal changes in affective state measured prospectively and retrospectively. *British Journal of Psychiatry,* **168**:627–32.

Palinkas, L.A., Cravalho, M., and Browner, D. (1995). Seasonal variation of depressive symptoms in Antarctica. *Acta Psychiatrica Scandinavica,* **91**:423–9.

Raheja, S.K., King, E.A., and Thompson, C. (1996). The seasonal pattern assessment questionnaire for identifying seasonal affective disorders. *Journal of Affective Disorders,* **41**:193–9.

Rosen, L.N., Targum, S.D., Terman, M., Bryant, M.J., Hoffman, H., Kasper, S.F., *et al.* (1990). Prevalence of seasonal affective disorder at four latitudes. *Psychiatry Research,* **31**:131–44.

Rosenthal, N.E., Sack, D.A., Gillin, C., Lewy, A.J., Goodwin, F.K., Davenport, Y., *et al.* (1984). Seasonal affective disorder: a description of the syndrome and preliminary findings with light therapy. *Archives of General Psychiatry,* **41**:72–80.

Rosenthal, N.E., Genhart, M., Sack, D.A., Skwerer, R.G., and Wehr, T.A. (1987). Seasonal affective disorder: relevance for treatment and research of bulimia. In *Psychobiology of bulimia* (ed. J.I. Hudson and G. Pope II), pp. 205–8. American Psychiatric Press, Washington DC.

Sakamoto, K., Nakadaira, S., Kamo, K., Kamo, T., and Takahashi, K. (1995). A longitudinal follow-up of seasonal affective disorder. *American Journal of Psychiatry,* **152**:862–8.

Schlager, D., Schwartz, J.E., and Bromet, E.J. (1993). Seasonal variations of current symptoms in a healthy population. *British Journal of Psychiatry,* **163**:322–6.

Schwartz, P.J., Brown, C., Wehr, T.A., and Rosenthal, N.E. (1996). Winter seasonal affective disorder: a follow-up study of the first 59 patients of the National Institute of Mental Health Seasonal Studies Program. *American Journal of Psychiatry,* **153(3)**:1028–36.

Smith, T.W. (1979). Happiness: time trends, seasonal variations, intersurvey differences, and other mysteries. *Social Psychology Quarterly,* **42(1)**:18–30.

Spoont, M.R., Depue, R.A., and Krauss, S.S. (1991). Dimensional measurement of seasonal variation in mood and behavior. *Psychiatry Research,* **29**:269–84.

Stiles, W.B., Barkham, M., and Shapiro, D.A. (1993). Lack of synchronized seasonal variation in the intensity of psychological problems. *Journal of Abnormal Psychology,* **102(3)**:388–94.

Suhail, K. and Cochrane, R. (1997). Seasonal changes in affective state in samples of Asian and white women. *Social Psychiatry and Psychiatric Epidemiology,* **32**:149–57.

Terman, M. (1988). On the question of mechanism in phototherapy for seasonal affective disorder: considerations of clinical efficacy and epidemiology. *Journal of Biological Rhythms*, **3**(2):155–72.

Terman, M., Botticelli, S.R., Link, B.G., Link, M.J., Quitkin, F.M., Hardin, T.E., *et al.* (1989). Seasonal symptom patterns in New York: patients and population. In *Seasonal affective disorder* (ed. C. Thompson and T. Silverstone), pp. 77–95. CNS Publishers, London.

Thompson, C., Stinson, D., Fernandez, M., Fine, J., and Isaacs, G. (1988). A comparison of normal, bipolar and seasonal affective disorder subjects using the Seasonal Pattern Assessment Questionnaire. *Journal of Affective Disorders*, **14**:257–64.

Thompson, C., Raheja, S.K., and King, E.A. (1995). A follow-up study of seasonal affective disorder. *British Journal of Psychiatry*, **167**:380–4.

Watson, D., and Clark, L.A. (1997). Measurement and mismeasurement of mood: recurrent and emergent issues. *Journal of Personality Assessment*, **68**(2): 267–97.

Watson, D., Clark, L.A., and Tellegen, A. (1988). Development and validation of brief measures of positive affect and negative affect: the PANAS scales. *Journal of Personality and Social Psychology*, **54**(6):1063–70.

Watson, D., Wiese, D., Vaidya, J., and Tellegen, A. (1999). The two general activation systems of affect: structural findings, evolutionary considerations, and psychobiological evidence. *Journal of Personality and Social Psychology*, **76**(5):820–38.

Wicki, W., Angst, J., and Merikangas, K.R. (1992). The Zurich Study XIV: epidemiology of seasonal depression. *European Archives of Psychiatry and Clinical Neuroscience*, **241**:301–6.

Williams, D.G. (1989). Personality effects in current mood: pervasive or reactive? *Personality and Individual Differences*, **10**(9):941–8.

Williams, D.G. (1990). Effects of psychoticism, extraversion, and neuroticism in current mood: a statistical review of six studies. *Journal of Personality and Individual Differences*, **11**(6): 615–30.

Zuckerman, M. (1991). *Psychobiology of personality*. Cambridge University Press, Cambridge (England).

Treatment

Chapter 7

Light therapy

Timo Partonen

7.1 Introduction

The treatment of SAD is similar to that of other forms of affective disorder, except that bright-light therapy is recommended as the first-line option for winter SAD. Light therapy, also called light treatment or phototherapy, involves exposure to artificial light.

Bright-light therapy conventionally means the administration of visible light producing at least 2500 lx at eye level. Important parameters for light therapy generally include the intensity, duration, and timing of daily light exposure. The intensity of light is usually expressed in lux (lx), a unit of illuminance corrected for the visual spectral responsiveness of the eye, or in candela (cd), a unit of luminance (see Table 7.1). The dose is composed of two factors: the intensity of light and the duration of exposure to light. If these parameters were changed, the dose would be adjusted.

The therapeutic use of light in winter SAD arose from basic research showing that exposure to ordinary room light (less than 500 lx) could alter circadian and seasonal rhythms in animals. Some circadian effects of light are mediated via the suppression of nocturnal melatonin secretion. In 1980, it was shown that light of high intensity (more than 2000 lx) was required to suppress the melatonin secretion in humans. This observation, with the heuristic idea of extending the period of daylight in winter to correspond with that in summer, led to the first clinical study of light therapy in SAD in 1981 (Rosenthal *et al.* 1984). Recent evidence, however, has pointed out that light of relatively low intensity can also alter human secretion of melatonin (Brzezinski 1997).

As a point of reference, indoors there is typically 100 lx or less at home, and 300 to 500 lx at the workplace. Outdoors, the level of illumination varies greatly by latitude, season, time of

---

Table 7.1 Units of light

Light is electromagnetic radiation to which organs of sight react, ranging in wavelength from about 380 to 760 nm, propagated at a speed of about 300 000 km per second and considered variously as a wave, corpuscular, or quantum phenomenon.

- Candela (cd) is a unit of luminous intensity and equal to 1/60 of the luminous intensity of a 1 cm² of a black body heated to the temperature of the solidification platinum.
- Lumen (lm) is a unit of luminance and equal to the luminous flux emitted in a unit solid angle by a point source of 1-candle intensity (1 lm = 1 cd × sr).
- Lux (lx) is a unit of illuminance and equal to the illumination produced by luminous flux of 1 lumen (lm) falling perpendicularly on a surface of 1 m² (1 lx = 1 lm / m²).

day, and local weather conditions, ranging roughly from 2000 lx or less on a rainy winter day to 10 000 lx or more (usually 50 000 to 100 000 lx) in direct sunshine.

7.2 **Efficacy**

Many controlled studies of light therapy have been conducted by researchers around the world. Although there are limitations of design to these studies, several qualitative overviews have concluded that bright-light therapy is an effective treatment for winter SAD. In addition, two meta-analyses also confirm the efficacy of bright-light therapy against placebo controls — one using a pooled clustering technique and the other applying the Cochrane systematic review method (see the chapter by Thompson and, for information about the method, the website at *http://www.update-software.com/cochrane/cochrane-frame.html*).

The best evaluated treatment regimes are those using 2500 lx of artificial light exposure in the morning. Applying high-threshold measures for remission of depressive episodes, a meta-analysis of data derived from controlled trials on a total of 332 winter SAD patients revealed that light of 2500 lx administered via a light-box device in 2-hour, daily morning sessions for 1 week improved 67 per cent of patients with mild, and 40 per cent with moderate to severe depressive episodes (Terman *et al.* 1989). Recently, the use of higher intensities (up to 10 000 lx) and shorter exposures (down to 30 minutes) has yielded equal response rates. In selected samples, a good treatment response has been achieved in 80 per cent or more of the patients.

7.3 **Dose**

The dose of light exposure can be measured with the intensity and duration of the exposure. Illuminance, measured in terms of quanta or the intensity of light falling at a given place on a surface, was the first light therapy variable studied systematically. The distance of the subject from the light source is of critical importance to illuminance measurement. Originally, researchers used a set of fluorescent light lamps in a metal fixture placed 90 cm from the subject to achieve the illuminance of 2500 lx measured at the level of the eye. Light therapy devices emitting less than 500 lx were less effective than more intense units in the initial series of controlled studies (Rosenthal *et al.* 1985; James *et al.* 1985; Wirz–Justice *et al.* 1986; Isaacs *et al.* 1988; Winton *et al.* 1989).

Since the first documentation, the usual dose used in studies of light therapy has been 2500 lx for 2 hours per day, and there have been few experiments on how efficacy is affected by varying the intensity or the daily duration of light exposure (Grota *et al.* 1989; Magnusson and Kristbjarnarson 1991; Wirz–Justice *et al.* 1987; Partonen 1994). Because of the convenience of shorter daily treatment sessions, the light-box emitting fluorescent light of 10 000 lx has become the clinical standard in the United States and Canada. The intensity–response curve for the efficacy of light therapy has not been defined in detail though.

Response to daily sessions of bright-light therapy generally occurs within 2 to 4 days, and marked improvement is usually observed within 1 to 2 weeks. Trials of longer periods of time have shown increasing response after 2 weeks of bright-light therapy (Labbate *et al.* 1995) and a definite clinical response at 3 or 4 weeks (Bauer *et al.* 1994). The duration–response curve for the efficacy of light therapy has not been fully defined either.

The effect persists for varying periods of time after stopping the treatment, but symptoms ultimately return for most patients (Terman *et al.* 1994). Interestingly, there are reports showing that, in some patients, the improvement achieved with the administration of bright-light therapy for 5 to 6 days only may last for the remaining part of the winter season (Meesters *et al.* 1991, 1993*a*; Lingjærde *et al.* 1993). If the light therapy is effective, it is however advisable to continue it, in order to optimize the outcome throughout the winter, until the patient can gain sufficient natural daily light through exposure to sunshine the following spring. Daily continuation treatment after the initiation period (1 to 2 weeks) is not necessary, since remission can be maintained by exposures given 5 times a week (Partonen and Lönnqvist 1995).

Those patients who live in a climate with extended spells of cloudy or rainy weather often find that light therapy is helpful at any time of the year. Following the summer, it is often beneficial to resume the bright-light therapy near (for example, a week before) the calendar date when the patient's past depressive episodes have usually started, and to continue the administration of light on a regular basis. There is some evidence that the prophylactic use of light therapy can prevent the development of a depressive episode during the following winter months (Partonen and Lönnqvist 1996). However, there is no evidence that the preventive use of light therapy for 5 days only at a symptom-free period at the beginning of autumn is successful (Meesters *et al.* 1994).

7.4 **Time of day**

There has been controversy about the importance of timing of light exposure. Some controlled trials have found that the morning is the most effective time for light therapy (Lewy *et al.* 1987; Avery *et al.* 1990; Sack *et al.* 1990; Avery *et al.* 1991), whereas several studies have shown efficacy following light exposure in the evening or in the middle of the day (Hellekson *et al.* 1986; Wehr *et al.* 1986; Jacobsen *et al.* 1987; Meesters *et al.* 1993*b*, 1995; Wirz–Justice *et al.* 1993; Lafer *et al.* 1994; Thalén *et al.* 1995). The most recent experiment on this specific topic has confirmed that morning bright-light therapy has greater efficacy than exposure to light in the evening (Lewy *et al.* 1998).

Because there is no study that has proved the opposite, it is reasonable to start light therapy with exposure in the morning, if feasible. Otherwise, bright-light therapy can be administered at any time of day, except late in the evening when there is a risk of insomnia as an adverse effect.

7.5 **Wavelength**

The original series of studies of light therapy involved full-spectrum, white fluorescent light that largely reproduce the distribution and range of visible and ultraviolet light in the sky. There is though no evidence that any specialized spectral pattern of fluorescent light is important for efficacy in clinical practice for the treatment of SAD (Lewy *et al.* 1987; Bielski *et al.* 1992), and ongoing trials of light therapy use sources of white fluorescent light in equality. However, the sources emitting white light may have greater efficacy than those producing light of one colour or a limited range of wavelengths. Recent studies have also demonstrated the efficacy of white fluorescent light that is free of ultraviolet radiation (Lam *et al.* 1991, 1992). Wavelengths of the ultraviolet region of the electromagnetic spectrum are not necessary for the efficacy of light therapy, and current consensus is that they should in fact be avoided because of long-term toxicity.

Studies of the effects of different wavelengths may elucidate the mechanisms of action for the antidepressant effects of light. There is evidence that, for equal density of photons, light within the range of the green wavelengths has greater effect than red light and that white light is superior to both red and blue light (for more details, see the chapter by Leahy and Oren) (Brainard *et al.* 1990; Stewart *et al.* 1991; Oren *et al.* 1991). As the retina absorbs light maximally in the green region of the visible spectrum, these findings suggest that light therapy acts primarily via the activation of the common photoreceptors and pigments in the eye.

7.6 Route of administration

The effects of bright-light therapy are thought to be mediated exclusively by the eyes, not the skin — although this assumption has not been thoroughly verified (Wehr *et al.* 1987). Recently, the method of extraocular light exposure, using light source units that exploit fibre optics technology, has been introduced to manipulate the circadian clock (see the chapter by Campbell and Murphy). A light pad is placed in a disposable cover that is in contact with the skin (in the popliteal region), and the patient is exposed to visible light of high intensity in the 400 to 550 nanometres range. There are current research projects investigating the effects of extraocular light exposure on mood, but light pads are not yet part of clinical practice nor an option for the light therapy of SAD.

7.7 Adverse effects

Bright-light therapy usually results in no harm. However, some adverse effects include eye irritation (16 per cent), headache (14 per cent), and nausea (10 per cent) (Labbate *et al.* 1994; Kogan and Guilford 1998; Terman and Terman 1999). In general, they are well-tolerated and subside with time or by reducing the dose of light (by either increasing the distance from the light device or decreasing the duration of the therapy session). These adverse effects seldom lead to cessation. Other, less frequent adverse effects are, for example, agitation and sedation. Hypomania and mania have also been reported as uncommon but serious side-effects of bright-light therapy. Since a few reports exist of manic behaviour or suicidal tendencies being induced during bright-light therapy (Lam *et al.* 2000), patients who are using a light-therapy device at home without close supervision must be informed about health hazards and encouraged to keep in contact with their clinician.

Light devices with smaller illuminating surfaces, lamps of higher colour temperature with a balance toward the range of the blue wavelengths, and exposure to light from fixtures tilted upward to the eyes induce greater perceptual glare and visual disturbance. Specific filters blocking the blue light reduce glare and the increased perceptual brightness and improve visual acuity. Such filters can benefit those patients who are prone to headache or who find light exposure troubles their eyes.

7.8 Risks

Whilst the relatively steady head position reduces the usual variability in levels of direct light input relative to that experienced outdoors, fluorescent bright-light therapy is considered relatively safe for the eyes. A follow-up study did not show any ocular damage after several years of treatment, with a cumulative duration of exposure for up to 1250 hours (Gallin *et al.* 1995). There are no documented reports of induced ocular damage resulting from standard light therapy procedures. However, there is still a paucity of data and subthreshold photochemical damage cannot be ruled out when the lights are being used for long periods. Therefore, patients at risk of light-induced lesions, such as those with progressive retinal conditions or risk factors for light toxicity, need to be monitored by an ophthalmologist (for more details, see the chapter by Remé *et al*).

7.9 Placebo effect

As the ideal standard of a double-blind design is impossible in studies with light therapy, designs of bright-light trials have been compromised by a lack of control for plausible placebo and blinding. Many attempts have been made to control for placebo effects of light therapy. Some of the controlled trials have, in elegant ways, managed to show that the effect of active bright-light therapy exceeded the impact of a placebo (Eastman *et al*. 1992, 1998; Terman *et al*. 1998). However, doubts remain about the possibility of a marked placebo response to bright-light exposure for winter SAD, as for any condition in which patients sincerely expect the treatment to help them. Although the efficacy of bright-light therapy for winter SAD has been accepted by clinicians, there is a continuous need to find adequate methods to quantify the placebo effect in randomized clinical trials of light therapy (see the chapter by Eastman).

7.10 Outcome

Atypical depressive symptoms, rather than the overall severity of a depressive episode, best predict a good response, and of those, increased sleeping, increased eating, and carbohydrate craving specifically (Oren *et al*. 1992; Kräuchi *et al*. 1993; Lam 1994; Terman *et al*. 1996). Rating scales (objective, subjective, or both) measuring the severity of depression should be used before and during light therapy and periodically thereafter (for more information, see the chapter by Terman and Williams). Because of the rapid response and relapse with bright-light therapy, patients should be actively involved in determining their own optimal dose of light, whilst maintaining regular contact with their clinician.

Comorbid anxiety disorders promote, whereas comorbid personality disorders compromise, the benefit from bright-light therapy (Reichborn–Kjennerud and Lingjærde 1996; Levitt *et al*. 1993). Younger age also predicts a good treatment response (Lam 1994), and light therapy appears to be an effective option for patients with childhood and adolescent SAD (Sonis *et al*. 1987; Swedo *et al*. 1997). Except for some case reports, there are no data on the efficacy of light therapy among elderly patients thus far.

7.11 Practical tips

Bright-light therapy may be administered in a room that is furnished for this particular purpose, with light fittings or devices that are designed to deliver the adequate intensity of light to the eyes (Fig. 7.1), or with a number of extra fluorescent ceiling fixtures (Fig. 7.2). In both set-ups, levels of illuminance reached at the face need to be measured to ascertain the adequacy of settings.

The evidence-based data on light therapy have been reviewed recently and are summarized in Table 7.2 (for more information, see the chapter by Partonen and Magnusson). The optimum setting for the light therapy is to have the patient sitting, facing light of 2500 lx for

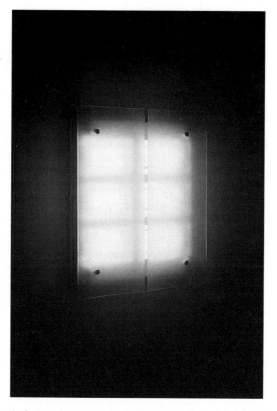

Fig. 7.1 A lamp that is designed as both a furnishing and a device for administration of bright-light therapy.

2 hours or light of 10 000 lx for 30 minutes each morning (preferably between 6.00 a.m. and 10.00 a.m.), for the period of time needed to reduce symptoms and induce remission. Alternatively, the patient may be allowed to move around or be involved in fitness training, if the light therapy is administered in a room with extra ceiling fixtures to produce the adequate illumination at eye level.

It is essential to monitor the initial effects of bright-light therapy on the patient, for example, by administering it at a well-equipped out-patient facility. If either of the regimens just outlined fails to produce a good response within a week, both extending the length of each session and dividing the extended daily exposure between morning and evening need to be considered. Patients used to be instructed to glance briefly at the light device approximately once a minute, but such direct glances are not necessary, certainly if the patient is facing the lights directly or turned aside to no more than an angle of 60 degrees. It is advisable to encourage the patient, while seated, to engage in other activities on the illuminated tabletop surface, such as reading, in order to avoid disturbing perceptual glare.

Many social factors can interfere with the light therapy sessions and compromise the outcome. If the response to light therapy is incomplete, the clinician needs to monitor the patient's compliance with the instructions for the distance from and positioning to the device

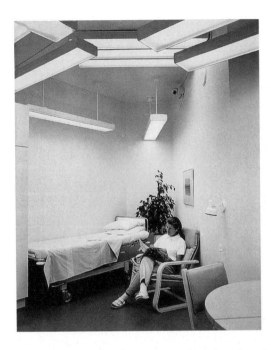

Fig. 7.2 A room furnished with extra ceiling fixtures to produce the adequate illumination for administration of bright-light therapy.

and the daily duration of light therapy sessions. Replacing worn light lamps in the light device with new ones, increasing the patient's levels of general lighting at home, or setting a timer to turn on bedroom or bedside lights before the usual wake-up time may all improve the outcome.

7.12 **Bright-light fixtures**

7.12.1 **Light-box**

The so-called 'light-box' — a metal box containing fluorescent lamps, with a reflector and a diffusing screen — is the particular lighting fixture that has been most thoroughly researched. It has been proven effective in nearly all studies and is thus regarded as the 'golden standard' by which other devices should be judged.

Commercial light devices are now widely available in stores or via mail order. A light device should meet electrical safety standards and have been tested in reputable clinical trials. Recommended light sources are those which emit no ultraviolet radiation or have that band of the spectrum filtered. In addition, an electronic ballast and a plastic diffuser in front of the lamps may make the light source more convenient to use. To enhance colour rendering and visual comfort, light sources that produce wide-band illumination encompassing the region of the green wavelengths, as found in most fluorescent and incandescent lamps, are recommended.

Patients need to be guided to maintain a proper distance and positioning to ensure the correct dose of light exposure. However, a light device should provide a reasonably wide and long field of illumination, so that there is no need for rigid positioning of the head in front of a beam of light nor for close proximity to the lamps in order to maintain effective levels of illuminance at the eyes. There are many ways to position the light fixture, for example,

Table 7.2 Evidence-based data on light therapy

Strong evidence
- Light therapy is an effective first-line treatment for seasonal disorder.
- The fluorescent light-box, with light intensities of greater than 2500 lx, is the preferred device for light therapy.
- The starting dose for light therapy using a fluorescent light box is 2500 lx for 2 hours per day.
- Alternatively, light-boxes emitting 10 000 lx require 30 min. of exposure per day.
- Light therapy should be started in the early morning, upon awakening, to maximize treatment response, but exposure at other times of the day may be helpful for some patients.

Fairly strong evidence
- Light-boxes should use white, fluorescent light with the ultraviolet wavelengths filtered out.
- Response to light therapy often occurs within 1 week, but some patients require 2 to 4 weeks to show a response.
- Common side-effects of light therapy include headache, eyestrain, nausea, and agitation, but these effects are generally mild and transient, or resolve with reducing the dose of light.

Reasonable evidence
- Correct positioning is important, for example, sitting close enough to the light-box to obtain the correct illumination.
- There are no absolute contraindications to light therapy and no evidence that light therapy is associated with ocular or retinal damage.

Fairly reasonable evidence
- None.

Some evidence
- Some patients may respond to other light devices such as light visors and dawn simulators.
- Patients can be encouraged to become active participants in establishing an optimal light protocol.
- Patients with ocular risk factors should have a baseline ophthalmologic consultation prior to starting light therapy, and periodic monitoring.

placing it horizontally on a table, suspending it diagonally above the patient, or hanging it on a wall next to a table.

It is better for the clinician to assess the benefits before the patient is advised to purchase a device for personal use. Patients are, in addition, advised to browse, for example at shops and cafés where available (see Figs. 7.3 to 7.5), and compare the commercially available light therapy devices before deciding which to purchase.

7.12.2 **Dawn simulators**

The dawn simulator is a recent development designed to save time spent in light therapy and to allow the patient to sleep during the treatment. The device has a lamp (usually an incandescent lamp or a fluorescent tube) and an alarm clock that is programmed to increase the room illumination slowly within 30 minutes, while subjects are sleeping, thus simulating a summer dawn during a winter morning.

Early results suggest a beneficial effect of dawn simulators in SAD, but other studies show greater effects with the standard light-boxes. Although the efficacy has not been established for dawn simulators, these devices may be helpful for some patients when light-boxes are not available or are inconvenient. The promising results with the dawn simulator originate from a couple of centres and need independent replication.

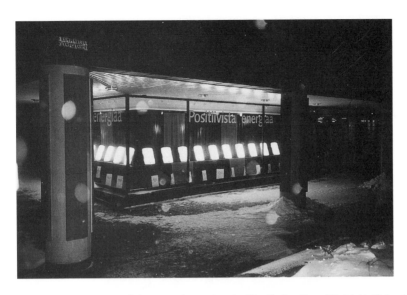

Fig. 7.3 Devices at a window of the Powerhouse head office in the City of Helsinki, Finland.

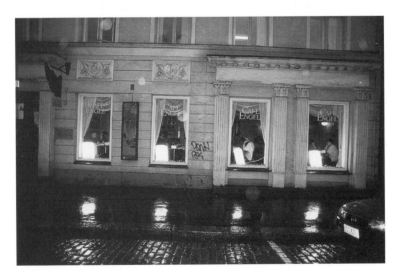

Fig. 7.4 Devices at a café by the Senate Square in the City of Helsinki, Finland.

7.12.3 **Portable devices**

Another recent development, portable, head-mounted devices can also save time spent in light therapy and allow the patient to move during the treatment. Studies of the efficacy of light visors or helmets have failed to show a relationship between the intensity of light and response rate. There are some data supporting the view that patients who are being treated

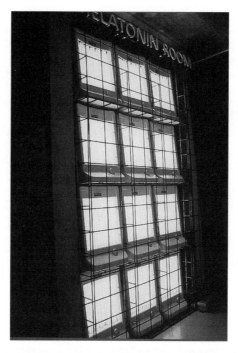

Fig. 7.5 Devices as an installation in a museum in Lausanne, Switzerland (Décosterd & Rahm)

with the standard light-box can switch to the light visor without relapse. This is useful information for patients who travel or for other reasons prefer using the light visor temporarily. However, the portable devices require further documentation of their clinical efficacy and other benefits.

References

Avery, D.H., Khan, A., Dager, S.R., Cox, G.B., and Dunner, D.L. (1990) Bright light treatment of winter depression: morning versus evening light. *Acta Psychiatr Scand* **82**:335–8.

Avery, D.H., Khan, A., Dager, S.R., Cohen, S., Cox, G.B., and Dunner, D.L. (1991) Morning or evening bright light treatment of winter depression? The significance of hypersomnia. *Biol Psychiatry* **29**:117–26.

Bauer, M.S., Kurtz, J.W., Rubin, L.B., and Marcus, J.G. (1994) Mood and behavioral effects of four-week light treatment in winter depressives and controls. *J Psychiatr Res* **28**:135–45.

Bielski, R.J., Mayor, J., and Rice, J. (1992) Phototherapy with broad spectrum white fluorescent light: a comparative study. *Psychiatry Res* **43**:167–75.

Brainard, G.C., Sherry, D., Skwerer, R.G., Waxler, M., Kelly, K., and Rosenthal, N.E. (1990) Effects of different wavelengths in seasonal affective disorder. *J Affect Disord* **20**:209–16.

Brzezinski, A. (1997) Melatonin in humans. *N Engl J Med* **336**:186–95.

Eastman, C.I., Lahmeyer, H.W., Watell, L.G., Good, G.D., and Young, M.A. (1992) A placebo-controlled trial of light treatment for winter depression. *J Affect Disord* **26**:211–22.

Eastman, C.I., Young, M.A., Fogg, L.F., Liu, L., and Meaden, P.M. (1998) Bright light treatment of winter depression: a placebo-controlled trial. *Arch Gen Psychiatry* **55**:883–9.

Gallin, P.F., Terman, M., Remé, C.E., Rafferty, B., Terman, J.S., and Burde, R.M. (1995) Ophthalmologic examination of patients with seasonal affective disorder, before and after bright light therapy. *Am J Ophthalmol* **119**:202–10.

Grota, L.J., Yerevanian, B.I., Gupta, K., Kruse, J., and Zborowski, L. (1989) Phototherapy for seasonal major depressive disorder: effectiveness of bright light of high or low intensity. *Psychiatry Res* **29**:29–35.

Hellekson, C.J., Kline, J.A., and Rosenthal, N.E. (1986) Phototherapy for seasonal affective disorder in Alaska. *Am J Psychiatry* **143**:1035–7.

Isaacs, G., Stainer, D.S., Sensky, T.E., Moor, S., and Thompson, C. (1988) Phototherapy and its mechanisms of action in seasonal affective disorder. *J Affect Disord* **14**:13–19.

Jacobsen, F.M., Wehr, T.A., Skwerer, R.A., Sack, D.A., and Rosenthal, N.E. (1987) Morning versus midday phototherapy of seasonal affective disorder. *Am J Psychiatry* **144**:1301–5.

James, S.P., Wehr, T.A., Sack, D.A., Parry, B.L., and Rosenthal, N.E. (1985) Treatment of seasonal affective disorder with light in the evening. *Br J Psychiatry* **147**:424–8.

Kogan, A.O. and Guilford, P.M. (1998) Side effects of short-term 10,000-lux light therapy. *Am J Psychiatry* **155**:293–4.

Kräuchi, K., Wirz–Justice, A., and Graw, P. (1993) High intake of sweets late in the day predicts a rapid and persistent response to light therapy in winter depression. *Psychiatry Res* **46**:107–17.

Labbate, L.A., Lafer, B., Thibault, A., and Sachs, G.S. (1994) Side effects induced by bright light treatment for seasonal affective disorder. *J Clin Psychiatry* **55**:189–91.

Labbate, L.A., Lafer, B., Thibault, A., Rosenbaum, J.F., and Sachs, G.S. (1995) Influence of phototherapy treatment duration for seasonal affective disorder: outcome at one vs. two weeks. *Biol Psychiatry* **38**:747–50.

Lafer, B., Sachs, G.S., Labbate, L.A., Thibault, A., and Rosenbaum, J.F. (1994) Phototherapy for seasonal affective disorder: a blind comparison of three different schedules. *Am J Psychiatry* **151**:1081–3.

Lam, R.W. (1994) Morning light therapy for winter depression: predictors of response. *Acta Psychiatr Scand* **89**:97–101.

Lam, R.W., Buchanan, A., Clark, C.M., and Remick, R.A. (1991) Ultraviolet versus non-ultraviolet light therapy for seasonal affective disorder. *J Clin Psychiatry* **52**:213–6.

Lam, R.W., Buchanan, A., Mador, J.A., Corral, M.R., and Remick, R.A. (1992) The effects of ultraviolet-A wavelengths in light therapy for seasonal depression. *J Affect Disord* **24**: 237–44.

Lam, R.W., Tam, E.M., Shiah, I-S., Yatham, L.N., and Zis, A.P. (2000) Effects of light therapy on suicidal ideation in patients with winter depression. *J Clin Psychiatry* **61**:30–2.

Levitt, A.J., Joffe, R.T., Brecher, D., and MacDonald, C. (1993) Anxiety disorders and anxiety symptoms in a clinic sample of seasonal and non-seasonal depressives. *J Affect Disord* **28**:51–6.

Lewy, A.J., Sack, R.L., Miller, L.S., and Hoban, T.M. (1987) Antidepressant and circadian phase-shifting effects of light. *Science* **235**:352–4.

Lewy, A.J., Bauer, V.K., Cutler, N.L., Sack, R.L., Ahmed, S., Thomas, K.H., *et al.* (1998) Morning vs evening light treatment of patients with winter depression. *Arch Gen Psychiatry* **55**:890–6.

Lingjaerde, O., Reichborn–Kjennerud, T., Haggag, A., Gärtner, I., Berg, E.M., and Narud, K. (1993) Treatment of winter depression in Norway: I. Short- and long-term effects of 1500-lux white light for 6 days. *Acta Psychiatr Scand* **88**:292–9.

Magnusson, A. and Kristbjarnarson, H. (1991) Treatment of seasonal affective disorder with high-intensity light: a phototherapy study with an Icelandic group of patients. *J Affect Disord* **21**:141–7.

Meesters, Y., Lambers, P.A., Jansen, J.H.C., Bouhuys, A.L., Beersma, D.G.M., and van den Hoofdakker, R.H. (1991) Can winter depression be prevented by light treatment? *J Affect Disord* **23**:75–9.

Meesters, Y., Jansen, J.H.C., Beersma, D.G.M., Bouhuys, A.L., van den Hoofdakker, R.H. (1993a) Early light treatment can prevent an emerging winter depression from developing into a full-blown depression. *J Affect Disord* **29**:41–7.

Meesters, Y., Jansen, J.H.C., Lambers, P.A., Bouhuys, A.L., ,Beersma, D.G.M., van den Hoofdakker, R.H. (1993b) Morning and evening light treatment of seasonal affective disorder: response, relapse and prediction. *J Affect Disord* **28**:165–77.

Meesters, Y., Jansen, J.H.C., Beersma, D.G.M., Bouhuys, A.L., van den Hoofdakker, R.H. (1994) An attempt to prevent winter depression by light exposure at the end of September. *Biol Psychiatry* **35**:284–6.

Meesters, Y., Jansen, J.H.C., Beersma, D.G.M., Bouhuys, A.L., van den Hoofdakker, R.H. (1995) Light therapy for seasonal affective disorder: the effects of timing. *Br J Psychiatry* **166**:607–12.

Oren, D.A., Brainard, G.C., Johnston, S.H., Joseph–Vanderpool, J.R., Sorek, E., and Rosenthal, N.E. (1991) Treatment of seasonal affective disorder with green light and red light. *Am J Psychiatry* **148**:509–11.

Oren, D.A., Jacobsen, F.M., Wehr, T.A., Cameron, C.L., and Rosenthal, N.E. (1992) Predictors of response to phototherapy in seasonal affective disorder. *Compr Psychiatry* **33**:111–4.

Partonen, T. (1994) Effects of morning light treatment on subjective sleepiness and mood in winter depression. *J Affect Disord* **30**:47–56.

Partonen, T. and Lönnqvist, J. (1995) The influence of comorbid disorders and of continuation light treatment on remission and recurrence in winter depression. *Psychopathology* **28**:256–62.

Partonen, T. and Lönnqvist, J. (1996) Prevention of winter seasonal affective disorder by bright-light treatment. *Psychol Med* **26**:1075–80.

Reichborn–Kjennerud, T. and Lingjærde, O. (1996) Response to light therapy in seasonal affective disorder: personality disorders and temperament as predictors of outcome. *J Affect Disord* **41**:101–10.

Rosenthal, N.E., Sack, D.A., Gillin, J.C., Lewy, A.J., Goodwin, F.K., Davenport, Y., *et al.* (1984) Seasonal affective disorder: a description of the syndrome and preliminary findings with light therapy. *Arch Gen Psychiatry* **41**:72–80.

Rosenthal, N.E., Sack, D.A., Carpenter, C.J., Parry, B.L., Mendelson, W.B., and Wehr, T.A. (1985) Antidepressant effects of light in seasonal affective disorder. *Am J Psychiatry* **142**:163–70.

Sack, R.L., Lewy, A.J., White, D.M., Singer, C.M., Fireman, M.J., and Vandiver, R. (1990) Morning vs evening light treatment for winter depression: evidence that the therapeutic effects of light are mediated by circadian phase shifts. *Arch Gen Psychiatry* **47**:343–51.

Sonis, W.A., Yellin, A.M., Garfinkel, B.D., and Hoberman, H.H. (1987) The antidepressant effect of light in seasonal affective disorder of childhood and adolescence. *Psychopharmacol Bull* **23**:360–3.

Stewart, K.T., Gaddy, J.R., Byrne, B., Miller, S., and Brainard, G.C. (1991) Effects of green or white light for treatment of seasonal depression. *Psychiatry Res* **38**:261–70.

Swedo, S.E., Allen, A.J., Glod, C.A., Clark, C.H., Teicher, M.H., Richter, D., *et al.* (1997) A controlled trial of light therapy for the treatment of pediatric seasonal affective disorder. *J Am Acad Child Adolesc Psychiatry* **36**:816–21.

Terman, M., Terman, J.S., Quitkin, F.M., McGrath, P.J., Stewart, J.W., and Rafferty, B. (1989) Light therapy for seasonal affective disorder: a review of efficacy. *Neuropsychopharmacology* **2**:1–22.

Terman, J.S., Terman, M., and Amira, L. (1994) One-week light treatment of winter depression near its onset: the time course of relapse. *Depression* **2**:20–31.

Terman, M., Amira, L., Terman, J.S., and Ross, D.C. (1996) Predictors of response and nonresponse to light treatment for winter depression. *Am J Psychiatry* **153**:1423–9.

Terman, M., Terman, J.S., and Ross, D.C. (1998) A controlled trial of timed bright light and negative air ionization for treatment of winter depression. *Arch Gen Psychiatry* **55**:875–82.

Terman, M. and Terman, J.S. (1999) Bright light therapy: side effects and benefits across the symptom spectrum. *J Clin Psychiatry* **60**:799–808.

Thalén, B-E., Kjellman, B.F., Mørkrid, L., Wibom, R., and Wetterberg, L. (1995) Light treatment in seasonal and nonseasonal depression. *Acta Psychiatr Scand* **91**:352–60.

Wehr, T.A., Jacobsen, F.M., Sack, D.A., Arendt, J., Tamarkin, L., and Rosenthal, N.E. (1986) Phototherapy of seasonal affective disorder: time of day and suppression of melatonin are not critical for antidepressant effects. *Arch Gen Psychiatry* **43**:870–5.

Wehr, T.A., Skwerer, R.G., Jacobsen, F.M., Sack, D.A., and Rosenthal, N.E. (1987) Eye versus skin phototherapy of seasonal affective disorder. *Am J Psychiatry* **144**:753–7.

Winton, F., Corn, T., Huson, L.W., Franey, C., Arendt, J., and Checkley, S.A. (1989) Effects of light treatment upon mood and melatonin in patients with seasonal affective disorder. *Psychol Med* **19**:585–90.

Wirz–Justice, A., Bucheli, C., Graw, P., Kielholz, P., Fisch, H-U., and Woggon, B. (1986) Light treatment of seasonal affective disorder in Switzerland. *Acta Psychiatr Scand* **74**:193–204.

Wirz–Justice, A., Schmid, A.C., Graw, P., Kräuchi, K., Kielholz, P., Pöldinger, W., *et al.* (1987) Dose relationships of morning bright white light in seasonal affective disorders (SAD). *Experientia* **43**:574–6.

Wirz–Justice, A., Graw, P., Kräuchi, K., Gisin, B., Jochum, A., Arendt, J., *et al.* (1993) Light therapy in seasonal affective disorder is independent of time of day or circadian phase. *Arch Gen Psychiatry* **50**:929–37.

Further reading

Bouhuys, A.L., Meesters, Y., Jansen, J.H.C., and Bloem, G.M. (1994) Relationship between cognitive sensitivity to (symbolic) light in remitted seasonal affective disorder patients and the onset time of a subsequent depressive episode. *J Affect Disord* **31**:39–48.

Geerts, E., Bouhuys, N., Meesters, Y., and Jansen, J. (1995) Observed behavior of patients with seasonal affective disorder and an interviewer predicts response to light treatment. *Psychiatry Res* **57**:223–30.

Kasper, S., Ruhrmann, S., Neumann, S., and Möller, H.J. (1994) Use of light therapy in German psychiatric hospitals. *Eur Psychiatry* **9**:288–92.

Lee, T.M.C., Chan, C.C.H., Paterson, J.G., Janzen, H.L., and Blashko, C.A. (1997) Spectral properties of phototherapy for seasonal affective disorder: a meta-analysis. *Acta Psychiatr Scand* **96**:117–21.

Lee, T.M.C. and Chan, C.C.H. (1999) Dose-response relationship of phototherapy for seasonal affective disorder: a meta-analysis. *Acta Psychiatr Scand* **99**:315–23.

Oren, D.A., Shannon, N.J., Carpenter, C.J., and Rosenthal, N.E. (1991) Usage patterns of phototherapy in seasonal affective disorder. *Compr Psychiatry* **32**:147–52.

Postolache, T.T., Hardin, T.A., Myers, F.S., Turner, E.H., Yi, L.Y., Barnett, R.L., *et al.* (1998) Greater improvement in summer than with light treatment in winter in patients with seasonal affective disorder. *Am J Psychiatry* **155**:1614–6.

Praschak–Rieder, N., Neumeister, A., Hesselmann, B., Willeit, M., Barnas, C., and Kasper, S. (1997) Suicidal tendencies as a complication of light therapy for seasonal affective disorder: a report of three cases. *J Clin Psychiatry* **58**:389–92.

Stinson, D. and Thompson, C. (1990) Clinical experience with phototherapy. *J Affect Disord* **18**:129–35.

Terman, M., Terman, J.S., and Rafferty, B. (1990) Experimental design and measures of success in the treatment of winter depression by bright light. *Psychopharmacol Bull* **26**:505–10.

Wirz–Justice, A., Graw, P., Kräuchi, K., Sarrafzadeh, A., English, J., Arendt, J., *et al.* (1996) 'Natural' light treatment of seasonal affective disorder. *J Affect Disord* **37**:109–20.

Dawn simulators

Avery, D.H., Bolte, M.A.P., Cohen, S., and Millet, M.S. (1992) Gradual versus rapid dawn simulation treatment of winter depression. *J Clin Psychiatry* **53**:359–63.

Avery, D., Bolte, M.A., and Millet, M. (1992) Bright dawn simulation compared with bright morning light in the treatment of winter depression. *Acta Psychiatr Scand* **85**:430–4.

Avery, D.H., Bolte, M.A., Dager, S.R., Wilson, L.G., Weyer, M., Cox, G.B., *et al.* (1993) Dawn simulation treatment of winter depression: a controlled study. *Am J Psychiatry* **150**:113–7.

Avery, D.H., Bolte, M.A.P., Wolfson, J.K., and Kazaras, A.L. (1994) Dawn simulation compared with a dim red signal in the treatment of winter depression. *Biol Psychiatry* **36**:181–8.

Avery, D.H., Bolte, M.A., and Ries, R. (1998) Dawn simulation treatment of abstinent alcoholics with winter depression. *J Clin Psychiatry* **59**:36–42.

Lingjærde, O., Føreland, A.R., and Dankertsen, J. (1998) Dawn simulation vs. lightbox treatment in winter depression: a comparative study. *Acta Psychiatr Scand* **98**:73–80.

Terman, M., Schlager, D., Fairhurst, S., and Perlman, B. (1989) Dawn and dusk simulation as a therapeutic intervention. *Biol Psychiatry* **25**:966–70.

Portable devices

Joffe, R.T., Moul, D.E., Lam, R.W., Levitt, A.J., Teicher, M.H., Lebegue, B., *et al.* (1993) Light visor treatment for seasonal affective disorder: a multicenter study. *Psychiatry Res* **46**:29–39.

Levitt, A.J., Joffe, R.T., Moul, D.E., Lam, R.W., Teicher, M.H., Lebegue, B., *et al.* (1993) Side effects of light therapy in seasonal affective disorder. *Am J Psychiatry* **150**:650–2.

Levitt, A.J., Joffe, R.T., King, E. (1994) Dim versus bright red (light-emitting diode) light in the treatment of seasonal affective disorder. *Acta Psychiatr Scand* **89**:341–5.

Levitt, A.J., Wesson, V.A., Joffe, R.T., Maunder, R.G., and King, E.F. (1996) A controlled comparison of light box and head-mounted units in the treatment of seasonal depression. *J Clin Psychiatry* **57**:105–10.

Meesters, Y., Beersma, D.G.M., Bouhuys, A.L., and van den Hoofdakker, R.H. (1999) Prophylactic treatment of seasonal affective disorder (SAD) by using light visors: bright white or infrared light? *Biol Psychiatry* **46**:239–46.

Rosenthal, N.E., Moul, D.E., Hellekson, C.J., Oren, D.A., Frank, A., Brainard, G.C., *et al.* (1993) A multicenter study of the light visor for seasonal affective disorder: no difference in efficacy found between two different intensities. *Neuropsychopharmacology* **8**:151–60.

Teicher, M.H., Glod, C.A., Oren, D.A., Schwartz, P.J., Luetke, C., Brown, C., *et al.* (1995) The phototherapy light visor: more to it than meets the eye. *Am J Psychiatry* **152**:1197–202.

Chapter 8

Lamp standards and ocular safety

Charlotte E. Remé, Christian Grimm, Farhad Hafezi, and Andreas Wenzel

8.1 Introduction

The effect of bright-light exposure to treat winter depression (SAD), sleep disturbances, maladaptation to shift work, and jet lag is most likely mediated through retinal photoreceptors. It remains unclear, however, whether this is performed by the classical, vision-mediating photoreceptors, the rods and cones. Novel circadian photoreceptors such as the cryptochromes or visual pigments residing in non-photoreceptor retinal neurons may be involved (van der Horst *et al.* 1999; Thresher *et al.* 1998; Freedman *et al.* 1999). Irrespective of the nature of those photoreceptors there is no doubt that ocular tissues receive high irradiance levels during light therapy (Terman *et al.* 1990). Therefore, consideration of ocular safety is mandatory for light therapies, especially those applied for extended time periods (Remé *et al.* 1996*b*).

8.2 Effects of bright light on the eye

UV and visible light not only damage ocular structures, but may also modify retinal morphology and function (Remé *et al.* 1998*a*). Under laboratory conditions, a change in habitat illuminance modifies photoreceptor visual pigment levels, phospholipid fatty acid composition, visual transduction proteins, antioxidant state, and other retinal parameters in rodents (for review, see Remé *et al.* 1998*c*).

There is widespread evidence from human and animal studies that both UV and visible light can damage the eye (for reviews, see Remé *et al.* 1996*a*, 1998*c*). Of primary importance in the context of light therapy are the lens and the retina. While lens chromophores mainly absorb UV, retinal chromophores are designed to absorb visible light. In juvenile eyes, there is a small transmission window for UV in the lens, around wavelengths of 360 nm. However, this window closes before puberty. After that, the lens acts as a UV filter shielding the retina from dangerous short-wavelength light. With increasing age, the lens transmission for visible light shifts towards longer wavelengths, reducing the violet–blue part of the spectrum, and an overall reduction of light transmission occurs (Remé *et al.* 1996*a*).

Exposure of the unprotected eye to UV over extended time periods may induce and/or accelerate the formation of cataracts. Exposure to high levels of visible light may damage or even destroy retinal photoreceptors and pigment epithelium. Furthermore, there is accumulating evidence that light exposure can accelerate some forms of retinal degeneration, especially age-related macular degeneration and inherited dystrophies such as retinitis pigmentosa (Cideciyan *et al.* 1998; Young 1988). An important common factor in dystrophies, degenerations, and light-induced lesions in the retina is cell death by apoptosis (Remé *et al.* 1998*b*).

8.3 The retinal chromophore for light damage

There are several potential chromophores that could mediate light-induced retinal lesions, including rod and cone visual pigments, mitochondrial cytochromes, prostaglandin synthesizing enzymes, lipofuscin, and opsins in the pigment epithelium. However, recent studies unequivocally demonstrate that the visual pigment rhodopsin is the primary mediator of light-induced lesions (Grimm *et al.* 2000). Furthermore, it is the availability of rhodopsin *during* light exposure which defines the number of photons absorbed and therefore light damage susceptibility (Wenzel *et al.* 2001). The level of available rhodopsin, in turn, depends on the rate of its regeneration after photobleaching. Rhodopsin molecules are provided by metabolic regeneration via the pigment epithelium on the one hand and, under certain conditions, by photoreversal of bleached molecules within the photoreceptor itself (see section 8.4).

8.4 Blue light causes cell death, green light does not

Of particular relevance for the design of therapy lamps are recent observations that the exposure to deep blue light causes distinct photoreceptor cell death, whereas exposure to green light of equal energy does not (Grimm *et al.* 2001) (see Fig. 8.1).

Blue light induces photoreversal of bleached rhodopsin intermediates (probably meta-rhodopsin II) back into rhodopsin's dark-adapted state so that one molecule of rhodopsin

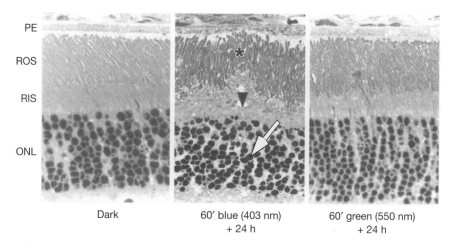

Fig. 8.1 Light micrographs illustrating the effects of different wavelengths on light-induced retinal lesions: a normal retina without light exposure (dark), which shows no signs of injury; a retina that has been exposed to deep blue light for 60 minutes (60′ blue), which shows distinct signs of lesions with apoptotic nuclei of the outer nuclear layer (ONL, white arrow) and disintegrated structures of rod inner (RIS) and outer segments (ROS) (arrowhead and star); and a retina which has been exposed to green light for 60 minutes (60′ green), which displays regular morphology. PE: pigment epithelium

epithelium can absorb more than one photon under experimental conditions. Green light, by contrast, leads to a rapid and almost complete bleach of rhodopsin which then is replenished through the much slower process of metabolic regeneration. Experiments clearly show that rhodopsin readily absorbs and bleaches blue light, but the bleach is partially reversed. This mechanism thus provides a relatively high level of unbleached pigment during a given light exposure period (see section 8.3).

8.5 Measurements of fluorescent tubes used for light therapy

We have performed detailed measurements of fluorescent tubes commonly used in light therapy lamps (Remé *et al.* 1996*b*). Details of this study can be found in the original publication. In brief, our analysis revealed significant differences between tubes in the emission of UV and of deep blue of the visible spectrum (see Fig. 8.2). In view of the already described lesions of the lens by UV and of the retina by blue light, one should obviously choose a type of fluorescent tube which does not emit UV and only a relatively small fraction of blue. Furthermore, a diffusing screen in front of the tubes would both reduce glare and provide UV and blue protection.

8.6 Cumulative doses during light therapy regimens

We have calculated cumulative doses for UVB, UVA, and blue light for different tubes, which reveal distinct differences as would be expected from variations in emission characteristics. For example, a daily 30-minute session with 10 000 lux white light emitted by tube B, for 5 months per year over a period of 10 years, would result in a cumulative dose of 800 J/cm^2 UVA and 2303 J/cm^2 blue. By contrast, the same regimen applied with tube D would result in a cumulative dose of 6 J/cm^2 UVA and 1372 J/cm^2 for blue (for details, see Remé *et al.* 1996*b*). The daily erythemally effective dose of radiant exposure (including UVA and B) for other SAD treatments has been calculated to be 40 J/m^2 (Diffey 1993). Such calculations support our claim to use only tubes with negligible (< 1 per cent) UV and reduced blue light emission. Lesions of the eye after chronic blue light exposure await investigations, whereas UV effects on the lens have been amply documented (Remé *et al.* 1996*a*). Alternative and/or additional protective measures are discussed in section 8.7.

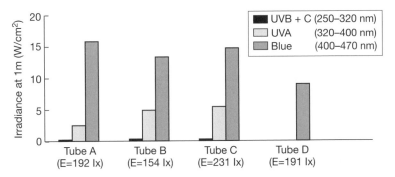

Fig. 8.2 Spectral emission (E) of selected therapy lamps. The emission of UVB, UVA, and blue light was measured and plotted in a histogram. All measured lamps show distinct blue emission, whereas UVA emission is most prominent in tube B and C. There is a small fraction of UVB emission in tube A, B, and C. These measurements indicate that indeed there are significant differences in emission and that tube D of our series is the most suitable one for light therapy.

8.7 **Safety recommendations**

8.7.1 **Therapy lamps**

Therapy lamps should use only fluorescent tubes with negligible (< 1 per cent) UV and reduced blue (< 10 per cent) emission. Furthermore, a diffusing screen in front of the tubes should be applied, which reduces glare and shields from UV. Ideally, other technical data of lamps should be standardized so that clinical studies using such lamps are comparable.

8.7.2 **Eye glasses**

As a safety measure in cases where lamps with unknown spectral emission are used or in patients with endangered eyes (see section 8.7.3), transparent eye glasses should be used, with a cut-off at 450 to 470 nm. Such glasses would also increase patient comfort by enhancing contrast vision and reducing glare. The advice of an optician on buying such glasses is necessary. There are therapeutic glasses for patients suffering from retinal degenerations such as retinitis pigmentosa.

8.7.3 **Ophthalmologic examinations**

For all patients scheduled for light therapy it is of primary importance to inquire about any medication they are taking, because a large number of drugs can potentially act as photosensitizers for UV and/or visible short-wavelength blue light, depending on the type of molecule involved. Examples include tetracyclines, sulfonamides, psoralens, and some antidepressants and neuroleptics (Terman *et al.* 1990) (Roberts *et al.* 1992) (Remé *et al.* 1988).

Furthermore, all patients should undergo ophthalmologic examination prior to light therapy. For those without eye disease, this examination can be brief and, when no side-effects to therapy are reported, a control every 2 to 3 years is sufficient. Patients with eye complaints and/or eye disease should have a careful ophthalmologic check-up before therapy is started and within 3 weeks after the end of therapy. When any side-effects occur, an immediate consultation of an ophthalmologist is necessary.

In cases of age-related macular degeneration and retinitis pigmentosa it is highly questionable whether those patients should receive light therapy, because light may be an accelerating factor for the diseases (Cideciyan *et al.* 1998; Young 1988). The decision should be made between the ophthalmologist and the light therapist in view of the most urgent needs of the patient.

Brief ophthalmologic examination of patients without eye disease

- Visual acuity without and with best correction

- Slit lamp examination of anterior segment and vitreous

- Intraocular pressure

- Ocular fundus with pupil dilation, centre, and periphery

Ophthalmologic examination of patients with pre-existing eye disease

Depending on the type of disease, additional tests may be necessary; this will be the decision of the ophthalmologist.

- Visual acuity without and with best correction

♦ Pupillary reactions; swinging flashlight test

♦ If indicated, orthoptic status

♦ Visual field

♦ Slit lamp examination of anterior segment and vitreous

♦ Intraocular pressure

♦ Ocular fundus with pupil dilation, optic nerve, macula, central 30°, periphery

♦ Amsler grid

♦ Fundus photography

8.8 Conclusion

The application of bright light to treat winter depression has brought significant improvement for many patients ever since the first clinical trials. The benefits for patients far outweigh ocular side-effects (Terman and Terman 1999), and a survey of patients during 3 to 5 years did not detect any serious ocular complications (Gallin *et al.* 1995). However, it remains to be seen whether higher cumulative doses over longer time periods could exacerbate ocular or retinal diseases. The time span of exposure to UV and the formation of cataracts, for example, is likely to be in the range of 10 to 20 years, depending on the individual exposure conditions. Similarly, age-related macular degeneration is a disease which develops almost over a lifetime (that is, within 40 to 60 years), again depending on the individual circumstances.

There are relatively few and simple measures which could prevent acute and chronic harmful effects of light exposure on the eyes. These are carefully designed lighting fixtures with no UV emission and reduced blue light, clear eye glasses with a cut off around 450 to 460 nm, and ophthalmologic surveillance of patients. To this end, the lighting manufacturer should adhere to standards and declare the emission spectra of their lamps, eye glasses should come with their transmission properties, and light therapists ought to collaborate with ophthalmologists for the greatest benefit of their patients.

References

Cideciyan, A.V., Hood, D.C., Huang, Y., Banin, E., Li, Z.Y., Stone, E.M., *et al.* (1998). Disease sequence from mutant rhodopsin allele to rod and cone photoreceptor degeneration in man. *Proc Natl Acad Sci USA* **95**:7103–8.

Diffey, B.L. (1993). A photobiological evaluation of lamps used in the phototherapy of seasonal affective disorder. *J Photochem Photobiol* **B 17**:203–7.

Freedman, M.S., Lucas, R.J., Soni, B., von Schantz, M., Munoz, M., David–Gray, Z. *et al.* (1999). Regulation of mammalian circadian behavior by non-rod, non-cone, ocular photoreceptors. *Science* **284**:502–4.

Gallin, P.F., Terman, M., Remé, C.E., Rafferty, A.B., Terman, J.S., and Burde, R.M. (1995). Ophthalmological examination of patients with seasonal affective disorder, before and after bright light therapy. *Am J Ophthalmol* **119**:202–10.

Grimm, C., Wenzel, A., Hafezi, F., Yu, Sh., Redmond, M., and Remé, C.E. (2000). Protection of Rpe65-deficient mice identifies rhodopsin as a mediator of light-induced retinal degeneration. *Nat Genet* **25**:63–6.

Grimm, C., Wenzel, A., Williams, T.P., Rol, P., Hafzei, F., and Remé, C.E. (2001). Rhodopsin-mediated blue-light damage to the rat retina: effect of photoreversal of bleaching. *Invest Ophthalmol Vis Sci* **42**:497–505.

Remé, C.E., Federspiel–Eisenring, E., Hoppeler, T., Pfeilschifter, J., and Dietrich, C. (1988). Chronic lithium damages the rat retina, acute light exposure potentiates the effect. *Clin Vision Sci* **3**:157–72.

Remé, C.E., Reinboth, J.J., Clausen, M., and Hafezi, F. (1996a). Light damage revisited: converging evidence, diverging views? *Graefe's Arch Clin Exp Ophthalmol* **234**:2–11.

Remé, C.E., Rol, P., Grothmann, K., Kaase, H., and Terman, M. (1996b). Bright light therapy in focus: lamp emission spectra and ocular safety. *Technology Health Care* **4**:403–13.

Remé, C.E., Bush, R., Hafezi, F., Wenzel, A., and Grimm, C. (1998a). Photostasis and beyond: where adaptation ends. In *Photostasis and related topics* (ed. T.P. Williams and A. Thistle), pp. 199–206. Plenum Press, New York.

Remé, C.E., Grimm, C., Hafezi, F., Marti, A., and Wenzel, A. (1998b). Apoptotic cell death in retinal deg enerations. In *Progress in Retinal and Eye Research 77* (ed. N.N. Osborne and G.J. Chader.), pp. 443–63. Elsevier Science, Oxford.

Remé, C.E., Hafezi, F., Marti, A., Munz, K., and Reinboth, J.J. (1998c). Light damage to retina and pigment epithelium. In *The retinal pigment epithelium, function and disease* (ed. M.F. Marmor and T.J. Wolfensberger), pp. 563–86. Oxford University Press, Oxford.

Roberts, J.E., Remé, C.E., Dillon, J., and Terman, M. (1992). Exposure to bright light and the concurrent use of photosensitizing drugs. Letter, *N Engl J Med* **326**:1500–1.

Terman, M., Remé, C.E., Rafferty, B., Gallin, P.F., and Terman, J.S. (1990). Bright light therapy for winter depression: potential ocular effects and theoretical implications. *Photochem Photobiol* **51**:781–92.

Terman, M. and Terman, J. (1999). Bright light therapy: side effects and benefits across the symptom spectrum. *J Clin Psychiatry* **60**:799–808.

Thresher, R.J., Hotz Vitaterna, M., Miyamoto, Y., Kazantsev, A., Hsu, D., Petit, C., *et al.* (1998). Role of mouse cryptochrome blue-light photoreceptors in circadian photoresponses. *Science* **282**:1490–4.

van der Horst, G.T.J., Muijtjens, M., Kobayashi, K., Takano, R., Kanno, S., Takao, M., *et al.* (1999). Mammalian cry1 and cry2 are essential for maintenance of circadian rhythms. *Science* **398**:627–30.

Wenzel, A., Remé, C.E., Williams, T.P., Hafezi, F., and Grimm, C. (2001). The Rpe 65 Leu450Met variation increases retinal resistance against light-induced degeneration by slowing rhodopsin regeneration. *J. Neurosci* **21**:53–8.

Young, R.W. (1988). Solar radiation and age-related macular degeneration. *Surv Ophthalmol* **32**:252–69.

Chapter 9

Drug therapy

Siegfried Kasper, Eva Hilger, Matthäus Willeit,
Alexander Neumeister, Nicole Praschak–Rieder,
Barbara Heßelmann, and Andreas Habeler

9.1 Introduction

Light therapy has become increasingly popular in various countries around the world in the last fifteen years and its usage for the indication of SAD is supported by a substantial number of studies (Terman *et al.* 1989). However, there are just a few investigations for non-seasonal depression or for other treatment indications (for a review, see Kasper *et al.* 1994).

Although light therapy is widely accepted by patients with SAD, there are some who object to its usage, since it is viewed as too time-consuming. The number of patients who do not seek treatment for this reason is hard to estimate since centres offering light therapy mainly attract patients who are seeking this type of treatment. There are no studies as yet in representative samples of the population which indicate the percentage of patients willing to comply with this treatment.

9.2 Role of serotonin and noradrenaline in the pathophysiology of SAD

Many neurovegetative functions, which seem to be disturbed in SAD, have a relationship to the serotonergic system (5-HT). Serotonergic mechanisms are thought to be involved, for instance, in the regulation of appetite and weight. It has further been discussed in the literature whether the frequently reported carbohydrate craving in SAD patients during fall/winter represents a behavioural–biochemical feedback loop in order to raise the available brain 5-HT content (Rosenthal *et al.* 1987). Other evidence that 5-HT might be involved in the pathophysiology of SAD is derived from the finding that seasonal fluctuations in brain serotonin content occur in healthy subjects as well as in depressed patients. These findings suggest that the serotonergic system is responsive to seasonal changes and that this physiological variation may in turn change into a pathological variant (Kasper *et al.* 1996).

The humoral and behavioural response to the administration of the serotonergic agent meta-chlorophenylpiperazine (m-CPP), before and after light therapy, implies that SAD patients may have an underlying dysregulation within the 5-HT system which seems to be influenced by light therapy. Furthermore, hormonal tests with serotonergic agents have resulted in blunted responses in SAD patients (Jacobsen *et al.* 1994; Coiro *et al.* 1993). Recent studies with the tryptophan depletion test indicate that the short-term availability of 5-HT is a necessary condition for the antidepressant efficacy of light therapy (Lam *et al.* 1995; Neumeister *et al.* 1997).

Several lines of evidence suggest therefore that a dysfunction of brain 5-HT function is involved in the pathophysiology of SAD and also in the mechanism of action of light therapy. However, it is obvious that a simple model of the pathophysiology of SAD and the underlying mechanism of action of light therapy is inadequate. The current results from the literature and our own findings support the hypothesis that disturbances in the brain 5-HT function contribute to the pathophysiology of SAD and that the short-term availability of 5-HT seems to be an important factor for the antidepressant treatment of SAD, either by light therapy or psychopharmacological approaches.

The catecholaminergic pathways have not been studied to the same extent as serotonergic mechanisms. One study, supporting the importance of noradrenergic mechanisms in the pathogenesis of SAD, showed resting plasma noradrenaline levels to be inversely correlated with the level of depression in untreated patients with SAD (Rudorfer *et al.* 1993). Furthermore, it has been shown that light therapy decreases the urinary output of noradrenaline and its metabolites (Anderson *et al.* 1992). The major metabolite of noradrenaline, 3-methoxy-4-hydroxy-phenylethyleneglykol (MHPG), did not distinguish depressed patients with SAD from either light-treated patients with SAD or healthy controls in the study of Rudorfer *et al.* (1993). Additionally, cerebrospinal fluid levels did not differentiate patients from controls in relation to either MHPG or the 5-HT-metabolite, 5-hydroxyindoleacetic acid (Rudorfer *et al.* 1993).

In a recent study by Neumeister *et al.* (1998), both the 5-HT and catecholamine systems were investigated using the monoamine-depletion paradigm. The authors compared the effects of tryptophan depletion with catecholamine depletion and sham depletion. Tryptophan depletion was achieved by ingestion of a tryptophan-free amino acid beverage plus amino acid capsules; catecholamine depletion was achieved by administration of the tyrosine hydroxylase inhibitor, α-methyl-paratyrosine. The effects of these interventions were evaluated with measures of depression, plasma tryptophan levels, and plasma catecholamine metabolites. This study of 16 SAD patients confirmed previous work showing that serotonin plays an important role in the mechanism of action of light therapy and additionally provided new evidence that brain catecholaminergic systems may also be involved.

9.3 Psychopharmacological treatments of SAD

Several compounds have been studied for the psychopharmacological treatment of SAD (see Table 9.1), and there is evidence that antidepressants with a serotonergic mechanism of action might be the preferable choice.

9.3.1 Open studies

Early studies (O'Rourke *et al.* 1989; Jacobsen *et al.* 1989; McGrath *et al.* 1990) used d-fenfluramine, fluoxetine, or L-tryptophan, and all of them indicated beneficial effects (obtained however in a small number of SAD patients).

The Department of General Psychiatry at the University of Vienna studied further candidates for treatment of SAD, including mirtazapine (Kasper *et al.* 1997) and reboxetine (Kasper 1999). In the mirtazapine open-label trial, the antidepressant efficacy was evaluated

Table 9.1 Antidepressant medication in patients with SAD

Author	No. of patients	Antidepressants
Open studies		
O'Rourke *et al.* 1989	7	d-fenfluramine
Jacobson *et al.* 1989	3	Fluoxetine, trazodone
McGrath *et al.* 1990	9	L-tryptophan
Dilsaver *et al.* 1990	47	Bupropion, desipramine, tranylcypromine
Dilsaver & Jaeckle 1990	14	Tranylcypromine
Teicher & Glod 1990	6	Alprazolam
Wirz-Justice *et al.* 1992	1	Citalopram
Lingjaerde & Haggag 1992	5	Moclobemide
Hesselmann *et al.* 1999	8	Mirtazapine
Hilger *et al.* 1999	16	Reboxetine
Controlled studies		
Martinez *et al.* 1994	20	Hypericum ± bright light
Partonen & Lönnqvist 1996	32	Fluoxetine vs. moclobemide
Ruhrmann *et al.* 1998	40	Fluoxetine vs. bright light
Placebo-controlled studies		
Rosenthal *et al.* 1988	19	Atenolol vs. placebo
Lingjaerde *et al.* 1993	34	Moclobemide vs. placebo
Oren *et al.* 1994*a*	25	Levodopa + carbidopa vs. placebo
Oren *et al.* 1994*b*	27	Cyanocobalamin vs. placebo
Schlager 1994	23	Propranolol vs. placebo
Lam *et al.* 1995	78	Fluoxetine vs. placebo
Blashko *et al.* 1997	187	Sertraline vs. placebo
Lewy *et. al.* 1998	10	Melatonin vs. placebo
Lingaerde *et al.* 1999	27	Ginkgo biloba vs. placebo
Thorell *et al.* 1999	8	Citalopram vs. placebo

in eight depressed and drug-naïve SAD patients who, over a 4-week drug surveillance period, received 30 mg of mirtazapine per day (Hesselmann *et al.* 1999). Mirtazapine is a novel antidepressant drug, providing a noradrenaline-serotonin-specific mechanism of action by blocking adrenergic α2-auto-and α2-heteroreceptors as well as 5-HT$_2$- and 5-HT$_3$-receptors (De Boer *et al.* 1994). As a result of the 5-HT$_2$- and 5HT$_3$-receptor blockage, serotonin stimulates other 5-HT-receptors including the 5-HT$_{1A}$-receptor, whose activation seems to produce antidepressant effects (De Vry *et al.* 1992).

Clinical response in the trial was assessed using the Structured Interview Guide for Hamilton Depression Rating Scale, Seasonal Affective Disorder Version (SIGH-SAD). This 4-week study proved mirtazapine to be effective and safe in the treatment of SAD. Side-effects were rare, generally mild, and mostly disappeared within the first week of treatment. Only one of eight patients discontinued the treatment due to side-effects. Sedation, as a side-effect, only appeared during the first week of treatment. Two patients reported increased appetite and one of them, consecutive weight gain. Since mirtazapine affects, as already described, the noradrenergic as well as the serotonergic system in a specific way, it appears that more than one neurotransmitter is involved in the pathophysiology of SAD, as has been shown by depletion studies investigating both noradrenergic and serotonergic pathways (Neumeister *et al.* 1998).

Reboxetine, another newly introduced antidepressant with a selective inhibition of the noradrenaline reuptake (Kasper 1999), was also studied by the Vienna group in 16 patients suffering from SAD (Hilger *et al.* 1999). Patients were treated with 8 mg reboxetine p.o.q.d. for 6 weeks as monotherapy. Of these 16 patients, 11 experienced full remission as indicated by a drop of the Hamilton Depression Rating Scale score from 19.1 to 1.6. Nine of these 11 patients suffered from severe atypical depressive symptoms (for example, hypersomnia, fatigue, hyperphagia) and they experienced rapid remission of their atypical symptoms within the first week of treatment. One patient, resistant to treatment regimens with bright light and selective serotonin reuptake inhibitors (SSRIs), fully recovered after 4 weeks. Two of these 16 patients discontinued reboxetine treatment due to side-effects. One male patient experienced moderate urinary retention which resolved after drug discontinuation and one patient reported insomnia and psychomotor agitation. The apparent side-effects in the responder group were transient and comprised dry mouth, constipation, and sweating — typical noradrenergic side-effects. Since loss of energy is one of the leading symptoms of SAD, the noradrenergic compound, reboxetine, seems to be an excellent candidate for pharmacotherapy of SAD and warrants further studies in a double-blind fashion.

9.3.2 Controlled studies

A few controlled treatment approaches, without using a placebo group, have been undertaken. These have compared either fluoxetine with light therapy (Ruhrmann *et al.* 1998), hypericine with bright-light treatment (Martinez *et al.* 1994), or fluoxetine versus moclobemide (Partonen and Lönnqvist 1996). In the study of Ruhrmann *et al.* (1998), 40 patients were exposed to either bright light and placebo capsules, or fluoxetine (20 mg daily) and dim-light conditions. This study revealed that after 4 weeks fluoxetine was as effective as bright-light treatment. However, the bright-light group had a faster onset of antidepressant action and suffered fewer side-effects than the fluoxetine group. Agitation was the main side-effect seen in the fluoxetine group.

In the controlled treatment approach used in the study by Martinez *et al.* (1994), hypericine (St John's wort, 900 mg daily) was used with bright-light or dim-light conditions. Both treatment conditions (each including 10 patients) exhibited good antidepressant efficacy, with no superiority of the hypericine plus bright-light condition.

Since only a small number of patients were included in this trial, it could well be that an existing difference was masked by the small number of patients which participated. A Finnish multi-centre trial of 32 SAD patients, in a comparative 6-week, randomized, double-blind trial with either moclobemide (300–450 mg daily) or fluoxetine (20–40 mg daily), resulted in no difference between these two treatment conditions (Partonen and Lönnqvist 1996). In this study, 151 depressed patients without seasonal pattern also participated. It emerged that 79 per cent of SAD patients benefited from either fluoxetine or moclobemide, whilst the authors believed moclobemide was somewhat better in terms of quality of life.

9.3.3 Placebo-controlled trials

To date, there are ten placebo-controlled trials of antidepressants in SAD. Since nine of these studies (Lingjærde *et al.* 1993; Schlager 1994; Oren *et al.* 1994*a*, 1994*b*; Lam *et al.* 1995; Rosenthal *et al.* 1988; Lewy *et al.* 1988; Lingjærde *et al.* 1999; Thorell *et al.* 1999) used just a small number of patients, only the study of Blashko *et al.* (1997) can be considered as confirmative.

In the study by Lingjærde *et al.* (1993), the authors followed up on their approach to elaborate whether moclobemide is effective in SAD and used 400 mg moclobemide daily, compared with placebo, in a double-blind parallel-group study lasting for up to 14 weeks. Whereas the total scores of the Montgomery–Asberg Depression Rating Scale and a Clinical Global Impressions Scale showed no significant difference between the moclobemide and placebo groups, it was apparent that the atypical score was reduced significantly more on moclobemide than placebo even after one week. When patients were dichotomized according to the median age (45 years) there was a somewhat better effect of moclobemide compared to placebo in the older age group.

In a later study, Lingjærde *et al.* (1999) studied the effect of Ginkgo biloba in 27 SAD patients who received, in a double-blind fashion, either placebo or Ginkgo biloba for 10 weeks in an attempt to prevent symptoms of winter depression. Patients were started on Ginkgo biloba during a symptom-free phase about one month before symptoms of winter depression were expected to emerge. In the study it was not possible to demonstrate that Ginkgo biloba was able to prevent the development of the symptoms of winter depression.

The multi-centre, placebo-controlled study of fluoxetine in SAD published by Lam *et al.* (1995) included 78 SAD patients treated with either fluoxetine (20 mg daily) or placebo over a 5-week period. At the end of the treatment both groups showed significant improvement, but the fluoxetine group had lower depression scores at termination than the placebo group, without exhibiting statistical significance. However, the rate of clinical response (50 per cent reduction in depression scores) in the fluoxetine group (59 per cent) was superior to that in the placebo group (34 per cent). Post-hoc analysis showed that the greatest fluoxetine responses were in the most markedly depressed patients and that overall response was greater for patients studied later in the season. The authors concluded that fluoxetine appears to be an effective, well-tolerated treatment for SAD, but that larger samples need to be studied to conclusively determine whether fluoxetine is efficacious in SAD (which seems to be the case based on our personal experience).

The only conclusive study to answer the question of whether antidepressants are effective in SAD is the multi-centre trial comparing sertraline (50–200 mg daily) with placebo (Blashko *et al.* 1997). Unfortunately this excellent study, first presented at the American Psychiatric Association meeting in 1995 as a new research finding, is still not available as a full-length paper. One hundred and eighty-seven patients participated in this 8-week, double-blind study, of whom 70 in the sertraline and 72 in the placebo group, respectively, completed the study. A significantly greater proportion of those receiving placebo (15 per cent) than those receiving sertraline (3 per cent) were withdrawn from double-blind therapy due to inadequate response. There was no significant difference between the number of sertraline (11 per cent) and placebo (4 per cent) patients who discontinued due to adverse events. Overall, sertraline proved significantly and clinically superior to placebo treatment. The mean final daily dose for sertraline was 111 mg. These results are the first to demonstrate statistical significance in the improvement of active drug over placebo in SAD. Furthermore, this study also supports the hypothesis that 5-HT may be important in the pathogenesis of SAD.

Another interesting approach has been undertaken by Thorell *et al.* (1997) using the SSRI, citalopram. A small but carefully studied group of 8 patients were treated with light therapy for 10 days; thereafter, 4 patients were allocated (double-blind) 4 mg citalopram and 4 patients were given a placebo. They were studied throughout a one-year period. It emerged that citalopram was statistically significantly more successful in preventing depressive symptoms than the placebo. This is the first study in SAD patients to study the long-term outcome with antidepressants. Furthermore, this study supports the notion that initial light therapy with continued SSRI treatment (citalopram) is a useful strategy to achieve beneficial long-term effects in patients with SAD.

The study by Oren *et al.* (1994*a*) aimed to establish if a dopaminergic deficiency plays a role in the pathogenesis of SAD and furthermore tried to test the efficacy of levodopa (up to 7 mg/kg daily) plus carbidopa (100 mg daily) as a treatment for SAD. Patients were treated for 2 weeks, after a 2-week 'wash-out' period, with the dopaminergic compounds, and the results were compared to placebo. At the end of the study there was no difference in the rates of responses between the active and the placebo group and there was also no evidence to support the use of levodopa for the treatment of SAD patients in general. The authors concluded that a model of systemic dopaminergic deficiency does not readily explain the pathology of SAD.

The NIMH group also studied the effect of 1.5 mg cyanocobalamin (vitamin B_{12}), 3 times daily, in a 2-week placebo-controlled design in 27 patients (Oren *et al.* 1994*b*). This approach was in response to a number of studies that had demonstrated that vitamin B_{12} can affect the circadian pacemaker, altering its sensitivity to light. However, this study showed that there was no significant difference between the two groups. The authors questioned if the methylated form of vitamin B_{12}, used extensively in related studies, might still be an option for treatment for SAD and the topic of a further study.

In an early study, Rosenthal *et al.* (1988) tested the hypothesis that the antidepressant effect of bright light is mediated by the suppression of melatonin. The authors studied 19 patients treated either with atenolol (which suppresses melatonin secretion) or placebo, in a double-blind, crossover study. There was no difference in the antidepressant efficacy between drug and placebo in the sample as a whole — a strong argument against the melatonin hypothesis of light therapy. However, the authors noted that in 3 of the patients treated with atenolol, there was marked and sustained relief of symptoms, suggesting that it may be useful in treating the winter depressive symptoms of some patients with SAD.

In another effort to better understand the pathophysiology of SAD, which might be linked to its therapeutic properties, Schlager (1994) used 60 mg or less of propranolol in 23 SAD patients in the hope of influencing nocturnal melatonin secretion, since propranolol effectively blocks melatonin secretion. Propranolol was administered daily between 5.30 a.m. and 6.00 a.m. with the intention to truncate nocturnal secretion in its final hours, which the author postulated should have an antidepressant effect. After open treatment with a mean dose of 33 mg propranolol daily, patients were switched either to the placebo condition or to continuation treatment with propranolol. Patients in the placebo condition relapsed significantly more often than in the propranolol condition. The author concluded that these findings are consistent with the hypothesis that duration of nocturnal melatonin secretion is the critical seasonal time queue in humans. However, the results of this study may only be true for a small subgroup of patients who respond to propranolol treatment. Therefore, these findings must be viewed with caution and need to be substantiated in further investigations.

To further test the melatonin hypothesis, Lewy *et al.* (1998) studied 10 patients with winter depression; 5 patients received low doses of melatonin in the afternoon (0.125 mg) and 5 patients received placebo capsules during a 3-week observation period. Compared to placebo, melatonin treatment significantly decreased depression ratings. The authors take this study as a confirmation of the melatonin hypothesis and they discuss their findings in line with those of Schlager *et al.* (1994) just mentioned. The authors emphasize that their treatment is capable of phase-resetting the disturbed endogenous rhythm in SAD patients. There is a need for replication of this finding and it is noteworthy that the authors comment, based on their experience, that SAD patients appear to be very sensitive to the sedating effect of melatonin.

9.4 Conclusion

Although light therapy is a popular treatment for SAD, it is now apparent that several pharmacological approaches can also be undertaken to treat this subgroup of major depressed patients. However, it seems not advisable to use antidepressants with a strong and enduring sedating component, as shown by tricyclic and tetracyclic antidepressants. So far, SSRIs, and possibly compounds with a distinct noradrenergic mechanism of action (like the noradrenaline reuptake inhibitor, reboxetine, or mirtazapine) seem to be the treatment of choice for SAD. However, the multi-centre, placebo-controlled trial of sertraline is the only one to confirm the effectiveness of an antidepressant. There is a need for controlled trials of antidepressants in SAD which share good antidepressant properties with negligible side-effects.

References

Anderson, J.L., Vasile, R.G., Mooney, J.J., Bloomingdale, K.L., Samson, J.A., and Schildkraut, J.J. (1992). Changes in norepinephrine output following light therapy for fall/winter seasonal depression. *Biol Psychiatry*, **32**:700–4.

Blashko, C.A., Moscovitch, A., Eagles, J.M., Darcourt, G., Thompson, C., and Kasper, S. (1997). A placebo-controlled study of sertraline in the treatment of outpatients with seasonal affective disorder. *Arch Gen Psychiatry* (submitted).

Coiro, V., Volpi, R., Marchesi, C., De Ferri, A., Davoli, C., Caffarra, P., *et al.* (1993). Abnormal serotonergic control of prolactin and cortisol secretion in patients with seasonal affective disorder. *Psychoneuroendocrinology*, **18**:551–6.

De Boer, T., Nefkens, F., and Van Helvoirt, A. (1994). The α_2-antagonist Org 3770 enhances serotonin transmission in vivo. *European Journal of Pharmacology*, **253**:R5–R6.

De Vry, J.M., Schreiber, R., Glaser, T., and Traber, J. (1992). Behavioral pharmacology of 5-HT$_{1A}$ agonists: animal models of anxiety and depression. In *Serotonin 1A receptors in depression and anxiety* (ed. S.M. Stahl), pp. 55–81. New York.

Dilsaver, S.C. and Jaeckle, R.S. (1990). Winter depression responds to an open trial of tranylcypromine. *J Clin Psychiatry*, **51**:326–9.

Dilsaver, S.C., Del Medico, V.J., Quadri, A., and Jaeckle, R.S. (1990). Pharmacological responsiveness of winter depression. *Psychopharmacol Bull*, **26**:303–9.

Hesselmann, B., Habeler, A., Praschak–Rieder, N., Willeit, M., Neumeister, A., and Kasper, S. (1999). Mirtazapine in seasonal affective disorder (SAD): a preliminary report. *Human Psychopharmacology*, **14**:59–62.

Hilger, E., Willeit, M., Praschak–Rieder, N., Neumeister, A., Stastny, J., Thierry, N., *et al.* (1999). Rapid remission of atypical depressive symptoms with the selective noradrenaline reuptake inhibitor reboxetine in SAD patients. *European Neuropsychopharmacology*, **9** (**Suppl. 5**):243.

Jacobsen, F.M., Murphy, D.L., and Rosenthal, N.E. (1989). The role of serotonin in seasonal affective disorder and the antidepressant response to phototherapy. In *Seasonal affective disorder and phototherapy* (ed. N.E. Rosenthal and M.C. Blehar), pp. 333–41. Guilford Press, New York.

Jacobsen, F.M., Mueller, E.A., Rosenthal, N.E., Rogers, S., Hill, J.L., and Murphy, D.L. (1994). Behavioral responses to intravenous meta-chlorophenylpiperazine in patients with seasonal affective disorder and control subjects before and after phototherapy. *Psychiatry Res*, **52**: 181–97.

Kasper, S. (1996). Klinische Wirksamkeit von Mirtazapin: Übersicht der gepoolten Daten aus Metaanalysen. *Jatros Neuro*, **11**:60–8.

Kasper, S. (1999). Treatment benefits of reboxetine. *International Journal of Psychiatry in Clinical Practice*, **3**(Suppl. 1):53–8.

Kasper, S., Ruhrmann, S., and Schuchardt, H.M. (1994). The effects of light therapy in treatment indications other than seasonal affective disorder (SAD). In *Biologic effects of light 1993*, (ed. M.F. Holick and E.G. Jung), pp. 206–18. Walter de Gruyter & Co, Berlin, New York.

Kasper, S., Neumeister, A., Rieder–Praschak, N., Ruhrmann, S., and Heßelmann, B. (1996). Serotonergic mechanisms in the pathophysiology and treatment of seasonal affective disorder. In *Biological effects of light 1995* (ed. M.F. Holick and E.G. Jung), pp. 325–31. Walter de Gruyter & Co, Berlin, New York.

Kasper, S., Praschak–Rieder, N., Tauscher, J., and Wolf, R. (1997). A risk–benefit assessment of mirtazapine in the treatment of depression. *CNS Drug Safety*, **17**(4):251–64.

Lam, R.W., Gorman, C.P., Michalon, M., Steiner, M., Levitt, A.J., Corral, M.R., *et al.* (1995). Multi-centre, placebo-controlled study of fluoxetine in seasonal affective disorder. *Am J Psychiatry*, **152**:1765–70.

Lewy, A.J., Bauer, V.K., Cutler, N.L., and Sack, R.L. (1998) Melatonin treatment of winter depression: a pilot study. *Psychiatry Res*, **77**:57–61

Lingjærde, O. and Haggag, A. (1992). Moclobemide in winter depression: some preliminary results from an open trial. *Nord J Psychiatry*, **46**(3):201–3.

Lingjærde, O., Reichborn–Kjennerud, T., Haggag, A., Gärtner, I., Narud, K., and Berg, E.M. (1993). Treatment of winter depression in Norway. II. A comparison of the selective monoamine oxidase A inhibitor moclobemide and placebo. *Acta Psychiatr Scand*, **88**:372–80.

Lingjærde, O., Føreland, A.R., and Magnusson, A. (1999). Can winter depression be prevented by Ginkgo biloba extract? A placebo-controlled trial. *Acta Psychiatr Scand* **100**:62–6.

Neumeister, A., Praschak–Rieder, N., Heßelmann, B., Rao, M.L., Glück, J., and Kasper, S. (1997). Effects of tryptophan depletion on drug-free patients with seasonal affective disorder during a stable response to bright light therapy. *Arch Gen Psychiatry*, **54**:133–8.

Neumeister, A., Turner, E., Matthew, J., Postolache, T., Barnett, R., Rauh, M., *et al.* (1998). Effects of tryptophan depletion versus catecholamine depletion in patients with seasonal affective disorder remitted on light therapy. *Arch Gen Psychiatry*, **55**:524–30.

Martinez, B., Kasper, S., Ruhrmann, S., and Möller, H.J. (1994). Hypericum in the treatment of seasonal affective disorders. *J Geriatr Psychiatry Neurol*, **7**:29–33.

McGrath, R.E., Buckwald, B., and Resnick, E.V. (1990) The effect of L-tryptophan on seasonal affective disorder. *J Clin Psychiatry*, **51**:162–3.

O'Rourke, D., Wurtman, J.J., Wurtman, R.J., Chebli, R., and Gleason, R. (1989). Treatment of seasonal affective disorder with d-fenfluramine. *J Clin Psychiatry*, **50**:343–7.

Oren, D.A., Mould, D.E., Schwartz, P.J., Wehr, T.A., and Rosenthal, N.E. (1994a). A controlled trial of levodopa plus carbidopa in the treatment of winter seasonal affective disorder: a test of the dopamine hypothesis. *J Clin Psychopharmacol*, **14**:196–200.

Oren D.A., Teicher, M.H., Schwartz, P.J., Glod, C., Turner, E.H. Ito Y.N., *et al.* (1994b). A controlled trial of cyanocobalamin (vitamin B_{12}) in the treatment of winter seasonal affective disorder. *J Affect Disord*, **32**:197–200

Partonen, T. and Lönnqvist, J. (1996). Moclobemide and fluoxetine in treatment of seasonal affective disorder. *J Affect Disord*, **41**:93–9.

Rosenthal, N.E., Genhart, M., Jacobsen, F.M., Skwerer, R.G., and Wehr, T.A. (1987). Disturbances of appetite and weight regulation in seasonal affective disorder. *Ann N Y Acad Sci*, **499**: 216–30.

Rosenthal, N.E., Jacobson, F.M., Sack, D.A., Arendt, J., James, S.P., Parry, B.L., *et al.* (1988). Atenolol in seasonal affective disorders: a test of melatonin hypothesis . *Am J Psychiatry*, **145**:1, 52–6.

Rudorfer, M.V., Skwerer, R.G., and Rosenthal, N.E. (1993). Biogenic amines in seasonal affective disorder: effects of light therapy. *Psychiatry Res*, **46**:19–28.

Ruhrmann, S., Kasper, S., Hawellek, B., Martinez, B., Höflich, G., Nickelsen, T., *et al.* (1998). Effects of fluoxetine versus bright light in the treatment of seasonal affective disorder. *Psychological Med*, **28**:923–33.

Schlager, D.S. (1994). Early-morning administration of short-acting ß-blockers for treatment of winter depression. *Am J Psychiatry,* **151**:1383–5.

Teicher, M.H. and Glod, C.A. (1990). Seasonal affective disorder: rapid resolution by low-dose alprazolam. *Psychopharmacol Bull,* **26**:197–202.

Terman, M., Terman, J.S., Quitkin, F.M., McGrath, P.J., Steward, J.W., and Rafferty, B. (1989). Light therapy for seasonal affective disorder. A review of efficacy. *Neuropsychopharmacology,* **2**:1–22.

Thorell, L–H., Kjellman, B., Arned, M., Lindwall–Sundel, K., Walinder, J., and Wetterberg, L. (1999). Light treatment of seasonal affective disorder in combination with citalopram or placebo with 1-year follow-up. *Int Clin Psychopharmacol,* **14(Suppl. 2)**:7–11.

Wirz–Justice, A., van der Velde, P., and Nil, R. (1992). Comparison of light treatment with citalopram in winter depression: a longitudinal single case study. *Int Clin Psychopharmacol,* **7**:109–16.

Chapter 10

Other therapies

Ybe Meesters

10.1 Introduction

Bright-light therapy is the treatment of first choice for patients suffering from winter depression. Also, some beneficial effects of psychopharmaceuticals have been reported. Besides those therapies there are other treatments for depression, mainly offered by alternative and complementary health services, that may or may not have benefits. Although there are no rigorous scientific data to support the efficacy of the majority of those treatments, there are some exceptions (Ernst *et al.* 1998). In this chapter these treatments for SAD will be discussed.

The effects of (very) low intensity light and natural light as treatment for SAD will be mentioned, and also the effects of the use of plant extracts, ions, magnetic fields, sleep deprivation, and psychotherapy.

10.2 Alternative light treatments

Bright artificial light is a powerful treatment for SAD. The efficacy of bright light is supported by the results of a great number of studies (see the chapter by Partonen). In some studies, the researchers assumed that artificial light with a low intensity could function as a placebo control condition. When light-boxes were used, the effects of bright light were mostly superior to those of dim light. Nevertheless, some beneficial effects of dim light exposure have been reported (Terman *et al.* 1989; Lee and Chan 1999). The superiority of the effects of bright light over those of a low or very low intensity disappeared when the light fixture used was a head-mounted unit or light visor.

In a number of studies positive effects of very low-intensity light are reported. There was no difference in effect after light with an intensity of 60, 600, or 3000 lux had been used (Joffe *et al.* 1993), or between 400 and 6000 lux (Rosenthal *et al.* 1993). In the latter study, a significantly greater relapse occurred after the low-intensity light as compared to the bright-light condition. Also, red light with a mean intensity of 96 lux was equally effective as red light with a mean intensity of 4106 lux (Levitt *et al.* 1994), and bright white light of 600 lux compared to red light of an intensity of 30 lux (Teicher *et al.* 1995). Even the effects of exposure to almost invisible infrared light with an intensity of 0.18 lux were not significantly different when compared to the effects of bright white light of 2500 lux (Meesters *et al.* 1999).

These findings question the role of visible light and its intensity when treating SAD. In some other studies, where light visors were used, the effects of placebo conditions were equal to the effects of light conditions. In the placebo conditions, subjects were given the suggestion that they were exposed to invisible infrared light (Levitt *et al.* 1996, Meesters *et al.* 1997). The effects of placebo treatment can be very strong (Eastman 1990; see also the chapter by Eastman). That the suggestion of light can be beneficial has been shown by Richter *et al.* (1992) who reported that the effects of imaginary light did not differ in a statistically significant way from the effects of bright light. However, the effects of bright light remained after the end of the treatment period, whereas the subjects who had been given imaginary light showed a relapse soon after the treatment. It was not possible to suppress the nightly melatonin production by using imaginary light (Byrne *et al.* 1992), so the underlying working mechanism of imaginary light might be different from that of light treatment.

In the classic article of Rosenthal *et al.* (1984), the authors report a case in which a patient who lived in North America recovered from her depressive state in a couple of days after arriving on sunny Jamaica (see also Mueller and Allen 1984). Wirz–Justice *et al.* (1996) compared the effects of a 30-minute, outdoor, morning walk of SAD patients, in 'natural' surroundings, with the effects of a low dose of artificial light (30 minutes of 2800 lux). The outdoor light condition was superior and could phase advance the onset and/or offset of melatonin secretion and lower morning cortisol levels. The artificial light did not affect melatonin or cortisol levels. It is unusual for SAD patients to walk outdoors in the morning in winter, but when taking the results of this study into account, it would be an (inexpensive) alternative treatment.

SAD patients do not receive less outdoor light than healthy controls. Women with SAD do not spend less time outdoors in winter than controls, but spend more time outdoors in summer. The susceptibility to winter depression may therefore arise not from lack of sufficient (outdoor) light exposure, but from an increased vulnerability to the amount of light received (Graw *et al.* 1999).

To summarize, light of a very low intensity, natural light, or even the suggestion of light can be beneficial in treating SAD.

10.3 **Herbal treatments**

Herbal treatments in psychiatric disorders are quite often used in alternative health services. There is little evidence to justify claims about their efficacy. St John's wort (Hypericum perforatum) is an exception (Wong *et al.* 1998). This herb is well known for his antidepressant effect. In a meta-analysis Linde *et al.* (1996) showed that hypericum extracts are more effective than placebo and just about as effective as standard antidepressants in the treatment of depressions.

Martinez *et al.* (1994) compared the effects of hypericum combined with dim light (< 300 lux) with the effects of hypericum combined with bright light (3000 lux) treatment for SAD. The findings were clinically relevant and the results of both conditions did not differ significantly. Another study reported almost no differences in results after the use of hypericum as compared with the use of hypericum combined with light treatment for SAD. Only improvement in sleep was greater in the light plus hypericum condition (Wheatley 1999). The authors of both studies conclude that hypericum is beneficial in the treatment of SAD. The weakness of these studies is the absence of a placebo control group. According to Kasper (1997) the effect of hypericum is comparable to that of fluoxetine in treating SAD and might be an efficient treatment for SAD (see the chapter by Kasper *et al.*).

The possibility that hypericum is beneficial in treating SAD might be a real alternative for light treatment, but doctors should be aware of some serious possible side-effects of hypericum. Some cases have been described of depressed patients who became manic after using hypericum (Schneck 1998; O'Breasail and Argouarch 1998; Nierenberg *et al.* 1999). Increased photosensitivity has also been reported (Miller 1998; Lieberman 1998) — a side-effect that may be especially important if the use of hypericum is combined with light treatment.

Recently, several papers have been published about the interaction of hypericum with drugs. For example, mild serotonin syndrome in patients who combine hypericum with serotonin-reuptake inhibitors, decreased bioavailability of digoxin when combined with hypericum, and lowering of serum warfarin when combined with hypericum have been reported (Ernst 1999; Lantz *et al.* 1999; Fugh–Berman 2000; Yue *et al.* 2000). Even heart transplant rejection due to the interaction of hypericum and ciclosporin has been described (Ruschitzka *et al.* 2000) as well as a negative influence of the use of hypericum on the effects of drug treatment of HIV (Piscitelli *et al.* 2000).

Clinicians should be aware not only of these interactions and side-effects, but also of the beneficial effects of hypericum, and balance the benefits against the possible harm. An untreated resistant depression can be fatal and is often treated with combinations of different antidepressants with a risk of possible interaction effects (Wheatley 2000).

Besides hypericum, the effects of another plant extract in treating SAD have been studied. In an attempt to find a way to prevent the symptoms of winter depression, extracts from the leaves of the Maidenhair tree, Ginkgo biloba, were used in a study. No differences were found between a placebo condition compared to a condition in which Ginkgo biloba was used (Lingjærde *et al.* 1999).

10.4 Ion treatment

It is hard to find a plausible and invisible placebo condition to compare with light treatment for SAD; Eastman *et al.* (1992) describes one. They found that the results after light treatment were similar to those after treating patients with a deactivated ion generator. In their study the effects of an active ion generator were not studied. Terman and Terman (1995) compared the effects of negative ions at two exposure densities (1×10^4 ions/cm^3 or 2.7×10^6 ions/cm^3) in treating SAD. In the high-density condition, 58 per cent of the SAD patients improved by at least 50 per cent, against 15 per cent in the low-density treatment.

In another study, the effects of low- and high-density ion treatments in the morning were compared to the effects of light treatment at different times of the day. Low-density ion treatment was inferior to all other conditions, but the effects of high-density, negative air ionization treatment were no different from those of light treatment in SAD sufferers. If these results can be replicated, high-density, negative air ionization could be an alternative to light therapy or medication (Terman *et al.* 1998).

10.5 Magnetism

There are indications that the pineal gland is a magnetosensitive system and that changes in the ambient magnetic field can change the melatonin secretion and synchronize the circadian system. The environmental light and magnetic fields are subject to diurnal and seasonal variations and influence the activity of the pineal gland. It has been suggested that the simultaneous application of light and magnetic field treatment may increase the beneficial effects of light treatment alone (Sandyk *et al.* 1991). Partonen (1998) hypothesized that in

SAD patients specialized photoreceptors modulate the response of the photoreceptive system to light and the pineal response to a magnetic stimulus.

Transcranial magnetic stimulation (TMS) may become a new way of treating mood disorders. TMS is a non-invasive method of brain stimulation that uses strong magnetic fields. The results of the first studies are inconclusive. In some studies an improvement of mood is reported, in others no mood changes are seen at all after TMS (George *et al.* 1999; Berman *et al.* 2000; Loo *et al.* 2000; Little *et al.* 2000; Mosimann *et al.* 2000).

Further research about the role of magnetism is needed and may lead to a clinical application.

10.6 Physical exercise

There is some evidence that physical exercise is beneficial in treating depression (North *et al.* 1990; Ernst *et al.* 1998; Blumenthal *et al.* 1999). As treatment for SAD, some positive results of exercise are described. Mood improved by about 50 per cent in SAD patients after 2 weeks of practice on a home bicycle trainer (Koehler *et al.* 1993). Response in winter-depressed patients was seen to be equal after 1 week of physical exercise or 1 week of bright light (Pinchasov *et al.* 2000). Early morning aerobic exercises resulted in a significant reduction of depression scores in SAD patients (Kurz *et al.* 1995). Partonen *et al.* (1998) found that the results of exercise combined with bright light when compared to exercise in ordinary room light were superior in reducing atypical depressive symptoms in employees recruited from five workplaces. The combination of exercise and light might also be part of the explanation of the positive results in SAD patients after an outdoors, morning walk in 'natural' light conditions (Wirz–Justice *et al.* 1996).

10.7 Sleep deprivation

Sleep deprivation has been shown to be beneficial in treating depressed patients (Leibenluft and Wehr 1992); positive response rates of 50–60 per cent after sleep deprivation have been reported (Van den Hoofdakker 1994). The effects of sleep deprivation are usually temporary. The use of bright-light treatment after partial sleep deprivation might be an effective way of preventing the relapse after sleep deprivation (Neumeister *et al.* 1996*a*; 1996*b*). In a comparison between the effects of bright-light treatment and partial sleep deprivation in patients with affective disorders, bright light was superior to partial sleep deprivation (Heim 1988).

There is some discussion about the role of sleep deprivation in SAD. In a longitudinal single case study by Wirz–Justice *et al.* (1992), the positive effects of light treatment and of citalopram in treating a SAD patient are described. Light in the morning advanced and improved sleep, citalopram delayed sleep and induced intermittent awakenings. According to the authors, these opposite patterns suggest that sleep deprivation is not crucial to eliciting a therapeutic response. The same conclusion is drawn by Brunner *et al.* (1996) after a 40-hour constant routine experiment in which the role of sleep regulation in SAD was studied by means of recording a sleep electroencephalogram at baseline and after total sleep deprivation before and after light treatment. The authors conclude that the robust antidepressant effect of light treatment in SAD is unlikely to be mediated by changes in sleep. Another 40-hour constant routine study found that the response of SAD patients to total sleep deprivation was similar to the response of non-seasonal depressives to total sleep deprivation. Sleep deprivation, therefore, can be an additional treatment option to light therapy (Graw *et al.* 1998).

10.8 Psychotherapy

There is no evidence that psychotherapy is a useful treatment tool for SAD. If SAD is treated successfully by means of light treatment within a couple of days, there is little necessity to start more time-consuming psychotherapy. If there is some comorbidity with SAD as personality disorders or panic and anxiety disorders, these disorders can be treated with psychotherapy (Lam *et al.* 1999). This can be useful too if families and relations are disturbed as a consequence of the SAD complaints of one member of the family. But there is no evidence that psychotherapy is useful as a treatment of the SAD syndrome.

In a preliminary investigation Hodges and Marks (1998) found some indications that SAD sufferers had negative cognitions, so cognitive therapy might be useful. Another study also emphasized the role of cognitions in SAD. Subjects were exposed to symbolic light, to ensure that only cognitive processes were involved. The perception of the symbolic light was assessed at the end of the summer in a symptom-free episode in SAD patients. These perceptions were related to the starting point of the next depressive episode in the subsequent autumn/winter (Bouhuys *et al.* 1994). A ruminative response style was a predictor of severity in SAD and equally associated with vegetative and cognitive symptoms (Young and Azam 1999) — another indication that cognitions play a role in SAD. On the other hand, Levitan *et al.* (1998) found that the negative attributions of SAD sufferers were no predictor of a good result after light treatment.

Observed behaviour of a SAD patient and an interviewer during an interview seems to be related to the response to light therapy. This result suggests that behavioural processes may play a role in the mechanism underlying the response to light treatment in SAD (Geerts *et al.* 1995). If it becomes clear that this is the case, behavioural therapy may be an optional treatment. Amir and Stewart (1996) reported that the biological clock could be reset by means of conditioning. It is unclear if the biological clock plays a role in the underlying mechanism of winter depression but, if it is so, conditioning might be helpful.

10.9 Conclusions

Bright-light treatment is a powerful treatment for SAD. The effects of very low intensities of light are shown in studies using light visors. Also, in 'natural light' surroundings beneficial effects in treating SAD are described. If light treatment is not sufficient or unavailable, there are some alternative treatments besides drugs. The scientific evidence of the results of those treatments for SAD is unclear, weak, or absent. High-density ions, hypericum, and exercise treatments might be effective; so far, psychotherapy is not an evidence-based option. Further research is needed to establish these treatments as real alternatives to light in treating SAD.

Acknowledgements

I am grateful to J.S. Borger for her improvement of my English in this chapter.

References

Amir, S. and Stewart, J. (1996) Resetting of the circadian clock by a conditioned stimulus. *Nature* **379**:542–5.

Berman, R.M., Narasimhan, M., Sanacora, G., Miano, A.P., Hoffman, R.E., Hu, X.S., *et al.* (2000) A randomized clinical trial of repetitive transcranial magnetic stimulation in the treatment of major depression. *Biological Psychiatry* **47**:332–7.

Blumenthal, J.A., Babyak, M.A., Moore, K.A., Craighead, W.E., Herman, S., Khatri, P., *et al.* (1999) Effects of exercise training on older patients with major depression. *Archives of Internal Medicine* **159**:2349–56.

Bouhuys, A.L., Meesters, Y., Jansen, J.H.C., and Bloem G.M. (1994) Relationship between cognitive sensitivity to (symbolic) light in remitted seasonal affective disorder patients and the onset time of a subsequent depressive episode. *Journal of Affective Disorders* **31**:39–48.

Brunner, D.P., Kräuchi, K., Dijk, D.J., Leonhardt, G., Haug, H.J., and Wirz–Justice, A. (1996) Sleep electroencephalogram in seasonal affective disorder and in control women: effects of midday light treatment and sleep deprivation. *Biological Psychiatry* **40**:485–96.

Byrne, B., Gaddy, J.R., Doghramji, K., Maldonado, L., Margolis, C.G., Rollag, M.D., *et al.* (1992) Can hypnotic suggestion mimic the effect of bright light on melatonin production? *Abstracts of Society for Light Treatment and Biological Rhythms* **4**:12.

Eastman, C.I. (1990) What the placebo literature can tell us about light therapy for SAD. *Psychopharmacology Bulletin* **26**:495–504.

Eastman, C.I., Lahmeyer, H.W., Watell, L.G., Good, G.D., and Young, M.A. (1992) A placebo controlled trial of light treatment for winter depression. *Journal of Affective Disorders* **26**:211–22.

Ernst, E. (1999) Second thoughts about safety of St John's wort. *The Lancet* **354**:2014–16.

Ernst, E., Rand, J.I., and Stevinson, C. (1998) Complementary therapies for depression. An overview. *Archives of General Psychiatry* **55**:1026–32.

Fugh–Berman, A. (2000) Herb–drug interactions. *The Lancet* **355**:134–8.

Geerts, E., Bouhuys, N., Meesters, Y., and Jansen, J. (1995) Observed behavior of patients with seasonal affective disorder and an interviewer predicts response to light treatment. *Psychiatry Research* **57**:223–30.

George, M.S., Avery, D., Nahas, Z., Molloy, M., Oliver, N.C., Risch, S.C., *et al.* (1999) rTMS studies of mood and emotion. *Electroencephalography and Clinical Neurophysiology* **Suppl. 51**:304–14.

Graw, P., Haug, H.J., Leonhardt, G., and Wirz–Justice, A. (1998) Sleep deprivation response in seasonal affective disorder during a 40-h constant routine. *Journal of Affective Disorders* **48**:69–74.

Graw, P., Recker, S., Sand, L., Kräuchi, K., and Wirz–Justice, A. (1999) Winter and summer outdoor light exposure in women with and without seasonal affective disorder. *Journal of Affective Disorders* **56**:163–9.

Heim, M. (1988) Zur efficienz der bright-light therapie bei zyklothymen achsensyndromen — eine cross-over studie gegenüber partiellem schlafentzug. *Psychiatry, Neurology and Medical Psychology* **40**:S269–77.

Hodges, S. and Marks, M. (1998) Cognitive characteristics of seasonal affective disorder: a preliminary investigation. *Journal of Affective Disorders* **50**:59–64.

Joffe, R.T., Moul, D.E., Lam, R.W., Levitt, A.J., Teicher, M.H., Lebegue, B., *et al.* (1993) Light visor treatment for seasonal affective disorder: a multicenter study. *Psychiatry Research* **46**:29–39.

Kasper, S. (1997) Treatment of seasonal affective disorder (SAD) with hypericum extract. *Pharmacopsychiatry* **30 (Suppl. 2)**:89–93.

Koehler, W.K., Fey, P., Schmidt, K.P., Fleisner, G., and Pflug, B. (1993) Feedback loops in the circadian system: experiences with physical exercise in the treatment of SAD. *Journal of Interdisciplinary Cycle Research* **24**:298–99.

Kurz, B., Giedke, H., Grupe, O., Dickhuth, H–H., and Erkert, H.G. (1995) Early morning exercises (aerobic) reduce depression scores in 'winter-depressed' women (SAD/S-SAD). *Abstracts of the Society for Light Treatment and Biological Rhythms*, **7**:35.

Lam, R.W., Levitt, A.J., Kraus, R.P., Bowen, R.C., Morehouse, R.L., Hasey, G., *et al.* (1999) Management issues. In *Canadian consensus guidelines for the treatment of seasonal affective disorder* (ed. R.W. Lam and A.J. Levitt), pp. 96–114. Clinical & Academic Publishing, Canada.

Lantz, M.S., Buchhalter, E., and Giambanco, V. (1999) St John's Wort and antidepressant drug interactions in the elderly. *Journal of Geriatric Psychiatry and Neurology* **12**:7–10.

Lee, T.M.C. and Chan, C.C.H. (1999) Dose–response relationshi p of phototherapy for seasonal affective disorder: a meta-analysis. *Acta Psychiatrica Scandinavica* **99**:315–23.

Leibenluft, E. and Wehr, T.A. (1992) Is sleep deprivation useful in the treatment of depression? *American Journal of Psychiatry* **149**:159–68.

Levitan, R.D., Rector, N.A., and Bagby, M. (1998) Negative attributional style in seasonal and nonseasonal depression. *American Journal of Psychiatry* **155**:428–30.

Levitt, A.J., Joffe, R.T., and King, E. (1994) Dim versus bright red (light-emitting diode) light in the treatment of seasonal affective disorder. *Acta Psychiatrica Scandinavica* **89**:341–5.

Levitt, A.J., Wesson, V.A., Joffe, R.T., Maunder, R.G., and King, E.F. (1996) A controlled comparison of light box and head mounted units in the treatment of seasonal depression. *Journal of Clinical Psychiatry* **57**:105–10.

Lieberman, S. (1998) Nutriceutical review of St John's Wort (Hypericum perforatum) for the treatment of depression. *Journal of Women's Health* **7**:177–82.

Linde, K., Ramirez, G., Mulrow, C.D., Pauls, A., Weidenhammer, W., and Melchart, D. (1996) St John's wort for depression — an overview and meta-analysis of randomised clinical trials. *British Medical Journal* **313**:253–8.

Lingjærde, O., Føreland, A.R., and Magnusson, A. (1999) Can winter depression be prevented by Ginkgo biloba extract? A placebo-controlled trial. *Acta Psychiatrica Scandinavica* **100**:62–6.

Little, J.T., Kimbrell, T.A., Wasserman, E.M., Grafman, J., Figueras, S., Dunn, R.T., *et al.* (2000) Cognitive effects of 1- and 20-Hertz repetitive transcranial magnetic stimulation in depression: preliminary report. *Neuropsychiatry and Behavioral Neurology* **13**:119–24.

Loo, C.K., Taylor, J.L., Gandevia, S.C., McDarmont, B.N., Mitchell, P.B., and Sachdev, P.S. (2000) Transcranial magnetic stimulation (TMS) in controlled treatment studies: are some 'sham' forms active? *Biological Psychiatry* **47**:325–31.

Martinez, B., Kasper, S., Ruhrmann, S., and Möller, H.J. (1994) Hypericum in the treatment of seasonal affective disorders. *Journal of Geriatric Psychiatry and Neurology* **7** (**suppl. 1**):S29–S33.

Meesters, Y., Van Os, T.W.D.P., Grondsma, K., Veneman, F., Beersma, D.G.M., and Bouhuys, A.L. (1997) Light box vs light visor; bright white vs infrared or placebo light. *Abstracts of the Society for Light Treatment and Biological Rhythms* **9**:27.

Meesters, Y., Beersma, D.G.M., Bouhuys, A.L., and Van den Hoofdakker, R.H. (1999) Prophylactic treatment of seasonal affective disorder (SAD) by using light visors: bright white or infrared light? *Biological Psychiatry* **46**:239–46.

Miller, A. (1998) St John's Wort (Hypericum perforatum). Clinical effects on depression and other conditions. *Alternative Medicine Review* **3**:18–26.

Mosimann, U.P., Rihs, T.A., Engeler, J., Fisch, H.U., and Schlaepfer, T.E. (2000) Mood effects of repetitive transcranial magnetic stimulation of left prefrontal cortex in healthy volunteers. *Psychiatry Research* **94**:251–6.

Mueller, P.S. and Allen, N.C. (1984) Diagnosis and treatment of severe light-sensitive seasonal energy syndrome (SES) and its relation to melatonin anabolism. *Fair Oaks Hospital Psychiatry Letter* **2**:1–5.

Neumeister, A., Goesler, R., Lucht, M., Kapitany, T., Bamas, C., and Kasper, S. (1996a) Bright light therapy stabilizes the antidepressant effect of partial sleep deprivation. *Biological Psychiatry* **39**:16–21.

Neumeister, A., Lucht, M., and Kasper, S. (1996b) Kombination von schlafentzug un lichttharapie zur behandlung depressiver störingen. In *Therapeutischer schlafentzug. Klinik und wirkmechanismen* (ed. S. Kasper and H–J. Möller), pp. 69–80. Springer, Wien, New York.

Nierenberg, A.A., Burt, T., Matthews, J., and Weiss, A.P. (1999) Mania associated with St Johns's Wort. *Biological Psychiatry* **46**:1707–8.

North, T.C., McCullagh, P., Tran, Z.V. (1990) Effect of exercise on depression. *Exercise and Sport Science Review* **18**:379–415.

O'Breasail, A.M. and Argouarch, S. (1998) Hypomania and St John's Wort. *Canadian Journal of Psychiatry* **43**:746–7.

Partonen, T. (1998) Short note: magnetoreception attributed to the efficacy of light treatment. *Medical Hypotheses* **51**:447–8.

Partonen, T., Leppämäki, S., Hurme, J., and Lönnqvist, J. (1998) Randomized trial of physical execise alone or combined with bright light on mood and health related quality of life. *Psychological Medicine* **28**:1359–64.

Pinchasov, B.B., Shurgaja, A.M., Grischin, O.V., and Putilov, A.A. (2000) Mood and energy regulation in seasonal and non-seasonal depression before and after midday treatment with physical exercise or bright light. *Psychiatry Research* **94**:29–42.

Piscitelli, S.C., Burstein, A.H., Chaitt, D., Alfaro, R.M., and Falloon, J. (2000) Indinavir concentrations and St John's wort. *The Lancet* **355**:547–8.

Richter, P., Bouhuys, A.L., Van den Hoofdakker, R.H., Beersma, D.G.M., Jansen, J.H.C., Lambers, P.A., *et al.* (1992) Imaginary versus real light for winter depression. *Biological Psychiatry* **31**:534–6.

Rosenthal, N.E., Sack, D.A., Gillin, J.C., Lewy, A.J., Goodwin, F.K., Davenport, Y., *et al.* (1984) Seasonal affective disorder. A description of the syndrome and preliminary findings with light therapy. *Archives of General Psychiatry* **41**:72–80.

Rosenthal, N.E., Moul, D.E., Hellekson, C.J., Oren, D.A., Frank, A., Brainard, G.C., *et al.* (1993) A multicenter study of the light visor dor seasonal affective disorder: no difference in efficacy found between two different intensities. *Neuropsychopharmacology* **8**:151–60.

Ruschitzka, F., Meier, P.J., Turina, M., Lüscher, T.F., and Noll, G. (2000) Acute heart transplant rejection due to St John's Wort. *The Lancet* **355**:548–9.

Sandyk, R., Anninos, P.A., and Tsagas, N. (1991) Magnetic fields and seasonality of affective illness: implications for therapy. *International Journal of Neuroscience* **58**:261–7.

Schneck, C. (1998) St John's Wort and hypomania. *Journal of Clinical Psychiatry* **59**:689.

Terman, M., Terman, J.S., Quitkin, F.M., McGrath, P.J., Stewart, J.W., and Rafferty, B. (1989) Light therapy for seasonal affective disorder. A review of efficacy. *Neuropsychopharmacology* **2**:1–22.

Terman, T. and Terman, J.S. (1995) Treatment of seasonal affective disorder with a high-output negative ionizer. *Journal of Alternative and Complementary Medicine* **1**:87–92.

Terman, M., Terman, J.S., and Ross, D.C. (1998) A controlled trial of timed bright light and negative air ionization for treatment of winter depression. *Archives of General Psychiatry* **55**:875–82.

Teicher, M.H., Glod, C.A., Oren, D.A., Schwartz, P.J. Luetke, C., Brown, C., *et al.* (1995) The phototherapy light visor: more to it than meets the eye. *American Journal of Psychiatry* **152**:1197–202.

Van den Hoofdakker, R.H. (1994) Chronobiological theories of nonseasonal affective disorders and their implications for treatment. *Journal of Biological Rhythms* **9**:157–83.

Wheatley, D. (1999) Hypericum in seasonal affective disorder (SAD). *Current Medical Research and Opinion* **15**:33–7.

Wheatley, D. (2000) Safety of St John's wort (Hypericum perforatum). *The Lancet* **355**:576.

Wirz–Justice, A., Van der Velde, P., Bucher, A., and Nil, R. (1992) Comparison of light treatment with citalopram in winter depression: a longitudinal single case study. *International Clinical Psychopharmacology* **7**:109–16.

Wirz–Justice, A., Graw, P., Kräuchi, K., Sarrafzadeh, A., English, J., Arendt, J., *et al.* (1996) 'Natural' light treatment of seasonal affective disorder. *Journal of Affective Disorders* **37**:109–20.

Wong, A.C., Smith, M., and Boon, H.S. (1998) Herbal remedies in psychiatric practice. *Archives of General Psychiatry* **55**:1033–44.

Young, M.A. and Azam, O. (1999) Ruminative response style as a predictor of SAD severity. *Abstracts of the Society for Light Treatment and Biological Rhythms* **11**:20.

Yue, Q.Y., Bergquist, C., and Gerdén, B. (2000) Safety of St John's wort (Hypericum perforatum). *The Lancet* **355**:576–7.

Chapter 11

Is bright-light therapy a placebo?

Charmane I. Eastman

11.1 Are placebo controls still necessary in SAD bright-light treatment studies?

Over 10 years ago we studied bright-light treatment for patients with winter depression or SAD. Patients sat in front of a light-box upon waking each morning. After two weeks of treatment, 28 per cent of the patients responded (defined as a 50 per cent or greater decrease in depression scores). In a subsequent similar study, we found that 49 per cent of the patients responded (also after two weeks of treatment and using the same criterion for response). What could be responsible for this dramatic increase in response rate?

Most researchers and clinicians would first consider the four basic parameters of light treatment: intensity, duration, timing, and wavelength or spectrum (Rosenthal *et al.* 1988). Because we used the same light-box in both studies, wavelength was not changed. The light-box was 65 cm wide and 43.5 cm tall and contained six horizontally mounted cool-white fluorescent lamps (Apollo Light Systems, Orem, Utah). In the first study patients sat at a desk or table with the light-box directly in front of them. They used a 12-inch wooden ruler (which we provided) to measure exactly 12 inches (30 cm) from their nose to the middle of the plexiglass screen of the light-box. Patients usually read and ate during light treatment, and the light intensity they received, while looking down at reading material, averaged about 7000 lux. In the second study, the light-box was used in the same way, except that we gave the patients 15-inch wooden rulers, so they sat 37.5 cm from the box, and the light intensity was reduced to about 6000 lux. Could this decrease in light intensity from about 7000 to 6000 lux be responsible for the increase in response rate from 28 to 49 per cent? Probably not. Most people expect higher intensities to work better, and in fact current recommendations are to use 10 000 lux (Lam and Levitt 1999).

The third parameter, duration, was increased from 1 hour to 1.5 hours each morning. This increase in 'dose' would appear to be a logical reason for the increased response rate. The timing of the light treatment was also changed slightly. In both studies, patients woke up earlier than usual to have time to use the light-box in the morning and adhered to a fixed wake-up time throughout the study, including weekends. Morning wake time, and the start of morning light treatment 5–10 minutes later, was slightly earlier in the second study compared to the first (6.08 a.m. as opposed to 6.26 a.m.). If phase advancing the circadian clock is a mechanism contributing to the antidepressant response of light treatment (Lewy *et al.* 1987), then earlier bright light should produce a larger response rate.

In summary, there were changes in three of the four basic parameters of light treatment from study 1 to study 2. Most people would conclude that these changes were the reason for the dramatic increase in antidepressant response. One can imagine numerous subsequent studies that could be performed to tease apart these factors, and thus to hone the most effective light treatment regimen.

However, because we also ran placebo control groups, we know that the changes in these light parameters had little or no effect. The increase in response rate can be entirely accounted for by an increase in the magnitude of the placebo response. The preceding examination of the four light treatment parameters was just an exercise designed to illustrate the pitfalls of studies that have no placebo control groups. Figure 11.1 shows that the increase in response rate to light treatment (28 to 49 per cent) was almost exactly the same as the increase in response to placebo treatment (14 to 36 per cent). In other words, the placebo component of the bright-light treatment increased, which in turn produced an increase in the total antidepressant response to bright light.

I believe that the increase in placebo response from study 1 to study 2 was primarily produced by a change in the attitude of the staff who saw the patients, which in turn increased the patients' expectations for improvement (Eastman *et al.* 1993). In study 1 (Eastman *et al.* 1992) our attitude was slightly cautious and pessimistic. Some of the staff were reluctant to promise too much to the patients for fear they would be disappointed. We also inadvertently stressed the experimental aspect of the treatments by often referring to it as 'research' rather than 'treatment' and by calling our participants 'subjects' instead of

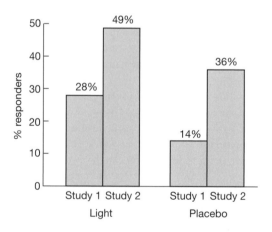

Fig. 11.1 Comparison of response rates to morning bright-light treatment and morning placebo treatment (sham negative ion generator) in two studies of patients with winter depression: study 1 (Eastman *et al.* 1992), study 2 (Eastman *et al.* 1998). Bars show the percentage of responders after 2 weeks of treatment. A responder was defined as a patient whose SIGH-SAD score was reduced to at least 50 per cent of the baseline score. We used the first 24 items of the scale, which comprises the original 17-item Hamilton Depression Rating Scale plus 7 items for rating the atypical depression symptoms which are common in winter depression. Each study lasted 5 weeks — a baseline week followed by 4 treatment weeks. Study 1 had a crossover design; study 2 had a parallel design. Therefore, to directly compare the studies, we only used the data from study 1 that were collected before the crossover and data from the corresponding time in study 2. The number of patients in each group were: study 1: light (n = 18), placebo (n = 14); study 2: light (n = 33), placebo (n = 31).

'patients'. In that study we were not able to demonstrate that light treatment produced a significantly better antidepressant response than placebo.

After studying the placebo literature (as reviewed in Eastman 1990), I decided that for study 2 we should try to increase the magnitude of the placebo effect. One reason is the possibility that the placebo effect may actually be necessary to help release the specific pharmacological effect of a drug or the specific effect of other treatments. Another reason was to overcome a common misconception about our first study: that there was something wrong with our light treatment because it produced a relatively low response rate.

The largest component of an antidepressant treatment can be the placebo component. Thus, response rates can be mainly determined by the size of the placebo component. The absolute magnitude of the response rate to a bright-light treatment does not tell us anything about how much the bright light, *per se*, helped the patients. Nevertheless, it is difficult to convince people that a light treatment is worthwhile unless the absolute magnitude of the response rate is large. Therefore, to increase the placebo response, I coached the staff to be more enthusiastic and optimistic with the patients when talking about the treatments, and to use the words 'treatment' and 'patient'. I myself also acted more positively and confidently when interacting with the patients and staff about the treatments. (For more on how knowledge of placebo effects should affect the design and interpretation of SAD light studies see Eastman 1990.)

Most researchers believe that bright light is more effective than a placebo, and that they can ignore the placebo component and concentrate their studies on the active, more interesting component of the treatment — that is, the bright light. In fact, eminent researchers (Thompson *et al.* 1999) stated: 'Future studies of light therapy should be concerned less with designing "plausible" placebos and more with improving other aspects of trial methodology.' However, if we had not included placebo control groups in our two studies, we would not have known that the improvement from study 1 to study 2 was due to an increase in the placebo response, and we might have gone on a wild goose chase to find out what aspects of the bright-light treatment accounted for the improved antidepressant response.

If light treatment studies do not include plausible controls, then we cannot know if or when the presumed active light treatment reaches the point of becoming superior to placebo. It may take weeks for light to produce a greater antidepressant effect than placebo (see my earlier comments). If there is no placebo control, then researchers could inadvertently be studying the light treatment when it is still working entirely through a placebo mechanism.

11.2 Components of the placebo response in SAD bright-light studies

Several factors contribute to the placebo response including anxiety reduction and expectations for improvement. Patients are usually relieved to receive an official diagnosis of SAD, to hear that their troubling behaviours (for example, sleeping too much, being less productive, eating too much) are not their fault, and that they are not just lazy or not trying hard enough. They are heartened to learn that the doctors believe that there are treatments that can help them. They feel good about finally 'doing something' about their problem by enrolling in a study. Light treatment requires considerable time and effort (compared to taking antidepressant drugs) and this investment and sacrifice may contribute to the placebo effect. Patients usually have weekly (or more) visits to a clinic or hospital where they are seen by staff who care about their symptoms and their progress.

Many studies require that patients wake up earlier than usual for light treatment. Some studies require a fixed, regular wake-up time. These changes in the sleep schedule can lead to better sleep or, conversely, can result in less sleep because of the earlier time for rising. Although these types of interventions might be antidepressant, they do not depend on the presence of bright light and for our purposes are considered non-specific factors which can contribute to the placebo response.

Finally, there may be spontaneous remissions or improvement due to the natural course of the disorder. Many patients are studied after the winter solstice on 21 December, when the photoperiod is gradually lengthening. Thus, it is important to run light and placebo groups concurrently, so that any natural improvement will be the same in both groups.

11.3 Placebo controls for bright-light treatment of SAD

The most vexing problem for SAD light treatment studies is devising an appropriate placebo control treatment. The placebo treatment should be similar to the light treatment in every way possible (except for the light itself), and should generate in patients the same expectations for success as the light treatment. A placebo pill is not an appropriate placebo control for light for several reasons including the fact that it does not require the same investment of time as light treatment.

The most common control for bright light has been dim light. However, patients usually expect bright light to work better, especially in light-box studies with crossover designs in which patients see both the bright and dim intensities. If patients expect bright light to work better than dim, then there will be a larger placebo response to the bright light, and any difference in antidepressant response between bright and dim light could be entirely due to the disparate placebo effects. However, dim light has been a valid control in studies of head-mounted visors, because patients did not have higher expectations for the presumed active visor than for the placebo (Joffe *et al.* 1993; Rosenthal *et al.* 1993; Levitt *et al.* 1994; Teicher *et al.* 1995). Additionally, the visors place the light source so close to the eyes that it is difficult for patients to judge whether their visor is supposed to be bright or dim. In one study, patients were not even told that one of the visors was the placebo control (Rosenthal *et al.* 1993). Furthermore, all these visor studies employed parallel designs, in which patients only used one visor and could not compare it to one with another intensity.

If dim light controls are to be used in future studies, then patient expectations must be assessed to show that they do not have greater expectations for the brighter light. Expectation ratings should be made after the patient sees the equipment that she or he will use, and as close as possible in time to the start of treatment. Expectations can change as patients learn more about the design of their particular study and about light treatment in general.

An ingenious placebo control for bright light treatment was devised by Levitt *et al.* (1996). Patients were told that the purpose of the experiment was to study infrared light, which is not visible to the human eye. The placebo light-box actually emitted no light of any kind, but when it was 'on' it made a hum and a pilot LED light indicated that the unit was operating. Careful instructions read to patients were devised to make them believe that even if their light-box did emit visible light, that was not important. However, this was actually a test of bright visible light vs. no light. Expectation ratings were made after the patients sat in front of the light-box with the unit 'on'. There was no difference in expectation ratings between the light and placebo groups, showing that the deception was successful. This study also included two groups assigned to wear light visors which either emitted bright light or no light. The same 'infrared deception' was successfully employed.

We used sham negative ion generators in our two studies of bright-light treatment for SAD (Eastman *et al.* 1992, 1998). We gave our patients literature about the mood-enhancing effects of negative ions and of bright light. We explained that people are exposed to more of both of these environmental factors in the summer than in the winter. Although negative ion generators are clearly not light-boxes, they are another type of electrical device that delivers a natural environmental factor that travels through the air to impinge upon the patient. We designed our studies so that light-box treatment and generator treatment would both require the same time commitment and regular period of inactivity spent sitting by the equipment. Both treatments required the same change in sleep schedule, that is, a more regular schedule and an earlier morning wake-up time.

In both of our studies we measured expectations at the end of the baseline week. Patients were told which equipment they would receive (light-boxes or negative ion generators), and when they would use it, at the beginning of the baseline week. Thus, they had time to think about it and read the literature we provided. Unfortunately, in study 1 (Eastman *et al.* 1992), we did not achieve our goal of equal expectations. Patients expected to improve with both treatments, but they expected to feel slightly better after light treatment than after negative ion treatment.

For study 2 we needed to increase patient expectations for negative ion treatment. The ion generators from study 1, which could be bought in retail stores as air cleaners, were not as large and did not look as impressive as the light-boxes. Therefore, we had grander-looking ion generators built. Furthermore, each patient was given two units instead of one. The new generators were large (32-cm tall), shiny black cylinders with three tiny indicator lights that flashed red and green in random patterns. The real ion generators made a slight hissing noise, so we had white noise generators put inside all the units so no one could tell by listening which were real and which were shams. Several other features were built into the units, so that even the research assistants who dispensed the equipment could not tell which were shams. (The generators were labelled with code numbers.) We coached the patients to use the word 'equipment' rather than light-box or ion generator so that they wouldn't reveal their treatment condition to the staff who performed the depression ratings. The raters were in another building and did not see patients carrying equipment, which also helped to maintain the blind. We coached all staff to be equally enthusiastic about both light and ion treatment in general. The media helped by covering both treatments in news stories. This time we achieved our goals of high expectations and no difference in expectations for light-box vs. negative ion generator treatment (Eastman *et al.* 1998).

Sham negative ion generators could be used as placebo controls in future studies of bright-light treatment for SAD. However, all the details of interactions with patients and the public should be carefully planned and controlled in order to achieve equal patient expectations for light and negative ion treatment. This goal should be easier to achieve now that there is a study showing that high-density negative ions are an effective antidepressant for SAD (Terman and Terman 1995). Patients could be given a copy of this publication.

11.4 Is bright light better than a placebo for SAD?

There are very few studies that used an appropriate placebo control treatment for bright light *and* that presented data to show that patients did not have higher expectations for the light than placebo. I only know six studies that meet these criteria, and I will call them the 'good efficacy studies'. Four of these studies used head-mounted light visors and compared brighter to dimmer light (Joffe *et al.* 1993; Rosenthal *et al.* 1993; Levitt *et al.* 1994; Teicher *et al.* 1995); one employed light-boxes and visors and used the infrared deception described in this chapter (Levitt *et al.* 1996); and the sixth was one of ours, using sham negative ion generators as the placebo (Eastman *et al.* 1998). Only one of these six good efficacy studies (ours) was able to demonstrate a significantly greater antidepressant effect of light compared to placebo.

Other studies have been cited in support of the efficacy of bright-light treatment, but the patients had higher expectations for light than for placebo. For example, the first formal study of SAD patients (Rosenthal *et al.* 1984) found bright light more antidepressant than dim, but the majority of patients expected the bright white light to work better than the dim yellow light. A more recent study (Terman *et al.* 1998) found bright light more antidepressant than a low-density negative ion placebo. However, patient expectation ratings were higher for light than for ions. A pooled cross-centre analysis (Terman *et al.* 1989) and a Cochrane meta-analysis (Thompson *et al.* 1999) have also been cited as evidence for light-box efficacy. However, these analyses are also doomed by the problem of unequal patient expectations. The finding that bright light was more antidepressant than dim light is not good evidence for bright-light efficacy if patients expected the bright light to work better. Similarly, the finding that longer durations work better than shorter is meaningless if patients expect a larger 'dose' to work better than a smaller one.

Why was our study (Eastman *et al.* 1998) the only good efficacy study that was able to show light treatment superior to placebo? One possible reason stems from the fact that the difference between light and placebo did not reach statistical significance until the third week of treatment. A time lag of three or more weeks is common in antidepressant studies (for example, Janicak *et al.* 1997). In the other five good efficacy studies, treatment lasted only one to two weeks. Perhaps if treatment had been continued, significance would have emerged. These five studies included head- mounted visors, and the tendency in our field has been to accept the idea that light visors may be placebos, but to maintain the faith that light-boxes are more effective than placebos. However, I believe the evidence for the efficacy of light-boxes is also weak, since it is based on only one study — our study. One study, however carefully planned and executed, should never be enough to satisfy the scientific community that an antidepressant is more effective than a placebo.

Kirsch and Sapirstein (1998) performed a meta-analysis of antidepressant drug studies in non-seasonal depression. They made the distinction between placebo response and placebo effect:

> The placebo response is the change that occurs following administration of a placebo. However, change might also occur without administration of a placebo. It may be due to spontaneous remission, regression toward the mean, life changes, the passage of time, or other factors. The placebo effect is the difference between the placebo response and changes that occur without the administration of a placebo.

In other words, the placebo effect does not include improvement due to the natural course of the disorder. In order to quantify the improvement due to natural history (that is, the change that might occur without the administration of a placebo pill), they analysed data from 'no-treatment' or 'waiting-list' control groups. Their conclusion was that the response to antidepressant drugs was composed of three elements in the following proportions: 24 per cent to natural history (spontaneous remission and other changes that occur without administration of the placebo), 51 per cent to placebo effects (obtained only after the placebo pill is administered), and 25 per cent to the pharmacological properties of the drug. In other words, 75 per cent of the benefit from the antidepressant drug would have also been obtained after giving an inactive placebo.

Kirsch and Sapirstein suggest that the apparent antidepressant drug effect (25 per cent) may actually be due to an enhanced placebo effect produced by the side-effects of these drugs. For more detail, see the series of controversial papers (including the paper by Kirsch and Sapirstein) in the American Psychological Association on-line journal *Prevention and Treatment* (*www.journals.apa.org/prevention/volume 1*).

The meta-analysis of Kirsch and Sapirstein (1998) was done by calculating the pre- to post-effect sizes using mean depression scores. Effect sizes were 1.55 for drug, 1.16 for placebo pill, and 0.37 for no-treatment. Thus, for example, the proportion of the response due to the pharmacological properties of the drug was (1.55–1.16)/1.55 × 100, or 25 per cent. If we do the same calculations on our data (Eastman *et al.* 1998) using the mean 24-item SIGH-SAD depression scores at baseline and after 4 weeks of treatment, the effect size for morning bright light is 2.0 and compares favourably with drugs. However, the effect size for the morning placebo ion generator — 1.8 — is almost as large. Thus only 10 per cent of the antidepressant response to bright-light treatment can be attributed to the bright light, and 90 per cent would be attributed to the placebo response. (The placebo response is composed of placebo effects, plus non-specific effects including effects of sleep schedules and other protocol requirements, plus natural history.)

Thus, 90 per cent of the antidepressant effect of bright light can be duplicated by the placebo treatment, when mean scores are considered. Our previous analysis (Eastman *et al.* 1998) also showed little difference between light and placebo, when using averages. The mean SIGH-SAD scores for morning light and morning placebo at week 4 of treatment were similar (10.0 vs. 11.9), and there was no significant difference between light and placebo. However, the mean scores were not a good indication of the antidepressant response because the distribution was not normal for the light group, with a cluster of scores at the bottom of the scale — a floor effect (see Fig. 3D in Eastman *et al.* 1998). Therefore, we performed statistical analyses using the categories 'responders' vs. 'non-responders'. When we used the response criteria common in drug studies (a 50 per cent reduction in depression ratings), there was no statistically significant difference between light and placebo. However, when we used stricter remission criteria (that the SIGH-SAD score had to be reduced to at least 50 per cent of baseline *and* to less than or equal to 8 — that is, a complete or almost complete remission), then light was significantly better than placebo (Fig. 11.2). The benefit of light over placebo grew larger during the first 3 weeks of treatment, and reached significance in the third and fourth treatment weeks.

If we use these response rates to estimate the proportion of bright-light treatment that can be achieved by the placebo, then Fig. 11.2 shows that eventually about half of the response to bright light was due to the placebo response. In other words, if the patients who had complete, or almost complete remissions from the bright-light treatment had been given the placebo treatment instead, then about half of them would have achieved equivalent robust remissions.

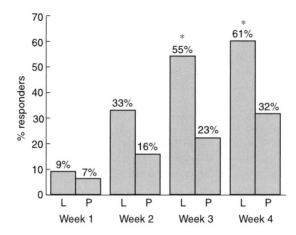

Fig. 11.2 Comparison of response rates to morning bright-light treatment (L) and morning sham negative ion generator placebo treatment (P) from study 2 (Eastman *et al.* 1998). Bars show the percentage of responders after each treatment week. Strict remission criteria were used. A responder was defined as a patient whose SIGH-SAD score was reduced to at least 50 per cent of the baseline score and to less than or equal to 8. Asterisks indicate a significant difference between light and placebo ($p < 0.05$) by chi-square tests. For light, $n = 33$; for placebo, $n = 31$.

These calculations may have led you to believe that the case for bright-light efficacy for SAD is weak or strong, depending on the amount of cognitive dissonance to which you have been subjected and whether you see the glass as half empty of half full. In any case, remember these facts about bright-light treatment of SAD:

1. Only one good efficacy study (that is, one with an appropriate placebo control treatment and no difference in patient expectations for bright light vs. placebo) showed a superior antidepressant response to bright light.

2. The superiority only emerged when considering the patients who achieved robust remissions.

3. Bright light was only significantly better than placebo after 3 weeks of treatment.

I, for one, think more good studies of bright-light treatment are necessary to more firmly establish efficacy for bright-light treatment of SAD.

Acknowledgements

Research supported by NIH grant MH42768. Thanks to Louis F. Fogg, Ph.D. for advice on statistics and human nature.

References

Eastman, C.I. (1990). What the placebo literature can tell us about light therapy for SAD. *Psychopharmacology Bulletin*, **26**:495–504.

Eastman, C.I., Lahmeyer, H.W., Watell, L.G., Good, G.D., and Young, M.A. (1992). A placebo-controlled trial of light treatment for winter depression. *Journal of Affective Disorders*, **26**:211–22.

Eastman, C.I., Young, M.A., and Fogg, L.F. (1993). A comparison of two different placebo-controlled SAD light treatment studies. In *Light and Biological Rhythms in Man* (ed. L. Wetterberg), pp. 371–83. Pergamon Press, Oxford/New York/Seoul/Tokyo.

Eastman, C.I., Young, M.A., Fogg, L.F., Liu, L., and Meaden, P.M. (1998). Bright light treatment of winter depression: a placebo-controlled trial. *Archives of General Psychiatry*, **55**:883–9.

Janicak, P.G., Davis, J.M., Preskorn, S.H., and Ayd Jr., F.J. (1997). *Principles and practice of psychopharmacotherapy*, Williams & Wilkins, Baltimore.

Joffe, R.T., Moul, D.E., Lam, R.W., Levitt, A.J., Teicher, M.H., Lebegue, B., *et al.* (1993). Light visor treatment for seasonal affective disorder: a multicenter study. *Psychiatry Research*, **46**:29–39.

Kirsch, I. and Sapirstein, G. (1998). Listening to Prozac but hearing placebo: a meta-analysis of antidepressant medication. *Prevention and Treatment* (*www.journals.apa.org/prevention*), **1**:0002a.

Lam, R.W. and Levitt, A.J. (1999). *Canadian consensus guidelines for the treatment of seasonal affective disorder*. Clinical & Academic Publishing, Canada.

Levitt, A.J., Joffe, R.T., and King, E. (1994). Dim versus bright red (light-emitting diode) light in the treatment of seasonal affective disorder. *Acta Psychiatrica Scandinavica*, **89**:341–5.

Levitt, A.J., Wesson, V.A., Joffe, R.T., Maunder, R.G., and King, E.F. (1996). A controlled comparison of light box and head-mounted units in the treatment of seasonal depression. *Journal of Clinical Psychiatry*, **57**:105–10.

Lewy, A.J., Sack, R.L., Miller, L.S., and Hoban, T.M. (1987). Antidepressant and circadian phase-shifting effects of light. *Science*, **235**:352–4.

Rosenthal, N.E., Sack, D.A., Gillin, J.C., Lewy, A.J., Goodwin, F.K., Davenport, Y., *et al.* (1984). Seasonal affective disorder: a description of the syndrome and preliminary findings with light therapy. *Archives of General Psychiatry*, **41**:72–80.

Rosenthal, N.E., Sack, D.A., Skwerer, R.G., Jacobsen, F.M., and Wehr, T.A. (1988). Phototherapy for seasonal affective disorder. *Journal of Biological Rhythms*, **3**:101–20.

Rosenthal, N.E., Moul, D.E., Hellekson, C.J., Oren, D.A., Frank, A., Brainard, G.C., *et al.* (1993). A multicenter study of the light visor for seasonal affective disorder: no difference in efficacy found between two different intensities. *Neuropsychopharmacology*, **8**:151–60.

Teicher, M.H., Glod, C.A., Oren, D.A., Schwartz, P.J., Luetke, C., Brown, C., *et al.* (1995). The phototherapy light visor: more to it than meets the eye. *American Journal of Psychiatry*, **152**:1197–202.

Terman, M. and Terman, J.S. (1995). Treatment of seasonal affective disorder with a high-output negative ionizer. *The Journal of Alternative and Complementary Medicine*, **1**:87–92.

Terman, M., Terman, J.S., Quitkin, F.M., McGrath, P.J., Stewart, J.W., and Rafferty, B. (1989). Light therapy for seasonal affective disorder: a review of efficacy. *Neuropsychopharmacology*, **2**:1–22.

Terman, M., Terman, J.S., and Ross, D.C. (1998). A controlled trial of timed bright light and negative air ionization for treatment of winter depression. *Archives of General Psychiatry*, **55**:875–82.

Thompson, C., Rodin, I., and Birtwhistle, J. (1999). Light therapy for seasonal and nonseasonal affective disorder: a Cochrane meta-analysis. *Society for Light Treatment and Biological Rhythms Abstracts*, **11**:11.

Further reading

Berg, A.O. (1977). Placebos: a brief review for family physicians. *Journal of Family Practice*, **5**:97–100.

Brown, W.A. (1998). The placebo effect. *Scientific American*, January:90–5.

Gallimore, R.G. and Turner, J.L. (1977). Contemporary studies of placebo phenomena. In *Psychopharmacology in the practice of medicine* (ed. M.E. Jarik), pp. 47–57. Appleton–Century–Crofts, New York.

Greenberg, R.P. and Fisher, S. (1989). Examining antidepressant effectiveness: findings, ambiguities, and some vexing puzzles. In *The limits of biological treatments for psychological distress* (ed. S. Fisher and R.P. Greenberg), pp. 1–37. Lawrence Erlbaum Associates, Hillsdale, NJ.

Lundh, L.G. (1987). Placebo, belief, and health. A cognitive–emotional model. *Scandinavian Journal of Psychology*, **28**:128–43.

Rawlinson, M.C. (1985). Truth-telling and paternalism in the clinic: philosophical reflections on the use of placebos in medical practice. In *Placebo: theory, research and mechanisms* (ed. L. White, B. Tursky, and G.E. Schwartz), pp. 403–18. Guilford Press, New York.

Shapiro, A.K. and Shapiro, E. (1984). Patientprovider relationships and the placebo effect. In *Behavioral health: a handbook of health enhancement and disease prevention* (ed. J.D. Matarazzo, S.M. Weiss, J.A. Herd, N.E. Miller, and S.M. Weiss), pp. 371–83. John Wiley & Son, New York.

Talbot, M. (2000). The placebo prescription. *New York Times Magazine*, January 9.

Wall, P.D. (1992). The placebo effect: an unpopular topic. *Pain*, **51**:1–3.

Chapter 12

Guidelines for management

Timo Partonen and Andres Magnusson

12.1 Introduction

This chapter is meant to give a short and practically orientated guide on how to treat patients with winter SAD. The evidence for various modes of treatment for winter SAD is reviewed elsewhere in this book (see the chapters by Partonen, Kasper *et al.*, Meesters, and Thompson). In addition, there are two relatively recent overviews on the treatment issues of SAD (ed. Lam 1998; ed. Lam and Levitt 1999).

12.2 Bright-light therapy

Bright-light therapy is the treatment of choice for the management of patients with winter SAD (see Table 12.1). The response to bright-light therapy is often good or excellent, and no additional treatment is usually required. However, it is essential to monitor the initial effects of bright-light therapy, for example by administering it at a well-equipped out-patient facility. Rating scales measuring the severity of depression are encouraged to be used before

Table 12.1 Guidelines for bright-light therapy and beyond

- **Dose**: start the administration with the usual dose of 2500 lx for 2 hours daily. Depending on the initial response, this dose may need to be changed in order to increase or decrease the effect by increasing the intensity of light (up to 10 000 lx) or decreasing the time for exposure (down to ½ hour) respectively. Alternatively, the light-box emitting fluorescent light of 10 000 lx, that has become the clinical standard in the United States and Canada, may be used in the first place to improve compliance.
- **Repetition**: keep giving daily exposures. Daily continuation treatment after the initiation period of 1 to 2 weeks may not be essential; exposures given 5 times a week can be adequate. Alternatively, curative measures of bright-light exposure for 1 to 2 weeks may be repeated, when needed, during the winter.
- **Timing**: start the administration with exposure to light in the morning. Treatment sessions are best scheduled between 6.00 a.m. and 10.00 a.m., if feasible. Alternatively, some patients may benefit from the exposure at other times of the day. However, exposure after 8.00 p.m. should be avoided because of a risk of insomnia.
- **Wavelength**: give white fluorescent light. The sources emitting white fluorescent light that is free of ultraviolet radiation are effective and may have greater efficacy than those producing light of one colour or a limited range of wavelengths.
- **Monitoring**: monitor the initial effects of bright-light therapy. The administration may need to be started at a well-equipped out-patient facility.
- **Assessment**: if this regimen fails to produce any response within a week, new strategies employing other modes of treatment need to be considered in order to guarantee a good outcome.

and after the treatment and periodically thereafter. It is better for the clinician to assess the benefits before the patient is advised to purchase a device for personal use. Best would be if the response to light exposure can be assessed before the patient starts the self-administration at home.

Bright-light therapy may induce adverse effects, but they are usually mild and few (see the chapter by Partonen). Although rare, manic behaviour and suicidal tendencies have been reported during the initiation of light therapy. It is therefore preferable to contact a psychiatrist or a physician before light treatment is started. This is especially important for those who have a history of severe mental illness such as mania or severe depression or suicidal thoughts. It is also important to consult a doctor before starting the bright-light therapy if the individual is taking any medication.

Patients who are using a light-therapy device at home without close supervision must be informed about health hazards and encouraged to keep in contact with their clinician. A potential problem might exist now that individuals can buy these devices through the internet or from local stores and carry out the treatment with no prior consultation or supervision, and without having adequate instructions for use.

Some experts advise that an ophthalmologic check-up should be routinely performed on all individuals taking light treatment (see the chapter by Remé et al.), whereas others do not. Ophthalmologic consultation is recommended for patients with the following known risk factors for retinal toxicity to light exposure: a pre-existing retinal or eye disease (for example, retinal detachments, retinitis pigmentosa, and glaucoma), a systemic illness that affects the retina (for example, diabetes mellitus), previous cataract surgery and lens removal, and older age (with its inherent greater risk of age-related degeneration). It is advisable to consult a doctor before starting the bright-light therapy if the individual has any eye-related problems.

Patients taking medications that have photosensitizing effects also need ophthalmologic examination. The following medications are examples of drugs that may have these effects: chloroquine (antimalarial), hematoporphyrins (used in the photodynamic therapy for cancer), hypericum (St John's wort), lithium (mood stabilizer), melatonin (pineal hormone), methoxypsoralens (used in the ultraviolet phototherapy for psoriasis), and phenothiazines (antiemetics and antipsychotics). Animal studies show retinal changes with drugs such as beta blockers, tricyclic antidepressants, and L-tryptophan, but ophthalmologic monitoring for patients on these drugs is not required, according to current consensus, unless they have other ocular risk factors.

The best-documented and most common way of giving the bright-light therapy is a so-called light-box device. The device is usually placed on a table, or alternatively attached to a wall, and the patient sits in front of it, usually at a distance of 30 to 90 cm, depending on the intensity of light needed for treatment and the quality of the fixture. Intensities of 2500 to 10 000 lx are generally recommended. The light device should have a high output of visible light at eye level, a low output of ultraviolet and blue light irradiation (see the chapter by Remé et al.), be reasonably priced, and produce illuminance which is not very sensitive to changes in the position or angle of the patient relative to the light. The patient does not have to stare directly into the lights but can either relax in front of them (for instance, while having breakfast or reading a newspaper) or can get on with some work (perhaps using a personal computer).

Bright-light therapy can be administered either at home or at the workplace. It is best to have the treatment in the morning hours, but if this is not feasible, it can be taken at other times of the day, except for late in the evening. The patient usually needs to spend ½ to 2 hours a day in front of the lights, and to use the lights for 5 to 7 days a week. Treatment should continue for most of the winter. The higher the intensity, the shorter time is needed for the daily usage. Some clinicians feel that the dose can be reduced during the maintenance phase of the treatment after a good response has been achieved. However, the dosing has to be individually tailored. The patient may well himself or herself sense how much light is needed to remain in remission. A response to bright-light therapy will usually take only 2 to 4 days, but a full effect may be achieved only after 2 to 4 weeks.

12.3 **Medication**

When there appears to be no response to bright-light therapy, or the patient prefers another mode of treatment, prescription of an antidepressant drug needs to be considered. Based on current evidence, the best choice would then be one of the selective serotonin reuptake inhibitors (SSRIs) or reversible inhibitors of monoamine oxidase A (RIMAs). Most of the drug trials have included relatively few individuals, and only one trial with sertraline has included a fairly large number of subjects (see the chapter by Kasper *et al.*). If the patient suffers from insomnia, an antidepressant that improves sleep may be prescribed (see the chapter by Thompson). No harmful drug–light interactions have been reported in the context of bright-light therapy (for more information, see the chapter by Remé *et al.*). The dosages of antidepressants should be similar to those used in the treatment of major depressive disorder, but the duration of treatment in patients with winter SAD can often be shorter than that required for other conditions.

Other options for improving responses to medications include switching to another antidepressant, combining with psychological therapy, augmenting with another psychotropic drug (for example, with L-tryptophan), combining with other antidepressants, and, as with any life-threatening depressive episode, electroconvulsive therapy (ECT) should be considered for those SAD patients with psychotic symptoms. However, in these rare cases, SAD is likely to be a comorbid disorder of another condition. There are no specific data available on the efficacy of ECT in winter SAD.

12.4 **Psychotherapy**

The most effective psychological treatments are likely to include behavioural, cognitive, interpersonal, and problem-solving therapies — that is, treatments that have been used in the management of non-seasonally depressed patients. In particular, problem-solving therapy, with a short duration on average, could be useful for the clinician working in primary care. However, there are no studies on the efficacy of psychotherapies in patients with winter SAD.

12.5 **Poor response**

Patients showing a limited response to the treatment should be evaluated to guarantee that they have an adequate dosing of treatment, they are compliant with the treatment, and they do not have unrecognized comorbid conditions. The clinician may increase the daily duration of bright-light therapy, or increase the intensity by advising the patient to sit closer to the light source. Comorbid disorders influence the clinical picture of winter SAD by modulating the course of illness, and each may require specific intervention (see the chapter by Reichborn–Kjennerud). For patients with refractory illness, it is important to take a detailed medical history and to examine previous treatment responses.

Factors to consider when deciding on a first-line treatment for patients with winter SAD include the severity of depressive symptoms, patient preference, safety, patient compliance, adverse effects, and costs. As a rule of thumb, the patient needs to start with a single treatment only, and this would help with the evaluation of treatment response and eventual adverse effects. If needed, however, combinations of versatile strategies for treatment may need to be applied.

12.6 Consensus guidelines

The Society for Light Treatment and Biological Rhythms (see the website at *http://www.sltbr.org/*) was founded in 1988 to stimulate research and clinical applications of light therapy. The annual meeting of the Society in 1990 included work groups that evaluated the safety factors related to light therapy and the efficacy of light therapy for SAD, subsyndromal SAD, and non-seasonal depressive disorders. They concluded that light therapy had been demonstrated as clinically effective for SAD and that further research was required before a claim can be made for other indications. Their reports were formalized as the Society's recommendations to the Food and Drug Administration in the United States.

Recently, the Canadian Consensus Guidelines for the Treatment of Seasonal Affective Disorder (see the website at *http://www.fhs.mcmaster.ca/direct/depress/sad2.html*) were developed by a group of Canadian researchers and clinicians in 1998. The purpose of these consensus guidelines was to systematically review all available evidence regarding the diagnosis, clinical picture, epidemiology, pathophysiology, and treatment of SAD, and to produce a series of recommendations that were clinically practical and scientifically meaningful. As an example, Table 12.2 shows the recommendations for the length of treatment. Level 1 describes the highest level of evidence, and level 5 describes the lowest level.

12.7 Tips

A natural mode of treatment is to take as much outdoor light as possible during the winter. Regular walks or outdoor exercise, such as skiing and skating, can be of great benefit for patients with winter SAD. It is also important to try to receive sunlight while spending time indoors. One could examine the possibility of working in brightly lit surroundings and, for instance, move one's desk close to a window. At home, those suffering from winter SAD should also try to spend as much time as possible in the brightest areas, for instance by a window facing the sun. It is often a relief for many to travel to very sunny locations during the dark period of the year, and some individuals may be able to negotiate with their employer to take prolonged holidays during the winter rather than the summer.

However, these adjustments may be difficult to achieve. Furthermore, in regions at high northern latitudes and those with heavy overcast weather, the habitat may not provide enough light to relieve winter SAD. In this case, the administration of bright-light therapy or other options for treatment need to be considered.

12.7 Conclusion

The first-line option for the treatment of patients with winter SAD is bright-light therapy. This treatment is usually administered using a light-box. New innovative light devices have

Table 12.2 Recommendations for the length of treatment by the level of evidence for data*

Level 1
- None.

Level 2
- A therapeutic trial of light therapy should be at least 2 weeks in length.
- A therapeutic trial of antidepressants should be at least 6 weeks in length.
- Because of risk of relapse, patients should continue with treatment for the entire winter season, until the time of their natural spring or summer remission. Treatment is not generally recommended during the summer.

Level 3
- None.

Level 4
- None.

Level 5
- When possible, antidepressants should be tapered off instead of abruptly discontinued.
- Treatment should be restarted in the autumn, either with onset of mild symptoms or in advance of the usual onset of symptoms.
- Light therapy may be helpful during the summer for occasional transient symptoms.
- Preventative year-round antidepressant treatment including the summer should be considered in situations where patients:
  a) are poorly compliant or motivated
  b) take a long time to taper off and are on medications
  c) are unable to recognize early signs and symptoms of depression
  d) have very early onset or very late offset of symptoms
  e) experience symptoms during the summer

* Levels of evidence for data are as follows:

Level 1 Randomized, controlled trials with sufficient numbers or good-quality meta-analyses based on randomized, controlled trials.
Level 2 Randomized, controlled trials with smaller numbers and with insufficient power.
Level 3 Non-randomized, controlled or cohort studies; case series; case-controlled or cohort studies; cross-sectional or high-quality retrospective studies.
Level 4 Evidence based on the published opinion of expert committees, for example, consensus or guidelines committees.
Level 5 Evidence which expresses the opinion of the committee members who have reviewed the literature and guidelines, following discussion with peers.

been developed, but their efficacy and clinical advantages have not yet been established. Continuing treatment throughout the winter season is advisable to prevent relapses. Those patients at risk of light-induced eye damage should consult an ophthalmologist before the bright-light therapy is started and at regular intervals thereafter. Antidepressant drugs are a relatively unexplored treatment for winter SAD, but preliminary data from randomized, controlled trials suggest that several antidepressants may be effective. While the treatment of choice for winter SAD is bright-light therapy, all methods of treatment need to be considered when the treatment response is not optimal. In addition, patients should be encouraged to examine if they can change their present situation, both at home and at work, in a way that would enable them to receive more light from the environment.

References

Lam, R.W. (ed.) (1998) Seasonal affective disorder and beyond: light treatment for SAD and non-SAD conditions. American Psychiatric Press, Washington DC.

Lam, R.W. and Levitt, A.J. (ed.) (1999) *Canadian consensus guidelines for the treatment of seasonal affective disorder*. Clinical & Academic Publishing, Vancouver.

Further reading

Lam, R.W. (1998) Seasonal affective disorder: diagnosis and management. *Primary Care Psychiatry* **4**:63–74.

Lam, R.W. and Levitt, A.J. (ed.) (1998) Canadian Consensus Guidelines for the Treatment of Seasonal Affective Disorder: a summary of the report of the Canadian Consensus Group on SAD. *Canadian Journal of Diagnosis* **October (Suppl.)**:1–16.

Partonen, T. and Lönnqvist, J. (1998) Seasonal affective disorder: a guide to diagnosis and management. *CNS Drugs* **9**:203–12.

Partonen, T. and Lönnqvist, J. (1998) Seasonal affective disorder. *The Lancet* **352**:1369–74.

Key Notes

Chapter 13

Prevalence from population surveys

Peter Paul A. Mersch

13.1 Introduction

The prevalence of SAD has received considerable interest since the initial description of the syndrome. In the first place, the magnitude of the disorder in the population had to be established and the characteristics of the subjects suffering from SAD had to be verified. In the second place, the formulation of the photoperiod hypothesis of SAD has stimulated research on the prevalence of SAD in the population. In this chapter the results of prevalence studies in the general population will be discussed. Since the results of these studies rely on the applied methodology, some relevant issues on this subject will be discussed first.

13.2 Methodological issues

13.2.1 Selection bias

Population surveys can be divided roughly into two groups: surveys in a random sample of the general population and surveys performed on a selection of the population (a cluster). Unless stratified random sampling is employed, the latter method is a threat to the attempts to generalize these results. Estimates of the prevalence of SAD in the general population from one town or county cannot automatically be generalized to the general population of a country, as the latitude hypothesis (discussed later) shows.

In general, the more extreme the selected group, the less the results can be generalized to the general population. Especially studies performed in companies or organizations (Eagles *et al.* 1996; Hedge and Woodson 1996; Ito *et al.* 1992; Ozaki *et al.* 1995; Partonen *et al.* 1993) are prone to selection bias. First, it is not likely that the employees of a company are a random selection of the population. Secondly, uncertainty with the respondents about the confidentiality of the results may bias the results. In the Ozaki *et al.* (1995) study, for instance, the questionnaire was handed out at a work-related physical examination. The highest response of all prevalence studies (96 per cent) could be a sign of the pressure subjects felt to participate. Thirdly, absenteeism due to the illness itself may bias the results. In a prevalence study in the Netherlands (Mersch *et al.* 1999*a*), respondents who met the criteria of SAD were significantly more often unemployed or absent for long periods of time on sick leave than respondents who did not meet the SAD criteria.

Different sampling methods are employed. The most reliable method is the drawing of a random sample of the general population from community registers (Magnusson and Stefansson 1993; Mersch *et al.* 1999*a*). In this case, systematic sampling error is avoided. A second method is the random selection of subjects from the telephone directory (Muscettola *et al.* 1995; Rosen *et al.* 1990; Terman 1988). In this case, there is a risk of systematic error, because people without a telephone are excluded from the sample. Moreover, some people with a telephone are not listed in the directory. Kasper *et al.* (1989*a*) employed an elegant method to reduce the latter chance of error by random number dialling, a method also used by Levitt and Boyle (1997).

13.2.2 Survey method

Two ways of data gathering are used in prevalence studies on SAD: interview or questionnaire. Most often a questionnaire was mailed to the research population (for example, Broman and Hetta 1998; Hagfors *et al.* 1995; Magnusson and Stefansson 1993; Mersch *et al.* 1999*a*; Muscettola *et al.* 1995; Rosen *et al.* 1990; Terman 1988), while in some cases subjects were interviewed by telephone (for example, Hagfors *et al.* 1992; Kasper *et al.* 1989*a*; Levitt and Boyle 1997; Wirz–Justice *et al.* 1992). In one study (Booker and Hellekson 1992) it is unclear whether subjects were interviewed at home or by telephone.

Kasper and colleagues (1989*a*) preferred telephone interviews to mail-out procedures because of the higher response rate. According to these authors the literature on survey methodology provides evidence that both methods are equally valid. However, the results of some studies indicate that the mail-out procedure may result in higher prevalence figures. At two locations two studies were performed at each (Finland: Hagfors *et al.* 1992 and Hagfors *et al.* 1995; Montgomery County: Kasper *et al.* 1989*a* and Rosen *et al.* 1990) — one using telephone interviews; the other, a questionnaire. Both used the same instrument — the Seasonal Pattern Assessment Questionnaire (SPAQ) (Rosenthal *et al.* 1987). In both Finland and Montgomery County the prevalence figures for SAD (winter + summer) were higher for the mail-out procedure than for the telephone interview (Finland: 7.1 per cent versus 3.4 per cent; Montgomery County: 7.3 per cent versus 5.0 per cent). As expected, the studies using the interview method reported higher response rates than the mail-out procedure (Finland: 88 per cent versus 55 per cent; Montgomery County: 92 per cent versus 60.5 per cent, respectively). So, it is possible that response rates also influence prevalence figures. For instance, the probability of responding to the questionnaire may partly be a function of the presence of SAD symptoms. This was tested on a selection of prevalence studies in the Mersch *et al.* (1999*b*) study. An analysis of variance showed no significant interaction between response rate and SAD symptoms.

In all studies designed to estimate the prevalence of SAD, the same assessment instrument was used — the SPAQ (Rosenthal *et al.* 1987). On the one hand this is an advantage since it facilitates comparison of the results of the different studies. On the other hand, if all prevalence figures are based on one instrument it has to be ascertained that this instrument indeed measures SAD. Therefore, the available literature on the reliability and validity of the SPAQ criteria for SAD will be discussed.

13.3 The Seasonal Pattern Assessment Questionnaire (SPAQ)

It is remarkable that one instrument has such a prominent place in the study of SAD, while research in the psychometric qualities of the SPAQ is relatively scarce. Studies that have been performed show mixed results and do not unequivocally support the confidence in its reliability suggested by its widespread use. The SPAQ has two objectives. The original purpose of the SPAQ was to study a number of characteristics of SAD like seasonal variation in mood, food intake, and weight gain, seasonal sleep duration, and sensitivity to weather conditions. Although not developed as such, the SPAQ was also introduced as a diagnostic or screening instrument for SAD by Kasper *et al.* (1989*a*), who were the first to formulate the criteria for SAD on the SPAQ.

13.3.1 Criteria for SAD

The criteria for SAD on the SPAQ are based on data from 168 SAD patients (Kasper *et al.* 1989*a*; Hardin *et al.* 1991). It is not clear, however, how the cut-off scores for SAD on these criteria have been chosen. The SPAQ applies three criteria for SAD. The first is based on the Global Seasonality (GS) scale, providing a composite measure for change of mood, social activities, appetite, sleep, weight, and energy across the seasons. The scale for each item ranges from 0 ('no change') to 4 ('extremely marked change'); the total scale ranges from 0 to 24. The suggested cut-off score for SAD on this criterion is 10 for (telephone) interviews and 11 for the paper and pencil method.

A second criterion for SAD is based on one question — whether seasonal changes are considered a problem. The response possibilities are 0 = no problem, 1 = a mild problem, 2 = a moderate problem, 3 = a marked problem, 4 = a severe problem, and 5 = a disabling problem. A score of at least 2 is necessary to reach the SAD threshold.

The final criterion is the 'window', that is, the time interval within which the problems should recur. The timing of the problems is determined by asking in what months the subjects feel worst. The width of the window varies across studies and may thus be a confounding factor.

Subsyndromal-SAD (sub-SAD) (Kasper *et al.* 1989*b*) is defined as a cluster of seasonal complaints which are not severe enough for a diagnosis of SAD. The prevalence of sub-SAD, however, will be influenced by some confusion over the criteria — a GS score of 8 or 9 (9 or 10 for the self-report method) and 'seasonal changes are either a **problem or not**' (Kasper *et al.* 1989*a*, p. 829). In some studies (Booker and Hellekson 1992; Hagfors *et al.* 1992; Muscettola *et al.* 1995; Rosen *et al.* 1990; Terman 1988) this criterion was altered to become '**at least mild problems**' with the changes of season. In view of the way the criteria are formulated, this latter definition would indeed make more sense. It is clear that prevalence rates for sub-SAD are influenced by the use of different criteria.

13.3.2 Reliability of the criteria of the SPAQ

Global Seasonality score. In several studies, the test–retest reliability of the GS score was studied. It varied considerably across studies and samples, from 0.44 in subsyndromal winter SAD (interval 3.2 ± 0.8 months) and 0.61 in non-seasonal healthy subjects (interval 3.1 ± 0.6 months) (Kasper *et al.* 1989*b*) to 0.80 in winter SAD (interval 8.2 ± 7.1 months) (Hardin *et al.* 1991). Reliability appears to be better in the extreme samples (non-seasonal healthy subjects and winter SAD) than in the sub-SAD sample which can be expected to be more diffuse. In the latter group less than 20 per cent of the variance is explained.

In a study in Australia (Murray *et al.* 1993*a*), 297 subjects with either extremely high or extremely low seasonality scores were tested again after 17 months. The test–retest reliability on the GS score was 0.58. In a study by Wirz–Justice and colleagues (1993), 55 healthy women were tested in winter and in summer. The test–retest correlation was 0.65. Raheja *et al.* (1996) found a test–retest correlation of the GS score over a period of 5–8 years of 0.62.

Further analysis showed that there was better agreement between the first and second measurement for the higher GS scores than for the lower ones.

Thus far only one study has been published on the internal consistency and factor structure of the GS score (Magnusson et al. 1997). The alpha for the total scale was acceptable ($\alpha = 0.82$). Factor analysis showed a two-factor structure with the items sleep, social activity, mood, and energy loading on factor 1 (eigenvalue 3.14; explained variance $= 52.4$ per cent), while weight and appetite loaded on factor 2 (eigenvalue 1.06; explained variance $= 17.7$ per cent). The authors concluded that the GS scale 'is well co nstructed and that the 6 different items are coherent and act synergistically to measure the underlying concept' (p. 115). A two-factor structure was considered doubtful since the eigenvalue was relatively low; the GS items were coherent and deletion of weight and appetite did not improve the internal consistency.

Replication of the study of Magnusson and colleagues (1997) on the Mersch et al. (1999a) data showed virtually identical results (unpublished data). The preliminary results of a third study on this subject, examining contrast validity on four groups (discussed later), showed a higher alpha (0.85) and the same two-factor structure. The psychological factor explained 58.3 per cent of the variance and had a reliability coefficient of $\alpha = 0.87$. The vegetative factor explained 18.5 per cent of the variance, while Cronbach's $\alpha = 0.82$. So, in this case deleting the weight and appetite items increased the internal consistency. A two-factor structure should therefore not yet be ruled out (Mersch et al. 2000).

In the Mersch et al. (1999a) study the SPAQ was administered each month to approximately 200 different respondents from the general population, for 13 consecutive months, together with a depression scale (the CES-D). The GS score appeared to be sensitive to seasonal variation: there was a significant difference over the months of the year. The mean scores were significantly higher when the SPAQ was completed between December and May compared with completion between June and November. Also, the GS score was somewhat sensitive to mood at the moment of completion (see Fig. 13.1). There was a significant correlation between the GS score and a depression scale (CES-D) that measures depression at the moment of completion and the week before. But although the GS score was sensitive to month of completion, the estimation of SAD was not influenced due to the stability of the other two criteria.

An identical (preliminary) result was reported by Broman and Hetta (1998) who mailed sections of the SPAQ to 601 subjects in February and to 594 subjects in August, in Sweden. The GS score was significantly higher in the February sample than in the August sample, but there was no difference in the prevalence figure of winter SAD.

Degree of seasonal problems. The fact that an important part of the SAD criteria comprises only one question and the difference between the response categories is very subtle (mild severity = no SAD; moderate severity = SAD), endangers the reliability of the diagnosis. The diagnosis could be vulnerable to cultural differences in acceptance of admitting psychological problems and to mood at the moment of answering the SPAQ. The results of the Mersch et al. (1999a) study, however, show that the latter is not the case. Month of completion did not affect whether or not seasonal changes were experienced as a problem. Also, data on the test–retest reliability shows that this item appears to be stable over time. Correlations on the different studies are 0.79 (Thompson et al. 1988), interval = 50.5 ± 2 weeks; 0.80 (Rosenthal et al. 1987) for winter SAD; and 0.74 and 1.00 for sub-SAD and non-seasonal healthy subjects respectively (Hardin et al. 1991).

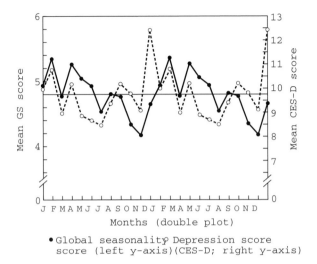

Fig. 13.1 Global seasonality score and CES-D score, measuring mood at the moment of completion, in the general population.

In a test–retest study by Murray *et al.* (1993*a*) the authors concluded that there was a clear relationship between responses in 1990 and 1992. Nevertheless, the finding that 44.9 per cent of the subjects who reported to have problems in the first assessment had no problems at the second, endangers the validity of the SPAQ diagnosis of SAD considerably. Of the 29 subjects diagnosed as having SAD in 1990, 12 subjects (41.4 per cent) were not diagnosed as such in 1992. WirzJustice *et al.* (1993) found that of the 6 subjects meeting winter-SAD criteria in the winter, only 3 received the same diagnosis in summer.

Months when subjects feel worst. In the Kasper *et al.* study (1989*a*), subjects who did not fall in the winter-SAD range (defined as 'feeling worst in December and/or January and/or February') or in the summer-SAD range (defined as 'feeling worst in June and/or July and/or August') were rejected for a diagnosis of SAD. In the same study however, it was advised to limit the threshold to the months of December and/or January (winter pattern) and June and/or July (summer pattern). This may have caused some confusion.

Although most of the prevalence studies followed one of these two versions, some however decided to skip this criterion altogether (Hagfors *et al.* 1992; Wirz–Justice *et al.* 1992), while one study stretched both the summer and winter period so that each encompassed six months (Mersch *et al.* 1999*a*). The problem with the criterion suggested by Kasper and colleagues (1989*a*) is that winter-SAD patients do not always have their depressive episode in December and/or January, but somewhere in a period that covers September through to March. Therefore, a two-month period may underestimate the SAD prevalence rate.

Only one study reported test–retest figures on this item (Murray *et al.* 1993*a*). In this version of the SPAQ, subjects answered in terms of seasons rather than months. Of the 143 responders who stated that winter was their worst time of year, 40 (28 per cent) did not do so 17 months later. Of the 18 subjects who met the criteria of winter SAD, 5 (27.8 per cent) no longer nominated winter as the most difficult season.

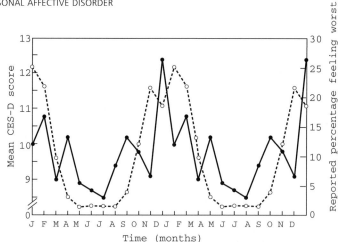

Fig. 13.2 Actual mood at the moment of completion measured by the CES-D and the percentage of subjects that reported in what months they felt worst.

In the Mersch *et al.* (1999*a*) study, the percentage of subjects that mentioned the months in which they felt worse corresponded fairly well with the mean depression score over the months (see Fig. 13.2).

13.3.3 **External validity**

Only a few prevalence studies have investigated the external validity of the SPAQ by interviewing a selection of the research population. Kasper and co-workers (1989*a*) interviewed 40 of the 416 respondents (9.6 per cent) with a structured psychiatric interview for the DSM-III-R and concluded that the SPAQ underestimated the number of subjects that met the SAD criteria with 100 per cent accordance (50 per cent false negatives, 0 per cent false positives). Magnusson (1996) interviewed 81 of the 587 respondents (13.8 per cent) of the Magnusson and Stefansson (1993) study. Of the 19 subjects who met the SPAQ criteria for winter depression, only 5 (26.3 per cent) were diagnosed as such by a clinical interview. Eleven were diagnosed as suffering sub-SAD, while 3 subjects received neither a SAD nor a sub-SAD diagnosis. On the other hand, the clinical interview identified 6 SAD cases in the 20 sub-SAD cases identified by the SPAQ. Extrapolation of the results led the author to conclude that the clinical interview and the SPAQ reached approximately the same number of SAD subjects (16 versus 19, respectively). In this case the SPAQ overestimated the SAD prevalence with approximately 0.5%. A methodologically weak point in both the Kasper *et al.* (1989*a*) and the Magnusson (1996) study is that the interviewers were not blind to the SPAQ diagnosis.

Preliminary results of the Levitt and Boyle (1997) study in Canada showed that the SPAQ detected four times as many SAD subjects (7.4 per cent versus 1.7 per cent) as a clinical interview based on the DSM-IV. Preliminary results of the Michalak (1998) study among 2000 residents of the United Kingdom showed comparable results. The prevalence of SAD estimated by the SPAQ was approximately 8 per cent while a DSM-IV interview with the subjects who met the SAD criteria on the SPAQ estimated the prevalence at approximately 1 per cent. This means that of the 109 subjects, no less than 95 (87 per cent) were false positives. Regretfully, only SPAQ-SAD cases (to detect false positives) were interviewed; no 'non-cases' (to detect false negatives) were interviewed. Preliminary results of a validity study on a selection of the respondents of the Mersch *et al.* (1999*a*) study showed that of the 38 respondents meeting the SPAQ criteria for winter SAD who were interviewed, 55.3 per cent appeared to be correctly classified by the SPAQ. This means that there were 44.7 per cent false positives.

The test–retest study by Raheja *et al.* (1996) showed that the ability of the SPAQ to identify SAD cases at the follow-up assessment after 5–8 years was low. It had a predictive value of 48 per cent and an efficiency of 57 per cent. There was a false positive rate of 51.7 per cent and a false negative rate of 27.8 per cent. The authors concluded that the SPAQ is unable to predict the seasonality of the future course of illness.

13.3.4 **Contrast validity**

A screening instrument like the SPAQ should be able to distinguish between different groups (for example, SAD and sub-SAD subjects and different patient groups and normal control groups), composed in a way other than by means of SPAQ criteria. In one study, the ratings of SAD patients were compared with those of sub-SAD subjects and normal controls (Kasper *et al.* 1989*b*). The mean seasonality score of SAD patients was significantly higher than that of sub-SAD and control subjects, while the rating of sub-SAD subjects was significantly higher than that of control subjects. None of the controls reported to have problems with the seasons (which is not surprising since this is one of the exclusion criteria), as opposed to 100 per cent of the SAD patients. Eighty per cent of the sub-SAD subjects reported experiencing seasonal problems, 55 per cent at least of moderate severity. Regretfully, no data are presented on how many subjects of the sub-SAD group met the SAD criteria on the SPAQ.

A study comparing SAD patients with bipolar patients treated with lithium and normal controls (Thompson *et al.* 1988) showed significant differences between the groups on GS score and severity of problems. The bipolar patients held an intermediate position, but differences between bipolar patients and healthy subjects were not significant on most variables.

Hardin and colleagues (1991) studied the SPAQ in six clinical populations and two normal populations (including the groups of the Kasper *et al.* 1989*b* study). The conclusion was that both the GS score and the severity of problem score of winter-SAD subjects were significantly higher than the other groups, with the exception of summer-SAD subjects. No figures are given on the ability of the SAD criteria to discriminate between groups.

In the Mersch *et al.* (2000) study, winter-SAD patients (n = 45) were compared with non-seasonal depressive out-patients (n = 48), non-depressive out-patients (n = 46) with other pathology, and normal controls (n = 37). Preliminary results show that of the SAD patients, most of whom had received treatment for their SAD, 20 were identified by the SPAQ criteria for SAD (44.4 per cent), while 5 subjects (11.1 per cent) met the 'Kasper criteria' for sub-SAD. None of the normal controls met the criteria of either SAD or sub-SAD. Of the non-seasonal depressives, who were measured at the moment they were depressed, 7 (14.6 per cent) met the criteria for SAD, while 7 others met the sub-SAD criteria. Of the non-depressive pathology group, one subject met the SAD criteria and two the sub-SAD criteria.

To study further the ability of the SPAQ criteria to discriminate between SAD patients and non-SAD subjects, discriminant analysis was performed on the SAD group and the other

3 groups of non-SAD subjects combined. When the GS score and the score on the question 'whether problems with the seasons are experienced' were entered in the analysis, 80.84 per cent of the subjects were correctly classified. If both seasonality factors (see p. 124) are entered in the analysis alone, the psychological factor (mood, sleep, social activity, and energy) is a better predictor than the vegetative factor (weight and appetite) — 77.27 per cent versus 67.05 per cent correctly classified, respectively. Combined with the variable 'problems with the seasons', the psychological factor predicted less well than the vegetative factor (77.84 per cent versus 80.24 per cent correctly classified, respectively). This means that the variables appetite and weight, combined with the 'problems' question, predicted almost as well as the total GS scale.

13.3.5 Conclusions

Evaluating the psychometric data on the SPAQ, it can be concluded that the test–retest reliability is reasonable. However, high test–retest correlations are of limited value in the conclusion of whether the criteria of the SPAQ are stable. If, for instance, in a winter-SAD group, every subject's rating is 3 points lower on the second assessment, the correlation is perfect, but it is likely that there are few winter depressives left. This may be the case in the studies of Murray *et al.* (1993*a*) and Wirz–Justice *et al.* (1993). In both studies, the seasons in which subjects were assessed were different: September and February (Murray *et al.* 1993*a*) and winter and summer (Wirz–Justice *et al.* 1993). That month of completion may influence results is shown in the Dutch prevalence study (Mersch *et al.* 1999*a*). It is interesting, however, that in both the Murray *et al.* (1993*a*) and the Wirz–Justice *et al.* (1993) studies, at the two points in time, different subjects received a diagnosis of SAD but the number of SAD subjects hardly differed. This confirms that the SPAQ may be acceptable as a screening instrument but that it is not suitable for use as a diagnostic instrument.

Another issue can limit the value of test–retest data. If stability over a long test–retest interval is expected, then SAD also has to be a stable, trait-like condition. Several follow-up studies have shown that, over time, SAD can either disappear or change into another mood disorder (Leonhardt *et al.* 1994; Raheja *et al.* 1996; Sakamoto *et al.* 1995; Schwartz *et al.* 1996; Thompson *et al.* 1995; Wicki *et al.* 1992). Although these longitudinal studies may be influenced by the treatments patients received (in most cases antidepressive medication and/ or light treatment), the results suggest that the diagnosis of SAD is not very stable over time. So, retesting has to take place within a limited time interval and subjects should not have received treatment between tests.

Concerning the external validity of the SPAQ, the results are mixed. One study concluded that the SPAQ underestimated the prevalence, while in another study, the SPAQ estimated quite accurately. Preliminary results from two studies show that the SPAQ may overestimate the prevalence with 400 per cent to 800 per cent. However, conclusions cannot be drawn until publication of these two studies. Contrast validity shows that the ability of the SPAQ to discriminate between different (patient) groups is fairly good.

13.4 Overview of prevalence studies in the general population

In the following section an overview is given of the prevalence studies that were performed in samples of the general population. Only studies of the adult population are reported here. Prevalence studies of children are discussed in Chapter 04.

13.4.1 **North America**

In an influential study, Kasper *et al.* (1989*a*) investigated the prevalence of SAD in Montgomery County, Maryland, USA, at latitude 39° N. In a random sample, 416 subjects of at least 21 years of age were interviewed by telephone. The response rate varied from 57 per cent to 92 per cent. Selection took place by random-digit dialling. On most demographic variables, the sample was representative of the total population of Montgomery County. Women had higher seasonality scores than men and younger women (between 21 and 40 years) had higher seasonality scores than older women. Figures for winter SAD and summer SAD were 4.3 per cent and 0.7 per cent, respectively. Three to four times more women than men met the winter-SAD criteria.

The study of Kasper *et al.* (1989*a*) was replicated by Terman (1988) in New York City (40° N) and extended by Rosen *et al.* (1990) to three other locations (Sarasota, 27° N; Montgomery County, 39° N; and Nashua, 42.5° N). They used the same methodology as Terman (1988) in order to allow for comparisons between the different latitudes. The SPAQ was mailed to a total sample of 3400 subjects, randomly selected from telephone directories at the four locations. The response rates varied from 40.1 per cent to 60.5 per cent. Prevalence rates of winter SAD, based on the 'Kasper criteria' (with the 'window' limited to January and February for a winter pattern and July and August for a summer pattern) varied from 1.4 per cent in Sarasoto, 6.3 per cent in Montgomery County, 4.7 per cent in New York, to 9.7 per cent in Nashua, and from 1.0 per cent in Montgomery County to 3.1 per cent in New York for summer SAD. Using the more conservative criteria than Kasper *et al.* (1989*a*), sub-SAD varied from 2.6 per cent in Sarasoto to 12.4 per cent in New York. There were large differences in mean age between the respondents at the four locations (from 40.5 per cent in Nashua to 58.7 per cent in Sarasota). It is remarkable that in Sarasota no cases of winter SAD below age 25 were found, while in New York all SAD cases were older than 34 years.

Booker and Hellekson (1992) interviewed 283 subjects at their homes in Fairbanks, Alaska (64° N) with the SPAQ. The criteria used to identify SAD and sub-SAD differed from those of Kasper *et al.* (1989*a*). Instead of a GS score of 10, the authors used 11 as the cut-off score. No motivation was given, but prevalence figures based on a GS score of 10 were given as well for both SAD and sub-SAD. All analyses were performed on the higher threshold. Furthermore, no 'window' was used to delineate a summer or winter type. Therefore, the number of SAD subjects may have been lower. Interpretation of the results is further complicated because the selection procedure of the sample was not described. The prevalence rates were high: 9.9 per cent SAD and 24.0 per cent sub-SAD on the basis of the 'Kasper criteria'. The higher threshold reduced the rates to 9.2 per cent and 19.1 per cent, respectively. More women (69.2 per cent) than men met the SAD criteria. Subjects who met the SAD criteria were younger and more often female than subjects who did not. Also, they showed a higher level of depression on the CES-D scale compared to the group without SAD/sub-SAD.

In a nationwide prevalence study in Canada (42° N to 50° N), Levitt and Boyle (1997) interviewed 1605 subjects (response rate 82 per cent) by telephone, selected by means of random-number dialling. With the SPAQ and the 'Kasper criteria' the number of SAD subjects in the population was estimated as 7.4 per cent, while a DSM-IV interview yielded a much lower figure (1.7 per cent).

Finally, Blazer *et al.* (1998) studied SAD in a sample of 8098 subjects from the 48 counterminous states of the USA by means of a structured interview (the CIDI), adjusted to include the DSM-III-R criteria for SAD. The study stretched over a period of 18 months and the response rate was 82.4 per cent. Only 0.4 per cent met the criteria for SAD. While 1.0 per cent met the criteria for a minor depression, which may be considered comparable to sub-SAD.

13.4.2 **Europe**

In Iceland (62° N to 67° N), Magnusson and Stefansson (1993) sent the SPAQ to a random sample of 1000 subjects of the Icelandic population between 17 and 67 years of age. The response rate was 61 per cent. With the 'Kasper criteria' applied (with the exception that subjects who felt worst in December were excluded), the prevalence rate for winter SAD was 3.8 per cent and 7.5 per cent for sub-SAD. None of the respondents met the criteria for summer SAD. Logistic regression showed age and gender to be significant predictors of SAD and sub-SAD combined. Residency, employment, and marital status were not significant predictors.

In Finland (60 to 70° N), Hagfors *et al.* (1992) used the SPAQ to interview, by telephone, a representative sample of 2015 subjects (response rate 88.5 per cent). Preliminary data, based on the 'Kasper criteria' (without the 'window' criterion), showed prevalence rates for SAD and sub-SAD of 3.4 per cent and 21.8 per cent, respectively.

The study in Finland was replicated and extended to Sweden using a mail-out procedure instead of a telephone interview (Hagfors *et al.* 1995). A sample of 3010 subjects in Sweden and 1200 subjects in Finland, aged 17 to 60, were randomly selected from the general population. The return rate was about 55 per cent. Preliminary results showed that, based on the 'Kasper criteria' for the self-report method, 7.1 per cent of the respondents in Finland and 3.9 per cent of the respondents in Sweden met the criteria for SAD (winter or summer pattern not specified). For sub-SAD the figures were 11.8 per cent and 13.9 per cent, respectively.

In a third study in Finland, Saarijärvi *et al.* (1999) mailed (a new translation of) the SPAQ to 3000 subjects in Finland between 16-64 years old, drawn from the national population register. Half of the subjects in this sample lived in the northern part of Finland (68°–70°N) and half in the south-western part (<61°N). The overall response rate was 59.3 per cent. The overall prevalence rates of winter-SAD and winter-sub-SAD was considerably higher in this study compared tho the Haglors *et al.* (1992 and 1995) studies: 9.5 per cent and 18.4 per cent, respectively. Summer-SAD and summer-sub-SAD criteria were met by 2.5 per cent and 8.7, respectively.

Wirz–Justice *et al.* (1992) studied the prevalence of SAD in Switzerland (47° N), by means of a telephone interview, with a representative sample of 989 subjects, using the SPAQ. With the 'Kasper criteria' (without the 'window') the prevalence rate of SAD was 2.2 per cent and 8.9 per cent for sub-SAD (preliminary data). Having seasonal problems was not correlated with living in sunny or overcast regions, or urban or rural areas.

In a prevalence study in the Netherlands (53° N) (Mersch *et al.* 1999*a*) a random sample of 5356 subjects, of whom the number of men and women were equal, was sent the Dutch version of the SPAQ. The sample was representative of the urban to rural residence ratio in the Netherlands. More than 400 questionnaires were sent each month for 13 consecutive months (March 1993 to March 1994 inclusive). The age range was 18 to 65 years; the response rate was 53.9 per cent. The 'Kasper criteria' were used with the exception that a summer pattern was delineated by April through September and a winter pattern by October through March. The prevalence rate for SAD was 3.1 per cent of which 3.0 per cent had a winter pattern, and for sub-SAD, 8.5 per cent of which 8.2 per cent showed a winter pattern. Women appeared to be significantly more sensitive to changes with the seasons than men, and a greater number of women than men reported to have problems with these changes.

The sex ratio in the SAD group was 3.6 to 1. For both men and women there was a significant negative relationship between seasonality and age. There was no relationship between having seasonal problems and age.

In a study by Broman and Hetta (1998), parts of the SPAQ were sent to a random sample of 1194 subjects in two urban areas in Sweden — Kiruna (67.8° N) and Trelleborg (54.4° N). The preliminary results revealed an overall prevalence rate of 3.5 per cent and no difference between the two regions. There was a negative relationship between age and sub-SAD. Also, there were twice as many possible anxiety cases among the subjects with SAD than among those without SAD.

At five locations in the South of Italy (39° N to 45° N), the SPAQ was sent to a total of 4000 subjects (Muscettola et al. 1995). The overall prevalence rate was 3.9 per cent for winter SAD, 2.1 per cent for summer SAD, and 4.8 for sub-SAD. The results of this study have to be interpreted with caution. Firstly, the response was extremely low (overall rate of 13.6 per cent). Secondly, there are some surprising results: the mean age of the respondents is high (49.6 years); more men than women responded (59.5 per cent versus 40.5 per cent); and, compared to other prevalence studies, a very high number of subjects reported problems with seasonal changes (52 per cent).

Eagles et al. (1996) investigated SAD in a sample of 443 nurses working in psychiatric services in Aberdeen (57°N), Scotland. Prevalence figures for SAD and sub-SAD are 2.9 per cent and 9.5 per cent respectively. No distinction between winter and summer-SAD is made. More women than men met the SAD criteria, while seasonality declined with age.

Michalak (1998) studied the prevalence of SAD in Wales, Great Britain (53° N), on a sample selected from local health authority databases. Of the 2000 SPAQs mailed, 68 per cent were returned. Preliminary results showed a prevalence rate for SAD of approximately 8 per cent. Figures for summer SAD and sub-SAD were not given. An interview yielded a SAD percentage of 1 per cent. Too little information on applied methodology is available to interpret these results.

13.4.3 Other countries

In the Philippines (Quezon City, 15° N), the SPAQ was handed out to 1441 employees of a department store (Ito et al. 1992). The response rate was 73.1 per cent, of whom no less than 84 per cent were female. Prevalence rates were 0 per cent winter SAD, 0.1 per cent summer SAD, and 0 per cent sub-SAD. Conclusions are hard to draw since the results may be influenced by selection bias and response bias due to the high response of females and possible privacy violations. Nevertheless, the complete lack of winter SAD is surprising and can tentatively be considered as support for the prevalencelatitude association.

A study was performed on a population of 526 adult female twins living across Australia (10° S to 40° S) (Murray et al. 1993b). Thirty-five subjects (6.7 per cent) were screened as 'potentially SAD'. Of these, 23 (4.4 per cent) met the criteria of winter SAD, while 4 (0.8 per cent) met the criteria of summer SAD. No information is given on the remaining 8 subjects. One of the objectives of the study — to estimate the prevalence of SAD in Australia — cannot be answered with the design used due to sampling bias. Another study in Australia (Morrissey et al. 1996) found conflicting results. Of the 800 SPAQs that were mailed to inhabitants of Townsville (19° S) only 176 were completed and returned (22 per cent). No information on sample selection is given. More respondents felt worst during summer (53.9 per cent) than during winter (7.9 per cent). The criteria for summer SAD were met by 9.1 per cent, while 1.7 per cent met the criteria for winter SAD.

In Nogoya, Japan, Ozaki *et al.* (1995) studied the prevalence in a random selected group of 1276 civil servants. Winter SAD was met by 0.86 per cent and summer SAD by 0.94 per cent. As discussed in the methodology section, these figures have to be interpreted with caution.

13.5 Characteristics of winter SAD

Several characteristics of SAD are remarkably consistent across studies. In the first place, women appear to be much more vulnerable to seasonal variation in mood than men. Prevalence figures show that two to four times as many women than men suffer from SAD. Also, vulnerability for seasonal variation declines with age. This is more pronounced in women, which may be due to regression effects. Most subjects who meet the criteria for SAD fall in the age range of 25 to 40 years. In none of those (few) studies where this was a subject of the study, did residency (urban versus rural), employment, or marital status have influence on prevalence figures (Wirz–Justice *et al.* 1992; Magnusson and Stefansson 1993).

Data on variables which are also part of the SAD criteria (for example, sleep duration, weight) are better studied in contrast with groups composed by means of other criteria and will not be discussed here.

13.6 Summer SAD

Wehr *et al.* (1987) were the first to describe a group of patients who experienced their recurrent depressive episode in summer. Compared to winter-SAD patients, summer-SAD patients did not show an increased need to sleep, more often had a decreased appetite and weight loss, and less often suffered carbohydrate craving (Boyce and Parker 1988; Wehr *et al.* 1989). Also, summer-SAD patients believed they were influenced by temperature rather than by light. Wehr *et al.* (1989) concluded that summer SAD is characterized by endogenous symptoms of depression and winter depression by atypical symptoms. Since then little knowledge has been gained. This is not surprising considering the very low prevalence figures. Also, the lack of a specific treatment for this summer-type of SAD does not stimulate research.

Although the prevalence rates are, in general, low, there is a considerable variation in reported summer-SAD figures. In Europe, for instance, the figures vary from negligible (0 per cent in Iceland: Magnusson and Stefansson 1993; 0.1 per cent in the Netherlands: Mersch *et al.* 1999*a*) to extremely high (10 per cent in Capri, Italy: Muscettola *et al.* 1995). In the USA, the variation between the figures is large as well, ranging from 0.5 per cent in Nashua to 3.1 per cent in New York (Rosen *et al.* 1990). This latter study, performed at four locations across the USA, shows percentages of summer SAD for New York and Sarasoto that are almost as high as winter SAD (3.1 per cent vs. 4.7 per cent and 1.2 per cent vs. 1.4 per cent, respectively).

In the study by Ozaki *et al.* (1995) in Nagoya, Japan, significantly more respondents reported feeling worse in summer (15 per cent) than in winter (10 per cent). This resulted in a somewhat higher percentage of summer SAD than winter SAD (0.94 per cent vs. 0.86 per cent). Significantly, more subjects with a summer type reported that they 'eat least', 'sleep least', and 'lose most weight' than subjects with a winter type, while more subjects with a winter type stated that they 'sleep most' and 'tend to gain most weight' compared to subjects with a summer type. There were no differences in age or GS score between respondents with a summer or winter type. In Australia, Morrissey *et al.* (1996) found 53.9 per cent of the respondents feeling worst in summer and only 7.9 per cent feeling worst in winter. According to the authors, light exposure is not the critical climatic mechanism in 'tropical-SAD' but rather, as shown in their study, a combination of heat and humidity.

It may be that in the case of summer SAD, local weather and social conditions play an even more important role than in winter SAD.

A most striking illustration of the situation in relation to research into summer SAD is the fact that many researchers did not report summer-SAD figures in their publications, only figures on winter SAD or the overall figures (Booker and Hellekson 1992; Broman and Hetta 1998; Eagles *et al.* 1996; Hagfors *et al.* 1992, 1995; Hedge and Woodson 1996; Ito *et al.* 1992; Levitt and Boyle 1997; Madden *et al.* 1996; Michalak 1998; Wirz–Justice *et al.* 1992).

13.7 Prevalence and latitude

A major hypothesis in the study of SAD is that the disorder is triggered by photoperiod variation. Since photoperiod variation over the seasons is greater closer to the poles, it is hypothesized that with an increase in latitude there is an increase in the prevalence of SAD. This association has been suggested by the outcome of two studies, one in the USA (Potkin *et al.* 1986) and one in Norway (Lingjærde *et al.* 1986). In both studies, a questionnaire comprising 15 symptoms of SAD was published in national newspapers with the request to return the questionnaire if 8 or more symptoms were present (criteria for SAD). Both studies showed a positive correlation between latitude and prevalence. This result is merely indicative; the characteristics of the readers of the newspaper are unknown and may have been different in different parts of the country. Also, it is unknown how many of the subjects who met the criteria of SAD (8 symptoms or more) returned their questionnaire. These percentages may have differed across the country due to cultural differences. Finally, since the questionnaire used in these studies was not validated, direct clinical assessment is more important in these studies than in those using a validated instrument.

Nevertheless, although both studies have their methodological limitations, they have stimulated more research into the relationship between prevalence and latitude. In the following, the evidence for the existence of such a relationship will be discussed.

13.7.1 Studies to test the prevalence–latitude association

Since the formerly discussed studies of Potkin *et al.* (1986) and Lingjærde *et al.* (1986) several studies have been designed to investigate the relationship between prevalence and latitude.

Rosen and colleagues (1990) studied the prevalence at four locations in the USA, applying the same methodology at every location. Positive correlations were found between the prevalence of winter SAD and of winter SAD and sub-SAD combined, and latitude. Recently, Levitt and Boyle (1997) studied the prevalence of SAD in the Province of Ontario, Canada across eight strata of 1 latitude (from 42° N to 50° N). They found no association between latitude and prevalence. Broman and Hetta (1998) came to the same conclusion. They sent sections of the SPAQ to a random sample of two urban areas in Sweden, one in the north (Kiruna at 67.8° N) and one in the south (Trelleborg at 54.4° N). There was no significant difference between the prevalence figures at the two latitudes (4.2 per cent and 5.2 per cent, respectively).

In a study in Italy (Muscettola *et al.* 1995), the prevalence rates at three of the five locations at which the study was performed were compared: Catanzaro (39° N), Napoli (41° N), and Trieste (46° N). The correlation was unexpected ($r = -0.50$). The results in this study may be biased, however, by the low response rates (13.6 per cent overall). Nevertheless, as the authors claim, comparison between the three locations in the study may have some value since the response rates were approximately the same. Murray and Hay (1997) studied SAD in a sample of 526 women (response rate of 52.8 per cent) across the latitudes of Australia. The correlation between latitude and the GS score of respondents with a winter type was not significant ($r = 0.06$, $p = 0.169$). According to these authors seasonality may have a broader psychological component.

In Japan (Sakamoto *et al.* 1993), the prevalence of SAD was assessed among patients with a mood disorder who contacted 53 out-patient university psychiatric clinics in Japan for the first time between 1 September 1990 and 31 March 1991. The clinics were located between 26° N and 44° N. The results showed a non-significant correlation between prevalence and latitude (Spearman's r = 0.33, p < 0.10). Okawa *et al.* (1996) studied seasonal variation in six cities in Japan at latitudes ranging from 32° N to 43° N. The global seasonality score showed a significant correlation with latitude. P artonen *et al.* (1993) assessed the frequency of depressive symptoms among 1000 subjects (801 women, 199 men) — all employees of a national bank in Finland. The SIGH-SAD self-rating scale was returned by 486 subjects, living between 60° N and 70° N. The results showed that depressive symptoms were not more common at higher latitudes than at lower latitudes. In a study among personnel wintering in three Antarctic stations (from 64° S to 90° S), Palinkas *et al.* (1996) did not find an association between seasonality and latitude. The sample was too small (n = 87) and the stay on Antarctica was too short, however, to draw conclusions on prevalence.

Finally, a study by Carskadon and Acebo (1993) on children allows for a prevalence–latitude comparison. The study sample was drawn from 78 schools that were grouped into three geographic zones: a northern zone (> 42° N), a central zone (between 36° N and 42° N), and a southern zone (< 36° N). The results showed a significant higher incidence of seasonal symptoms in the winter in the northern and central zones in comparison to the southern zone.

Summarizing the results, there is a balance between studies confirming and studies rejecting the latitude–prevalence hypothesis.

13.7.2 Comparison between prevalence studies

Another approach is to compare the results of the different prevalence studies in relation to the latitudes at which they were performed. For this purpose studies were selected that studied prevalence in the general population. Correlations between prevalence and latitude (Spearman r_s; p values are one-tailed) were calculated in North American studies (Booker and Hellekson 1992; Kasper *et al.* 1989*a*; Levitt and Boyle 1997; Rosen *et al.* 1990; Terman 1988) and in European studies (Hagfors *et al.* 1992, 1995; Magnusson and Stefansson 1993; Mersch *et al.* 1999*a*; Wirz–Justice *et al.* 1992). Compared to the Mersch *et al.* (1999*b*) study, the study of Broman and Hetta (1998) was added to the analyses. In Fig. 13.3 the prevalence rates are plotted as a function of latitude. The relationship is shown by regression lines.

The overall correlation between prevalence and latitude is almost zero: $r_{(n=15)} = 0.001$, $p = 0.482$. As shown by Fig. 13.3, there is a large difference between the North American and the European prevalence figures ($M_{NA} = 6.24$, sd = 3.06 and $M_{Eur} = 4.10$, sd = 1.50), which may explain the low correlation. Analysis of variance with latitude as covariate shows that the difference between the continents is significant ($F_{(1,12)} = 17.91$, $p = 0.001$). Correlations between prevalence and latitude for the North American and European data, separately, were $r_{(n=7)} = 0.90$, $p = 0.003$ and $r_{(n=8)} = 0.54$, $p = 0.085$, respectively, which may be considered as support for the prevalence–latitude hypothesis. But, if this is true, the difference between North America and Europe contradicts this, since, on the basis of the prevalence–latitude hypothesis, Europe ($M_{Eur} = 59.9°$ N) should have a higher mean prevalence estimate than North America ($M_{NA} = 42.5°$ N). The conclusion of the Mersch *et al.* (1999*b*) study was that 'if latitude influences prevalence this influence is only weak. Apparently, other factors contribute considerably to the variance' (p. 44). The inclusion of the results of the Broman and Hetta (1998) study does not change this conclusion.

13.8 Factors influencing prevalence

13.8.1 Prevalence and climate

The influence of climatic variables on the prevalence of SAD has received little attention. Although several studies mention (possible) meteorological influences on the prevalence of SAD, most of the attention of researchers has focused on the prevalence–latitude discussion. Nevertheless, climate seems to play a role. Potkin and colleagues (1986) reported high correlations between SAD and the weather in December in terms of sunshine, cloudiness, and temperature. The study in Japanese psychiatric clinics (Sakamoto *et al.* 1993) showed a weak relationship between prevalence and latitude, but a stronger negative correlation between prevalence and total hours of sunshine ($r = -0.66$, $p < 0.01$). In another study in Japan (Okawa *et al.* 1996), the SPAQ was sent to 1200 middle-aged parents (aged between 30 and 50 years) of high-school students in five cities. The global seasonality score correlated with latitude, but also with temperature and hours of sunshine.

In several studies the higher prevalence of summer SAD compared to winter SAD is attributed to climatic influences. In the Philippines study (Ito *et al.* 1992), more subjects reported feeling worst in summer (7.7 per cent) than in winter (4.2 per cent), with the highest peak on the item 'feeling worst' in April. The authors concluded that mood changes and seasonal problems were more related to the hot-dry season than to the winter season. In the study in Nagoya, Japan (Ozaki *et al.* 1995), the number of subjects with a summer pattern was

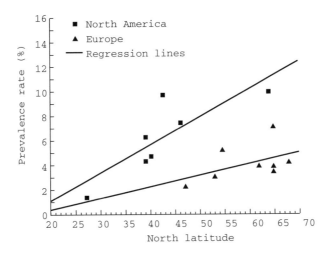

Fig. 13.3 Prevalence rates of winter SAD in North America and Europe in relation to latitude. The straight lines are regression lines.

20 per cent higher than subjects with a winter pattern. According to the authors, the weather may contribute to differences between results in their study and studies in western countries. A comparable result emerged in a prevalence study in Australia, in which Morrissey *et al.* (1996) found a high percentage of summer SAD (9.1 per cent) as opposed to winter SAD (1.7 per cent). A combination of heat and humidity apparently accounted for the high percentage of summer SAD. Only one study has investigated the role of climate (harsh winter weather) by comparing 45 healthy subjects from Minnesota with 42 healthy subjects from California during the winter (Garvey *et al.* 1988). There were no differences in the prevalence of depressive symptoms. The scale of the study is too small, however, to draw conclusions.

Four studies examined the role of climatic factors on energy or mood in SAD patients. Albert *et al.* (1991) followed patients over a mean period of 2.8 years. They concluded that 8 out of 10 SAD patients were influenced by weather in at least one season. Molin *et al.* (1996) followed 126 patients from September to May for four consecutive years. They found significant correlations between mood (measured by the BDI) and minutes of sunshine, global radiation, length of daylight, and temperature in 126 SAD patients. They concluded that this result is in accordance with the theoretical assumption that lack of light plays a role in SAD. Cloud cover, rainfall, or atmospheric pressure were not associated with mood. A study in Switzerland (Wirz–Justice *et al.* 1992) also found no relationship between 'seasonal problems' and living in sunny or overcast regions. Subjects with high GS scores appeared to spend less time outdoors than subjects with low GS scores. According to the authors seasonal problems may be less related to the amount of available sunshine than to the amount of exposure to outdoor light.

Young *et al.* (1997) investigated the role of environmental variables in the onset of a major depressive episode in SAD patients. In contrast with the Albert *et al.* (1991) and the Molin *et al.* (1996) studies, they found that the risk of onset of a depressive episode had a highly regular relationship with the photoperiod and appeared not to be related with hours of sunshine, mean daily temperature, or total daily radiation. Nevertheless, they concluded that other factors influence the annual variations in onset risk by moderating the effect of the photoperiod. As possible factors they mention other climatic variables, annually varying factors within the individual, and randomly varying factors like stressors. If stressors play a role in the aetiology of SAD, the anticipation of the winter and its harsh weather conditions may contribute to triggering a depressive episode in subjects with a predisposition for SAD. Also, weather conditions may in part explain the difference between North American and European prevalence figures.

13.8.2 Prevalence and genetics

Another factor that may play a role is genetics. Two studies on monozygotic and dizygotic twins investigated the percentage of the variance in seasonality that was explained by genetic influences. Madden *et al.* (1996) found that 29 per cent of the variance in seasonality in men and women (measured by the GS score) was explained by genetic influences. In a study by Jang *et al.* (1997), among 187 monozygotic and 152 dizygotic twins, the GS score appeared to be significantly inheritable, explaining 69 per cent (men) and 45 per cent (women) of the variance.

That genetic factors may influence prevalence figures is hypothesized by Magnusson and Stefansson (1993). On the basis of the low prevalence figure in Iceland compared to the figures in the United States (especially since Iceland lies farther to the North), it was hypothesized that a genetic adaptation to the long arctic winter had taken place within the Icelandic population. To test this, Magnusson and Axelsson (1993) studied the prevalence of SAD among the approximately 600 adults (20 to 74 years of age) who are wholly descended from Icelandic immigrants living in the Interlake District of Manitoba, Canada (50.5° N). The SPAQ was sent to

300 randomly selected subjects, of which a high number (82 per cent) responded. Applying the same criteria as were used in the Iceland study (Magnusson and Stefansson 1993), the SAD and sub-SAD prevalence figures were 1.2 per cent and 3.3 per cent. The lack of a control group from the same region prevents the drawing of conclusions concerning the role of genetic influences. Therefore, Axelsson *et al.* (1998) replicated the Magnusson and Axelsson (1993) study and extended it to include a group of non-Icelandic descendants living in the same area. The prevalence figure of SAD was significantly lower in the Icelandic descendants sample than in the non-Icelandic sample (4.8 per cent versus 9.1 per cent). The same was true for the combined SAD and sub-SAD figures (17.7 per cent versus 26 per cent). The authors interpreted these results as support for the genetic hypothesis.

Another study that shows the possible role of genetic factors is the study of Saarijärvi *et al.* (1999) in which a comparison was made between the prevalence of two ethnic groups, Finns and Lapps. The prevalence rate among Lapps, who lived in the North of Finland for about 10000 thousand years and who are genetically different from the Finns, was significantly lower than the prevalence rate of the Finns (6.4 per cent versus 11.1 per cent for winter-SAD and 12.7 per cent versus 18.2 per cent for winter-Sub-SAD). Nevertheless, according to the authors, social-cultural differences, i.e. the specialized life-style of the Lapps, may also play a role.

13.8.3 Prevalence and social-cultural factors

Scientific knowledge of the influence of social-cultural factors is scarce and most information is anecdotal. Firstly, translation of the SPAQ into different languages may influence outcome (cf. Picavet and van den Bos 1996). Secondly, the value of questions may be different in the different countries. For instance, differences in cultural acceptance of admitting psychological problems may influence the answer to the question 'are seasonal changes a problem'. According to Hagfors *et al.* (1992), people in Finland are less inclined to answer this question in the affirmative since 'having a problem' is associated with alcohol abuse. Comparing their data with the Kasper *et al.* (1989*a*) study they found approximately equal GS score distributions, but much lower percentages on the 'problem' question (15.7 per cent as compared to 27.0 per cent) (Hagfors 1993).

Thirdly, knowledge of SAD in the general population, which is likely to be greater in the USA than in Europe, may also influence ratings on the SPAQ and consequently prevalence figures. In the Montgomery County study (Kasper *et al.* 1989*a*), the question about whether respondents 'had heard of SAD' significantly contributed to the prediction of the difference between women with high and low seasonality scores. Fourthly, local social-cultural circumstances may influence prevalence figures. In the study by Muscettola *et al.* (1995), the high percentage of summer SAD (10 per cent) was explained by social factors. It was hypothesized that the major change in daily life activities during the summer may put high pressure on the inhabitants of Capri, a known holiday resort in Italy. Stressors like increased workload may have influenced the prevalence figures.

Nilssen *et al.* (1999) studied the prevalence of depression in two ethnically different populations, Norwegians (n = 517) and Russians (n = 450), living in Svalbard at 78° N latitude. Self-reported, one-year prevalence of depression for Russians was 2–3 times higher than for Norwegians, while during the polar night, the figures for Russians were 4–5 times higher. This study is interesting in several respects. In the first place, the level of depression in Norwegians during the polar night is lower at this extremely high latitude than in the general population in Norway. Also, it shows the possible influence of a number of differences between the Russian and Norwegian populations. Translation of the questionnaires into both languages may have influenced the answers. Furthermore, a different selection process of the populations may have taken place. The medium length of stay on Svalbard was 1.5 years for Russians and 4 years for Norwegians. More Russians than Norwegians were shift workers. A lower percentage of Russians participated in the screening and, finally, most Norwegians came from the North of Norway and were used to the climatic conditions on Svalbard, while most of the Russians normally lived in the south of Russia.

13.9 Symptoms of seasonality in the normal population

An important issue is whether SAD is a discrete illness or an extreme manifestation of phenomena present in the normal population as well (cf. Lacoste and Wirz–Justice 1989). Eastwood *et al.* (1985) studied this in a longitudinal study, recording daily measures of hours slept and energy, anxiety, and mood levels over a period of 14 months in a group of 30 patients with an affective disorder and a group of 34 normal controls. They concluded that affective symptoms show a periodic component in both patients and controls and that the pattern of cycles for the patients is defined by amplitude.

Terman (1988) compared the relative frequency distributions of seasonal mood changes of winter-SAD patients with the distribution in the general population. The pattern of the curves resemble each other except for a difference in amplitude and a summer dip in the general population, which of course is absent in the winter-SAD group. Thompson *et al.* (1988) compared SAD subjects with bipolar disorder patients and normal controls on the seasonal distribution of the GS items. All three groups showed the same seasonal curves with the greatest amplitude for the SAD group and a intermediate position for the bipolar disorder group. In two prevalence studies (Mersch *et al.* 1999a; Wirz–Justice *et al.* 1992), the same analyses were performed as employed by Thompson *et al.* (1988) on subjects with and without problems with the seasons. In both studies the curves were almost identical but for a smaller magnitude of the amplitude in the latter group.

Finally, in the Mersch *et al.* (1999a) study, the CES-D scale was sent to approximately 400 subjects each month for 13 consecutive months. For the total group of respondents there was a clear seasonal pattern with significant differences between the months: mood was significantly

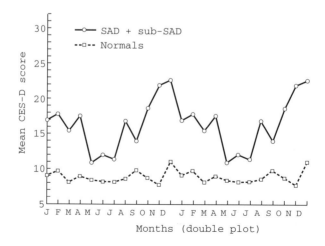

Fig. 13.4 Mood over the year as measured by the CES-D, for SAD and sub-SAD subjects combined and for healthy subjects.

more depressed in the winter compared to the summer (see Figs. 13.1 and 13.2). In Fig. 13.4 the mood score for winter SAD and sub-SAD combined and healthy subjects are plotted, separately.

One can see from Fig. 13.4 that the monthly fluctuation is largest for the SAD group. The difference between the months in this group is significant ($F_{(11,293)} = 3.64$, $p < 0.001$). Between the three winter months (December, January, February) and the three summer months (June, July, August) there is a significant difference ($M_{(winter)} = 19.08$ and $M_{(summer)} = 13.49$; $F_{(1,129)} = 9.64$, , $p = 0.002$). Although the variation between the months is much smaller for the normal group, differences between the months reach significance ($F_{(11,2451)} = 2.81$, $p = 0.001$). In this group too, there is a clear seasonal effect: there is a significant difference between the winter and summer months ($M_{(winter)} = 10.01$ and $M_{(summer)} = 8.37$; $F_{(1,1136)} = 11.48$, $p = 0.001$).

The conclusion from this short overview is that the evidence indicates that seasonal symptoms in SAD patients are present in the normal population as well, but at a less extreme level.

References

Albert, P.S., Rosen, L.N., Alexander, J.R., and Rosenthal, N.E. (1991) Effect of daily variation in weather and sleep on seasonal affective disorder. *Psychiatry Res* **36**:51–63.

Axelsson, J., Stefansson, J.G., Magnusson, A., and Karlsson, M.M. (1998) Seasonal affective disorders: the relevance of Icelandic and Icelandic–Canadian evidence to aetiological hypotheses. *Society for Research on Biological Rhythms Abstracts* **210**:144.

Booker, J.M. and Hellekson, C.J. (1992) Prevalence of seasonal affective disorder in Alaska. *Am J Psychiatry* **149**:1176–82.

Blazer, D.G, Kesoler , R.C and Swartz, M.S. (1998) Epideriology of recurrent major and minor depression with a seasonal pattern. The National Comorbidity Survey. *The British Journal of Psychiatry* **172**: 164–7.

Boyce, P. and Parker, G. (1988) Seasonal affective disorder in the Southern Hemisphere. *Am J Psychiatry* **145**:97–9.

Broman, J.E. and Hetta, J. (1998) Prevalence of seasonal affective disorders and related symptoms at two latitudes in Sweden. *Society for Research on Biological Rhythms Abstracts* **228**:162.

Carskadon, M.A. and Acebo, C. (1993) Parental reports of seasonal mood and behavior changes in children. *J Am Acad Child Adolesc Psychiatry* **32**:264–9.

Eagles, J.M., Mercer, G., Boshier, A.J., and Jamieson, F. (1996) Seasonal affective disorder among psychiatric nurses in Aberdeen. *J Affect Disord* **37**:129–35.

Eastwood, M.R., Whitton, J.L., Kramer, P.M., and Peter, A.M. (1985) Infradian rhythms. a comparison of affective disorders and normal persons. *Arch Gen Psychiatry* **42**:295–9.

Garvey, M.J., Goodes, M., Furlong, C., and Tollefson, G.D. (1988) Does cold winter weather produce depressive symptoms? *Int J Biometeorol* **32**:144–6.

Hagfors, C. (1993) 'Light sensitivity': real or expressiveness subscale on the SPAQ? *Society for Light Treatment and Biological Rhythms Abstracts* **6**:22–4.

Hagfors, C., Koskela, K., and Tikkanen, J. (1992) Seasonal affective disorder (SAD) in Finland: an epidemiological study. *Society for Light Treatment and Biological Rhythms Abstracts* **4**:24.

Hagfors, C., Thorell, L–H., and Arned, M. (1995) Seasonality in Finland and Sweden, an epidemiologic study, preliminary results. *Society for Light Treatment and Biological Rhythms Abstracts* **7**:22.

Hardin, T.A., Wehr, T.A., Brewerton, T., Kasper, S., Berrettini, W., Rabkin, J., *et al.* (1991) Evaluation of seasonality in six clinical populations and two normal populations. *J Psychiatry Res* **25**:75–87.

Hedge, A.L. and Woodson, H. (1996) Prevalence of seasonal changes in moo d and behaviour during the winter months in central Texas. *Psychiatry Res* **62**:265–71.

Ito, A., Ichihara, M., Hisanaga, N., Ono, Y., Kayukawa, Y., Ohta, T., *et al.* (1992) Prevalence of seasonal mood changes in low latitude area: Seasonal Pattern Assessment Questionnaire score of Quezon City workers. *Japanese J Psychiatry Neurol* **46**:249.

Jang, K.L., Lam, R.W., Livesley, W.J., and Vernon, P.A. (1997) Gender differences in the heritability of seasonal mood change. *Psychiatry Res* **70**:145–54.

Kasper, S., Wehr, T.A., Bartko, J.J., Gaist, P.A., and Rosenthal, N.E. (1989*a*) Epidemiological changes in mood and behavior. A telephone survey of Montgomery County, Maryland. *Arch Gen Psychiatry* **46**:823–33.

Kasper, S., Rogers, S.L.B., Yancey, A., Schultz, P.M., Skwerer, R.G., and Rosenthal, N.E. (1989*b*) Phototherapy in individuals with and without subsyndromal seasonal affective disorder. *Arch Gen Psychiatry* **46**:837–44.

Lacoste, V., Wirz–Justice, A. (1989) Seasonal variation in normal subjects: an update of variables current in depression research. In *Seasonal affective disorders and phototherapy* (ed. N.E. Rosenthal and M.C. Blehar), pp. 167–229. Guilford Press, New York.

Leonhardt, G., Wirz–Justice, A., Kräuchi, K., Graw, P., Wunder, D., Haug, H-J. (1994) Long-term follow-up of depression in seasonal affective disorder. *Comprehen Psychiatry* **35**:457–64.

Levitt, A.J. and Boyle, M.H. (1997) Latitude and the variation in seasonal depression and seasonality of depressive symptoms. *Society for Light Treatment and Biological Rhythms Abstracts* **9**:14.

Lingjærde, O., Bratlid, T., Hansen, T., and Götestam, K.G. (1986) Seasonal affective disorder and midwinter insomnia in the far north: studies on two related chronobiological disorders in Norway. *Clin Neuropharm* **9**:187–9.

Madden, P.A.F., Heath, A.C., Rosenthal, N.E., and Martin, N.G. (1996) Seasonal changes in mood and behavior. The role of genetic factors. *Arch Gen Psychiatry* **53**:47–55.

Magnusson, A. (1996) Validation of the Seasonal Pattern Assessment Questionnaire (SPAQ). *J Affect Disord* **40**:121–9.

Magnusson, A. and Axelsson, J. (1993) The prevalence of seasonal affective disorder is low among descendants of Icelandic emigrants in Canada. *Arch Gen Psychiatry* **50**:947–51.

Magnusson, A. and Stefansson, J. (1993) Prevalence of seasonal affective disorder in Iceland. *Arch Gen Psychiatryiatry* **50**:941–6.

Magnusson, A., Friis S., and Opjordsmoen S. (1997) Internal consistency of the Seasonal Pattern Assessment Questionnaire (SPAQ). *J Affect Disord* **42**:113–16.

Mersch, P.P.A., Middendorp, H., Bouhuys, A.L., Beersma, D.G.M., and Van den Hoofdakker, R.H. (1999*b*) Seasonal affective disorder and latitude: a review of the literature. *J Affect Disord* **53**:35–48.

Mersch, P.P.A., Vastenburg, N.C., Meesters, Y., Bouhuys, A.L., Beersma, D.G.M., and Van den Hoofdakker, R.H. (2000) The reliability and validity of the SPAQ: a comparison between patient groups. In preparation.

Michalak, E.E. (1998) Prevalence of seasonal affective disorder in a general population sample in the United Kingdom: final results. *Society for Research on Biological Rhythms Abstracts* **222**:156.

Molin, J., Mellerup, E., Bolwig, P., Scheike, T., and Dam, H. (1996) The influence of climate on development of winter depression. *J Affect Disord* **37**:151–5.

Morrissey, S.A., Raggatt, P.T.F., James, B., and Rogers, J. (1996) Seasonal affective disorder: some epidemiologic findings from a tropical climate. *Australian and New Zealand J Psychiatry* **30**:579–86

Murray, G., Armstrong, S., and Hay, D. (1993*a*) SPAQ reliability in an Australian twin sample. *Society for Light Treatment and Biological Rhythms Abstracts* **5**:32–3.

Murray, G., Armstrong, S., and Hay, D. (1993*b*) Seasonal affective variation in Australia: disorder or preference. *Society for Light Treatment and Biological Rhythms Abstracts* **5**:42.

Murray, G.W. and Hay, D.A. (1997) Seasonal affective disorder in Australia: is photoperiod critical? *Australian and New Zealand J Psychiatry* **31**:279–84.

Muscettola, G., Barbato, G., Ficca, G., Beatrice, M., Puca, M., Aguglia, E., *et al.* (1995) Seasonality of mood in Italy: role of latitude and sociocultural factors. *J Affect Disord* **33**:135–9.

Nilssen, O., Brenn, T., Hoyer, G., Lipton, R., Boiko, J., and Tkatchev, A. (1999) Self-reported seasonal variation in depression at 78 degree North. The Svalbard study. *Int J Circumpolar Health* **58**:14–23.

Okawa, M., Shirakawa, S., Uchiyama, M., Oguri, M., Kohsaka, M ., Mishima, K., *et al.* (1996) Seasonal variation of mood and behaviour in a healthy middle-aged population in Japan. *Acta Psychiatr Scand* **94**:211–16.

Ozaki, N., Ono, Y., Ito, A., and Rosenthal, N.E. (1995) Prevalence of seasonal difficulties in mood and behavior among Japanese civil servants. *Am J Psychiatry* **152**:1225–7.

Palinkas, L.A., Houseal, M., and Rosenthal, N.E. (1996) Subsyndromal seasonal affective disorder in Antarctica. *J Nerv Ment Dis* **184**:530–4.

Partonen, T., Partinen, M., and Lönnqvist, J. (1993) Frequencies of seasonal major depressive symptoms at high latitudes. *Eur Arch Psychiatry Clin Neurosci* **243**:189–92.

Picavet, H.S.J. and Van den Bos, G.A.M. (1996) Comparing survey data on functional disability: the impact of some methodological differences. *J Epidem Community Health* **50**:86–93.

Potkin, S.G., Zetin, M., Stamenkovic, V., Kripke, D., and Bunney, W.E. (1986) Seasonal affective disorder: prevalence varies with latitude climate. *Clin Neuropharm* **9**:181–3.

Raheja, S.K., King, E.A., and Thompson, C. (1996) The seasonal pattern assessment questionnaire for identifying seasonal affective disorders. *J Affect Disord* **41**:193–9.

Rosen, L.N., Targum, S.D., Terman, M., Bryant, M.J., Hoffman, H., Kasper, S.F., *et al.* (1990) Prevalence of seasonal affective disorder at four latitudes. *Psychiatry Res* **31**:131–44.

Rosenthal, N.E., Genhart, M., Sack, D.A., Skwerer, R.G., and Wehr, T.A. (1987) Seasonal affective disorder: relevance for treatment and research of bulimia. In *Psychobiology of bulimia* (ed. J.L. Hudson and H.G. Pope). American Psychiatric Press, Washington DC.

Saarijärvi, S., Laverna, H., Helenius, H., Saarieleto, S. (1999) Seasaonal affective disorders among rural Finns and Lapps. *Acta Psychiatry Scand* **99**: 95–101

Sakamoto, K., Kamo, T., Nakadaira, S., Tamura, A., and Takahashi, K. (1993) A nationwide survey of seasonal affective disorder at 53 outpatient university clinics in Japan. *Acta Psychiatr Scand* **83**:258–65.

Sakamoto, K., Nakadaira, S., Kamo, K., Kamo, T., and Takahashi, K. (1995) A longitudinal follow-up study of seasonal affective disorder. *Am J Psychiatry* **152**:862–8.

Schwartz, P.J., Brown, C., Wehr, T.A., and Rosenthal, N.E. (1996) Winter seasonal affective disorder: a follow-up study of the first 59 patients of the National Institute of Mental Health Seasonal Studies Program. *Am J Psychiatry* **153**:1028–36.

Terman, M. (1988) On the question of mechanism in phototherapy for seasonal affective disorder: considerations of clinical efficacy and epidemiology. *J Biol Rhythms* **3**:155–72.

Thompson, C., Stinson, D., Fernandez, M., Fine, J., and Isaacs, G. (1988) A comparison of normal, bipolar and seasonal affective disorder subjects using the Seasonal Pattern Assessment Questionnaire. *J Affect Disord* **14**:257–64.

Thompson, C., Raheja, S.K., and King, E.A. (1995) A follow-up study of seasonal affective disorder. *Br J Psychiatry* **167**:380–4.

Wehr, T.A., Sack, D.A., and Rosenthal, N.E. (1987) Seasonal affective disorder with summer depression and winter hypomania. *Am J Psychiatry* **144**:1602–3.

Wehr, T.A., Giesen, H., Schulz, P.M., Joseph–Vanderpool, J.R., Kasper, S., Kelly, K.A., *et al.* (1989) Summer depression: description of the syndrome and comparison with winter depression. In *Seasonal affective disorders and phototherapy* (ed. N.E. Rosenthal and M.C. Blehar), pp. 55–63. Guilford Press, New York.

Wicki, W., Angst, J., and Merikangas, K.R. (1992) The Zurich Study: XIV. Epidemiology of seasonal depression. *Eur Arch Psychiatry Clin Neurosci* **241**:301–6.

Wirz–Justice, A., Kräuchi, K., Graw, P., Schulman, J., and Wirz, H. (1992) Seasonality in Switzerland: an epidemiological survey. *Society for Light Treatment and Biological Rhythms Abstracts* **4**:33.

Wirz–Justice, A., Graw, P., and Recker, S. (1993) The seasonal pattern assessment questionnaire (SPAQ): some comments. *Society for Light Treatment and Biological Rhythms Abstracts* **5**:31–2.

Young, M.A., Meaden, P.M., Fogg, L.F., Cherin, E.A., and Eastman, C.I. (1997) Which environmental variables are related to the onset of seasonal affective disorder? *J Abnorm Psychology* **106**:554–62.

Chapter 14

Assessment instruments

Michael Terman and Janet B.W. Williams

14.1 **Introduction**

Research on SAD and its treatment — which has been prolific for nearly 20 years — benefits by a community effort using common protocols and measures. This has enabled direct comparisons of prevalence estimates and clinical trials worldwide, cross-centre pooling of early light-therapy data (Terman *et al.* 1989), and a Cochrane meta-analysis of efficacy (Thompson *et al.* 1999). Specialized instruments have been devised to assess seasonal symptom variation in patients and the general population, to diagnose the disorder, and to measure symptom severity and response to treatment.

The use of structured interview guides reduces variance of clinical data both within and between centres as well as inter-rater variance, and thus enhances the coherence and convergence of results. Structured interviews designed to enhance depression rating scales antedated SAD research (Williams 1988) and have been applied to diagnostic assessments for a wide scope of DSM-III and DSM-IV disorders (First *et al.* 1995). Related instruments have been tailored specifically for SAD. Raters read aloud a series of standardized, symptom-specific stem questions, and elaborate with designated probes if the patient's initial response is not clear-cut. Each response is scaled according to a series of ordinal, categorical anchor points that reflect symptom severity and frequency. The time frame may be retrospective or current (that is, focused on the past week). Total scores provide a global measure of clinical state and change in state with treatment or seasons of the year, while item analysis allows documentation of symptom-specific effects.

Structured interviews provide the additional advantage of feasible administration by raters who lack advanced clinical training and credentials, for example, research assistants who would be unqualified independently to assess clinical state. Training requires dual ratings with a clinician or another established interviewer, until inter-rater reliability converges to within a couple of points in the total score.

This chapter reviews a set of well-established and recent instruments for SAD research in three general formats: questionnaires, structured interviews for administration by a clinician or trained research assistant, and paper-and-pencil versions of structured interviews in a self-rating format. Although the latter format removes the clinical observer from the assessment, its reliability compared to interviewer ratings can be sufficiently high to serve as a measure in out-patient field studies and, indeed, as a check against interview results.

Our survey is divided into two sections: questionnaire instruments designed to measure seasonal variation and infer the presence of SAD, and structured instruments (in both interviewer and self-rating formats) designed for formal diagnosis and the scaling of syndromal severity.

14.2 **Seasonality and SAD**

Seasonal Pattern Assessment Questionnaire (SPAQ) (Rosenthal *et al.* 1984*a*, 1987*b*). The SPAQ provides a seven-part retrospective assessment of the degree of seasonal change in key variables of mood, sleep, energy, weight and appetite, and vulnerability to weather factors. The primary datum is based on a set of categorical scales of mood and behaviour change (none to extreme) that yields a global seasonality score (GSS) with a maximum of 24 points. 'Best' and 'worst' months of the year are rated separately, and by symptom, allowing identification of specific fall/winter exacerbation. Two items ask for estimates of sleep length in each of the four seasons and annual fluctuation of weight. Subjects then are asked whether the problems identified pose personal difficulties. In an expanded version (Wirz–Justice *et al.* 1993), subjects are also queried about morningness/eveningness (relative energy, alertness and mood), time spent outdoors, and specific dietary preferences.

The SPAQ has been widely used for generating community prevalence estimates of SAD. By the most commonly applied criteria, those who report at least a moderate problem and whose GSS is at least 11 are considered to have the disorder (Kasper *et al.* 1989). A more conservative criterion is a GSS of at least 17, which corresponds to the mean score of independently diagnosed SAD patients (Terman 1988) and minimizes score overlap with subsyndromal cases. Prevalence estimates of SAD based on the former criteria are approximately twice as high as those based on the latter criteria.

Regardless of the GSS cut-off point, the SPAQ must be credited for generating the finding — and realization by the public and the profession — of significant, bothersome seasonality in the general population, with a possible latitude dependency (Rosen *et al.* 1990; for contrasting data see the chapter by Mersch). Although the GSS correlates with independent diagnoses of SAD and subsyndromal SAD, the overlapping score distributions lack differential diagnostic utility and ratings are vulnerable to the season of SPAQ administration (for critique see Enns *et al.* 1999; Thompson and Cowan 2001). That said, however, the instrument provides a first-stage indication of clinically significant seasonal distress. The psychometric properties of the SPAQ are reviewed elsewhere in this volume (see the chapter by Mersch).

Personal Inventory for Depression and SAD (PIDS) (Terman and Williams 1998). The PIDS is a four-part instrument that combines two basic items of the SPAQ — global seasonality ratings and identification of best and worst months — with a DSM-IV-based assessment of a major depressive episode (during the past year) based on an algorithm from established self-report instrument (Spitzer *et al.* 1994, 1999) and a checklist for atypical neurovegetative symptoms with winter exacerbation. Developed as a primary-care doctor's office questionnaire, it is quickly rated and scored and useful as a preliminary screen for clinically significant seasonality that would merit light therapy or other treatment. A self-assessment version (PIDS-SA) includes a scoring and interpretation guide for the patient or consumer, with guidance on when physician referral is indicated. This version has been downloaded thousands of times from <*www.cet.org*> on the web.

Seasonal Health Questionnaire (SHQ) (Thompson and Cowan 2001). The SHQ seeks a provisional diagnosis of SAD by probing for symptoms of a major depressive disorder in the past 10 years, identifying the predominant season and number of consecutive years of occurrence, and identifying the number of non-seasonal episodes. Unlike the SPAQ and PIDS, it does not generate a global seasonality score, although subsyndromal SAD or minor depression might be inferred from reports of depressive symptoms that fall short of criteria for a major depressive episode. By comparison with the SPAQ, application of the SHQ in community samples and clinical groups may provide more valid prevalence estimates of SAD defined in terms of DSM and ICD criteria. Direct structured interview assessments (for example, Levitt *et al.* 1997) would, of course, go the extra mile toward establishing an epidemiological profile of the disorder.

14.3 **Diagnosis and symptom severity**

Structured Clinical Interview for DSM-IV Axis I Disorders (SCID) (First *et al.* 1995). The SCID provides a comprehensive, reliable assessment of primary psychiatric disorders including major depressive episodes (MDEs) in bipolar I and II disorders, and recurrent major depressive disorder. These specific diagnoses can earn a seasonal pattern specifier, which provides an operational definition of SAD that requires MDEs in the past two years. The research community has favoured a less restrictive definition (for example, Rosenthal *et al.* 1984*b*), considering that patients may have received successful treatment in the past two years or travelled toward the equator in winter, thus attenuating symptoms as gauged against a long-term, clinically severe history (Rosenthal and Terman 1993).

Diagnostic Interview for Atypical Depression (DIAD) (Terman *et al.* 1998*a*). Although atypical neurovegetative symptoms characterize most SAD patients, the items scrutinized by the SIGH-SAD (see next section) only partially overlap DSM-IV criteria for depression with atypical features, and indeed overlook the prerequisite indication of this classically chronic disorder — mood reactivity (transient positive response to pleasurable events). The DIAD includes 10 structured items that identify and scale all symptoms contributory to a DSM-IV diagnosis, with quantitative criteria for weight gain and hypersomnia, and delicate probing for rejection sensitivity which otherwise can be awkward to assess before a doctor/patient relationship has been well established. While the SIGH-SAD heavily scores fatigability among atypical symptoms, fatigability is indistinct from leaden paralysis (sensations of heaviness). The DIAD specifically identifies leaden sensations as contributory to the DSM-IV diagnosis.

Notably, the precision of questioning far exceeds that of the brief SCID survey of atypical features (First *et al.* 1995). DIAD inter-rater reliability, based on two independent ratings, is high (κ=0.77, n = 36). Importantly, raters agreed on whether patients were mood reactive in all cases (Rifkin *et al.* 1999). The instrument may serve to extend the phenomenology of SAD if patients are shown to have atypical features beyond the neurovegetative spectrum. For example, an unpublished study (M. Terman) using the instrument indicated that 94 per cent of a sample of SAD patients (n = 36) were mood reactive and 57 per cent met DSM-IV criteria for depression with atypical features.

Structured Interview Guide for the Hamilton Depression Rating Scale — Seasonal Affective Disorder Version (SIGH-SAD) (Williams *et al.* 1994). From the earliest studies of SAD (for example, Rosenthal *et al.* 1984*b*) it was apparent that the severity of winter depression could not adequately be described using the original Hamilton rating scale — which was designed to assess the severity of melancholic depression — when atypical symptoms often were prominent. The SIGH-SAD merged a structured interview for the 21-item Hamilton scale (SIGH-D) (Williams 1988) with eight additional items intended to describe atypical characteristics of SAD patients (expanded from Rosenthal *et al.* 1987*a*). The latter set emphasizes neurovegetative features of fatigability and afternoon slump, appetitive symptoms and weight gain, and hypersomnia. Although a further item on this subscale, social withdrawal, also characterizes patients with melancholia, the global ratio of 'atypical' symptom score to total SIGH-SAD score has been shown to be a strong statistical predictor of response to light therapy in SAD patients (Terman *et al.* 1996). Furthermore, the instrument shows a high intra-class correlation coefficient ($r = 0.95$, n = 318) based on two independent, same-day, live interviews (Terman *et al.* 1998*b*).

A self-report questionnaire version (SIGH-SAD-SR) is useful for time sampling of symptoms (for example, Terman *et al.* 1994) and out-patient monitoring in open treatment. This instrument also provides a valuable check on interviewer ratings. In protocols at the Columbia Clinical Chronobiology Program (for example, Terman *et al.* 1998*b*) patients complete both interview and self-report versions at each clinic visit. If there is an item score discrepancy of two points or more between these two versions, the interviewer is directed to continue questioning before the final SIGH-SAD score is established. With its more comprehensive assessment of depressive symptoms than the Hamilton scale, the SIGH-SAD is valuable for treatment assessment in patients with either seasonal or non-seasonal depression. In studies of light therapy for SAD, an entry score of 20 points or more (with a Hamilton score of at least 10 and an atypical symptom score of at least 5), and a remission criterion of 8 points or less, have been used effectively to discriminate active from placebo treatments (Terman *et al.* 1998*b*).

Hypomania Interview Guide (including Hyperthymia) (HIGH) (Williams *et al.* 1999). The structured HIGH instruments scrutinize a selected week (retrospectively, HIGH-R; current, HIGH-C) for 15 symptoms that typify hypomanic or manic episodes and subsyndromal hyperthymic episodes, measuring symptom severity on a 4-point scale. Current state also can be self-rated (HIGH-C-SR), allowing a check on interviewer ratings and facilitating time sampling outside the clinic to follow seasonal course. (These instruments supersede the HIGH-SAD used in earlier research.) A diagnostic algorithm based on 10 of the items allows a DSM-IV diagnosis of hypomanic episode. Additional items outside the scope of DSM-IV are increased energy, social activity, sexual thoughts and activity, sharpened and unusually clear thinking, and decreased eating.

The HIGH-R, focused on the 'highest week ever', shows excellent internal consistency ($\alpha = 0.75$), and the total score identifies unipolar, bipolar I, and bipolar II SAD patients in 75 per cent to 86 per cent of cases (n = 72) (Goel *et al.* 1999). In SAD treatment studies, the HIGH-C complements the SIGH-SAD for a thorough clinical evaluation of patients who show remission of depressive symptoms. Like the SIGH-SAD, the HIGH instruments are applicable for both seasonal and non-seasonal patients.

14.4 Note on instrument translations

With the international research effort into SAD, rating scale scores for the structured interviews — especially the SIGH-SAD — have been reported in the literature without qualification about the status of the translation. The reliability of ad hoc translations is open to question. Author-approved versions of the instruments require preparation according to a standard protocol: initial translation by a clinically knowledgeable colleague, independent back-translation into English, review of the back-translated version by the authors with suggested editorial changes, and re-translation into the target language. When interview scores or diagnostic summaries are reported in the literature, those based on ad hoc translations should include a statement such as 'Urdu version without back-translation'. Ideally, we should see 'Urdu version, author-approved with back-translation'.

14.5 Ancillary instruments

Daily sleep log and mood/energy ratings (Terman 1990). Patients maintain this chart by noting, upon awakening, their best recollection of time asleep the previous night and napping during the previous day, in 15-minute segments. They also enter global mood/energy ratings on an 11-point scale (worst ever = 0; normal = 5; best ever = 10), which is useful for tracking transient changes — sometimes marked, and which the SIGH-SAD cannot detect — during depressive episodes, under treatment, and during withdrawals. Sleep log data also often differ markedly from retrospective reports of sleep in the SIGH-SAD, both in day-to-day variability and average duration. In a recent application, 7-day averages of sleep onset and offset are computed during a depressive episode preceding light therapy. A normogram based on the derived sleep midpoint (Terman *et al.* 1998*c*) specifies an optimum morning treatment interval — about 3 hours after the sleep midpoint or 9 hours after melatonin onset — when circadian phase advances are maximized (Terman et al. 2001).

Columbia eye examination for users of light therapy (Gallin *et al.* 1993). Luckily for the field, extensive ophthalmologic examination of SAD patients before and after light therapy thus far has revealed no clinically significant changes (Gallin *et al.* 1995). However, the plethora of light-box types, with significant variation in radiation spectra within and outside the visible range, and potential concern about treatment for patients with pre-existing or suspected future retinal conditions, mandates continued vigilance (Remé *et al.* 1996). A structured eye examination chart was designed by a committee of ophthalmologists and SAD specialists to provide a basic comprehensive screening composed of conventional ocular tests, for completion by ophthalmologists or optometrists, with periodic follow-up as indicated.

Resources

The SPAQ form was published in Rosenthal *et al.* (1987*b*). The Columbia Clinical Assessment Tools Packet (PIDS, DIAD, SIGH-SAD, SIGH-SAD-SR, HIGH-R, HIGH-C, HIGH-C-SR, daily log and eye examination chart), with instructions and interpretation guides, is distributed by the Center for Environmental Therapeutics, 767 Broadway, Norwood, NJ 07648, USA; <www.cet.org>; e-mail <*info@cet.org*>.

Acknowledgements

Development of Columbia assessment tools was sponsored in part by grant MH42931 from the US National Institute of Mental Health.

References

Enns, M.W., Levitan, R.D., Levitt, A.J., Dalton, E.J., and Lam, R.W. (1999) Diagnosis, epidemiology, and pathophysiology. In *Canadian consensus guidelines for the treatment of seasonal affective disorder* (ed. R.W. Lam and A.J. Levitt), pp. 20–63. Clinical and Academic Publishing, Vancouver BC.

First, M.B., Spitzer, R.L., Gibbon, M., and Williams, J.B.W. (1995) *Structured Clinical Interview for DSM-IV Axis I Disorders — Patient Edition (SCID-P)*. New York State Psychiatric Institute, New York.

Gallin, P.F., Terman, M., Remé, C.E., Rafferty, B., and Burde, R.M. (1993) *The Columbia eye examination for users of light treatment*. New York State Psychiatric Institute, New York.

Gallin, P.F., Terman, M., Remé, C.E., Rafferty, B., Terman, J.S., and Burde, R.M. (1995) Ophthalmologic examination of patients with seasonal affective disorder, before and after bright light therapy. *American Journal of Ophthalmology* 119:202–10.

Goel, N., Terman, M., Terman, J.S., and Williams, J.B.W. (1999) Summer mood in winter depressives: validation of a structured interview. *Depression and Anxiety* 9:83–91.

Kasper, S., Wehr, T.A., Bartko, J.J., Gaist, P.A., and Rosenthal, N.E. (1989) Epidemiological findings of seasonal changes in mood and behavior: a telephone survey of Montgomery County, Maryland. *Archives of General Psychiatry* 46:823–33.

Levitt, A.J., Boyle, M., and Joffe, R.T. (1997) Latitude and the variation in seasonal depression and seasonality of depressive symptoms. *Society for Light Treatment and Biological Rhythms Abstracts* 9:14.

Remé, C.E., Rol, P., Kaase, H., and Terman, M. (1996) Bright light therapy in focus: lamp emission spectra and ocular safety. *Technology and Health Care* 4:403–13.

Rifkin, J.B., Terman, M., Williams, J.B.W., Stewart, J.W., Goel, N., and Terman, J.S. (1999) Assessment of atypical depression in seasonal affective disorder. *Society for Light Treatment and Biological Rhythms Abstracts* 11:23.

Rosen, L.N., Targum, S.D., Terman, M., Bryant, M.J., Hoffman, H., Kasper, S.F., *et al.* (1990) Prevalence of seasonal affective disorder at four latitudes. *Psychiatry Research* 31:131–44.

Rosenthal, N.E., Bradt, G.J., and Wehr, T.A. (1984a) *Seasonal Pattern Assessment Questionnaire (SPAQ)*. National Institute of Mental Health, Bethesda MD.

Rosenthal, N.E., Sack, D.A., Gillin, J.C., Lewy, A.J., Goodwin, F.K., Davenport, Y., *et al.* (1984b) Seasonal affective disorder: a description of the syndrome and preliminary findings with light therapy. *Archives of General Psychiatry* 41:72–80.

Rosenthal N.E., Genhart M., Jacobsen F.M., Skwerer R.G., Wehr T.A. (1987a) Disturbances of appetite and weight regulation in seasonal affective disorder. *Annals of the New York Academy of Sciences* 499:216–30.

Rosenthal, N.E., Genhart, M.J., Sack, D.A., Skwerer, R.G., and Wehr, T.A. (1987b) Seasonal affective disorder and its relevance for the understanding and treatment of bulimia. In *The psychology of bulimia* (ed. J.I. Hudson and H.G. Pope Jr), pp. 205–28. American Psychiatric Press, Washington DC.

Rosenthal, N.E. and Terman, M. (1993) DSM-IV debate continues. *Light Treatment and Biological Rhythms Abstracts* 6:18.

Spitzer, R.L., Williams, J.B.W., Kroenke, K., Linzer, M., deGruy III, F.V., Hahn, S.R., *et al.* (1994) Utility of a new procedure for diagnosing mental disorders in primary care. The PRIME-MED 1000 study. *Journal of the American Medical Association* 272:1749–56.

Spitzer, R.L., Kroenke, K., and Williams, J.B.W. (1999) Validation and utility of a self-report version of the PRIME-MD: the PHQ primary care study. *Journal of the American Medical Association* 282:1737–44.

Terman, M. (1988) On the question of mechanism in phototherapy for seasonal affective disorder: considerations of clinical efficacy and epidemiology. *Journal of Biological Rhythms* 3:155–72.

Terman, M. (1990) *Daily sleep log and mood/energy ratings*. New York State Psychiatric Institute, New York.

Terman, M. and Williams, J.B.W. (1998) Personal inventory for depression and SAD (PIDS). *Journal of Practical Psychiatry and Behavioral Health* 5:301–3.

Terman, M., Terman, J.S., Quitkin, F.M., McGrath, P.J., Stewart, J.W., and Rafferty, B. (1989) Light therapy for seasonal affective disorder: a review of efficacy. *Neuropsychopharmacology* 2:1–22.

Terman, J.S., Terman, M., and Amira, L. (1994) One-week light treatment of winter depression at its onset: the time course of relapse. *Depression* 2:20–31.

Terman, M., Amira, L., Terman, J.S., and Ross, D.C. (1996) Predictors of response and nonresponse to light treatment for winter depression. *American Journal of Psychiatry* 153:1423–9.

Terman, M., Rifkin, J.B., Stewart, J.W., and Williams, J.B.W. (1998a) *Diagnostic Interview for Atypical Depression (DIAD)*. New York State Psychiatric Institute, New York.

Terman, M., Terman, J.S., and Ross, D.C. (1998*b*) A controlled trial of timed bright light and negative air ionization for treatment of winter depression. *Archives of General Psychiatry* **55**:875–82.

Terman, M., Terman, J.S., and Williams, J.B.W. (1998*c*) Seasonal affective disorder and its treatments. *Journal of Practical Psychiatry and Behavioral Health* **5**:287–300.

Terman, J.S., Terman, M., Lo, E.-S., and Cooper, T.B. (2001) Circadian time of morning light administration and therapeutic response in winter depression, *Archives of General Psychiatry* **58**:69-75

Thompson, C., Rodin, I., and Birtwhistle, J. (1999) Light therapy for seasonal and nonseasonal affective disorder: a Cochrane meta-analysis. *Society for Light Treatment and Biological Rhythms Abstracts* **11**:11.

Thompson, C. and Cowan, A. (2001) The seasonal health questionnaire: a preliminary validation of a new instrument to screen for seasonal affective disorder. *Journal of Affective Disorders* (in press).

Williams, J.B.W. (1988) A structured interview guide for the Hamilton depression rating scale. *Archives of General Psychiatry* **45**:742–7.

Williams, J.B.W., Link, M.J., Rosenthal, N.E., Amira, L., and Terman, M. (1994) *Structured Interview Guide for the Hamilton Depression Rating Scale — Seasonal Affective Disorder Version (SIGH-SAD)* (revised edn). New York State Psychiatric Institute, New York.

Williams, J.B.W., Terman, M., Link, M.J., Amira, L., and Rosenthal, N.E. (1999) Hypomania interview guide (including hyperthymia), retrospective assessment version (HIGH-R). *Depression and Anxiety* **9**:92–100.

Wirz–Justice, A., Graw, P., and Recker, S. (1993) The seasonal pattern assessment questionnaire (SPAQ): some comments. *Light Treatment and Biological Rhythms* **5**:31–2.

Chapter 15

Evidence-based treatment

Chris Thompson

15.1 Introduction

Whenever a new medical syndrome is recognized, questions are inevitably raised about its validity. SAD has been no exception. There are a number of ways to counter sceptical voices in such a debate. Clinical features, such as the distinctiveness of the syndrome or a tendency to breed true in family histories, are helpful indicators. However, it is the syndrome's ability to predict a distinct prognosis, and an unusual response to a current or novel treatment that gives it clinical utility in everyday practice and transports the discussion from the sterile groves of academe to the consulting room and the clinical interface. In the case of SAD, the pattern of relapse and remission is distinctive and the response to light therapy appears to set it apart from non-seasonal depressions. Both of these propositions have been the subject of research, and it is the latter that forms the subject of this chapter.

This chapter will, therefore, explore the evidence that SAD responds to light therapy and that this response is specific; non-seasonal depression having either no response or a much smaller response to treatment. If the latter were true, it would further validate the syndrome of SAD, even though it might be disappointing to some psychiatrists and patients who would like to have an alternative treatment for the wider class of depression.

Two further questions will be addressed. First, does light therapy work better at certain times of day? If so, it might lend support to the circadian hypothesis of aetiology. Second, does SAD, like other forms of depression, respond to pharmacological antidepressants? If so, this would provide a useful second intervention should light therapy fail or be too inconvenient for the patient.

15.2 Light therapy

This section is based on the results of a meta-analysis of randomized controlled trials of bright light carried out at the University of Southampton).

The principle of randomization is now established as the foundation of modern trial methodology, since it removes many of the potential sources of bias. Randomized controlled trials (RCTs) are therefore recognized as the most appropriate design for therapeutic trials. However, many RCTs have methodological flaws that limit their validity, producing variability between the results of trials of the same treatment. For this reason, the highest tier of the hierarchy of evidence in medicine (Sackett *et al.* 1997) is a meta-analysis of several RCTs obtained from a systematic review of the literature, such as that to be described here.

Many aspects of bright-light treatment remain controversial, even after more than 15 years of research. The role of placebo mechanisms (patient expectations) and the optimum timing and daily duration of treatment have not been convincingly settled by any single study. Treatment trials have generally had small numbers, with widely varying designs and objectives, making them difficult to interpret.

As is often the case, the design of treatment trials of light has improved over time, and so three of the largest studies of bright-light treatment have been published most recently (Eastman *et al.* 1998; Terman *et al.* 1998; Lewy *et al.* 1998). Two of these found bright light to be superior to treatment with negative ion generators which were either inactivated or used at subtherapeutic doses (Terman *et al.* 1998; Eastman *et al.* 1998). All three studies found early-morning treatment to be superior to treatment in the evening. While there appeared to be general agreement across the three studies, their results were not consistent across all outcome measures. Most notably the duration of treatment and the definition of response varied. Two studies used only a 2-week treatment period (Lewy *et al.* 1998, Terman *et al.* 1998), but the third found that significant differences between phototherapy and placebo did not start emerging until 3 weeks and that morning light was only superior to evening light when a strict definition of response was used (Eastman *et al.* 1998).

In addition to individual studies, there have been four previous attempts to carry out systematic reviews and meta-analyses of phototherapy studies. Terman *et al.* (1989) pooled individual subject data from all studies completed by the end of winter 1986–87. Trials were identified through the authors' extensive knowledge of the field and individual trialists were approached for raw data. Bright light was found to be superior to dim light, with treatment in the morning being more effective than at other times of day. Tam *et al.* (1995) updated this approach by using MEDLINE to identify studies of 'Seasonal affective disorder, therapy' published between January 1989 and March 1995, but no attempt was made to pool data across studies. Lee *et al.* (1997*a* and *b*), in two articles, used an exhaustive search procedure to identify published and unpublished studies of light treatment in SAD up to August 1994. The main conclusions were that light given in the morning and evening was superior to light given at a single time each day and that blue, green, and yellow wavelengths, but not red or ultraviolet, were essential to the therapeutic effect of light treatment.

However, none of these reviews excluded non-randomized trials, thus introducing potentially powerful sources of bias and artificially increasing the apparent size of the clinical effect. Second, many of the trials included were crossover studies, which is a poor design for antidepressant studies (Sibbald and Roberts 1998). A particular problem in crossover studies is that order effects have been shown unequivocally, that is, the effect of the treatment depends on whether it is given first or second (Terman *et al.* 1998). All previous reviews have included data from both stages of the crossover trials, thus introducing this confounder.

15.2.1 A new systematic review and meta-analysis of RCTs of light treatment

In our study, we carried out a meta-analysis of only *randomized* controlled trials of light therapy identified through a systematic search strategy. Studies of both seasonal and non-seasonal affective disorders were included.

Four databases were searched: MEDLINE, January 1982 to February 1998, using the terms 'depressive disorders', 'seasonal affective disorder', 'season*', or 'winter' and 'phototherapy' or 'light'; EMBASE, January 1982 to February 1998, using the terms 'affective neurosis', 'depressi*', 'season*', or 'winter' and 'phototherapy' or 'light'; PSYCHLIT, 1990 to 1996, using the search terms 'depressi*', 'affective', 'season*', or 'winter' and 'phototherapy' or 'light'; and, finally, the Cochrane database of randomized controlled trials of depression, anxiety, and neurosis was searched.

Non-English language articles were included. The reference lists of the identified articles were also searched for otherwise missed articles, and key contributors to the literature were contacted for unexpressed data or missed articles. The results of the search were carefully screened in three stages. The first stage identified all original studies in which standardized assessment of symptoms had been performed in subjects with depressive disorders, before and after treatment with bright-light therapy. In the second stage, all articles were identified in which there was both random allocation of subjects and more than one treatment condition, at least one of which was bright-light therapy. Duplicate publications were removed. In the third stage, we identified studies from which we could extract the chosen outcome measure, which was the proportion of subjects responding to treatment according to their scores on the longest version of the Hamilton Depression Rating Scale (HDRS) used in each study. Response rates were defined in one or both of the following ways.

1. a reduction in HDRS score of at least 50 per cent ('responder');

2. a final HDRS score of 8 or less, as well as a reduction of at least 50 per cent ('remitter').

For each study, we recorded a range of quality indicators, such as the diagnostic criteria, crossover or parallel design, the treatments applied, the duration of the study, the 'blindness' of raters, the number of drop outs, and whether analysis was by intention to treat. We also recorded any evidence that randomization was concealed, since failure to conceal the randomization schedule from the researchers has been shown to artificially raise effect sizes in RCTs (Schulz et al. 1995).

Because of the order effects previously identified in crossover trials, only data for the first treatment received in such studies was included. This eliminated contaminated data from the second arm, but also allowed the inclusion of subjects who had completed the first treatment condition but dropped out in the second treatment.

We found 46 studies that unequivocally met our fundamental quality criterion of randomization. The full list will be included in an article currently in preparation and can be obtained from the author (see list of contributors for contact details). A preliminary overview showed that there were sufficient studies to allow five separate analyses.

1. 16 studies compared different amounts of light delivered by a light-box to SAD patients. This definition included comparisons of different intensities and different durations, as well as comparisons of phototherapy with a control condition predicted to be inactive. The higher 'dose' was entered as the experimental treatment with the other treatment condition(s) as the control.

2. 14 studies compared the light-box treatment of SAD patients with the same 'dose' at different times of day. Morning treatment was entered as the experimental condition with treatment at any later time in the day as the control.

3. 6 studies used a light-visor in SAD. Light of higher intensity was entered as the experimental treatment with light of lower intensity as the control.

4. 5 studies used a light-box in non-seasonal depressive disorder. Light of higher intensity was entered as the experimental treatment with light of lower intensity as the control.

5. 5 studies used dawn simulation, but these will not be described further.

The data were analysed by the Cochrane Collaborations Review Manager software package.

Treatment of SAD with a light-box

Only one of these studies described the method of concealing treatment allocation; 2 of the 16 studies of light 'dosing' were excluded because of insufficient data. Of the remaining 14 studies, 9 used a crossover design. They had widely variable washout arrangements (a period of no treatment between experimental conditions) 2 had a set period, 4 required relapse to a minimum HDRS score within a set period, 2 required relapse to a minimum HDRS score or a set period, and 1 had no washout period.

The difference in the dose of light was achieved broadly in three ways: a brighter vs. dimmer light source, a longer vs. shorter daily duration, or light therapy vs. a non-light comparator condition.

The responder analysis showed greater exposure to light to be more effective than less exposure with an odds ratio (OR) for active to control condition of 2.83 (CI 1.84 to 4.35). Only the longer vs. shorter subanalysis failed to show a difference between treatments. For the total sample, the absolute risk reduction (ARR) was 0.28, leading to a 'number needed to treat' (NNT) of 4. This means that four patients need to be treated with the experimental condition to get one extra responder compared to the control condition, which is a respectable effect size for a medical treatment.

Four of the studies of morning vs. later light were excluded from the analysis because of serious methodological flaws or insufficient data; 8 of the remaining 10 studies used a crossover design with variable washout arrangements (5 had a set period, 2 had no washout, and 1 required relapse to a minimum HDRS score after 2 weeks).

In the responder analysis, there was no significant difference between morning and other timings. However, when we took remission as the endpoint, morning light was superior to other times (OR 2.01; CI 1.27 to 3.18; ARR 0.15; NNT 7).

The question of timing was then explored further by comparing type 1 studies where light was given only in the morning or only in the evening, using the apparently less sensitive responder criterion. In the morning, active treatment was superior to control (OR 2.34, CI 1.37 to 4.00), but in the evening, it was not (OR 1.49, CI 0.82 to 2.69). Although this analysis further supports the superiority of morning light, it is a post-hoc comparison of two separate groups of studies, so the result may be explained by methodological variations.

Treatment of SAD with a light-visor

There were 6 studies of light-visors in SAD; 5 of these compared treatment with light of different intensities and were analysed. All had a parallel design with blind raters, but only one reported the method of allocation concealment. Light intensity fell into three groups (3500–7600 lx, 400–650 lx, and < 100 lx). None of the studies individually found a difference in therapeutic effect between these intensities. The combined statistical power of all 5 studies was insufficient to demonstrate a significant effect (OR 1.32, CI 0.78 to 2.25).

Only 2 studies compared light-visor and light-box treatment, and we were unable to combine the results, as one had a crossover design with insufficient data to calculate response rate to the first treatment received. The other study had a parallel design and found that 7 out of 12 patients responded to 7600-lux light-visor treatment and 3 out of 9 responded to 650-lux light-box treatment.

Treatment of non-seasonal depressive disorder with a light-box

Five studies of this type met the inclusion criteria, and 4 had sufficient data for pooling. The odds ratios decreased markedly with increasing sample size, and there was marked heterogeneity between study results. The pooled odds ratio was not significantly greater than 1 (OR 3.05, 95 per cent; CIs 0.86 to 10.82). Thus, even though the odds ratio appears high, these results do not support the efficacy of light therapy in non-seasonal affective disorder.

Summary of the effects of light therapy

1. In SAD, phototherapy by a light-box is superior to control treatments.

This finding appears to be robust, but the difficulty in blinding patients to treatment in phototherapy trials means that non-biological mechanisms, such as treatment expectations, may have contributed to it. If placebo effects can only be maintained over short treatment periods, this reinforces the need for longer duration trials lasting 6 to 12 weeks. Nevertheless, with an NNT of 4 to 5, the short-term effect of this form of light treatment in SAD is equivalent in importance to tricyclics for dysthymia (NNT 4) and clozapine induction of improvement in treatment-resistant schizophrenia (NNT 6).

2. Morning phototherapy may be superior to treatment later in the day.

Morning phototherapy is more likely to produce remission than phototherapy later in the day, with a trend in the same direction for responder rates. Why effect sizes should be greater for remission rather than responder rates is uncertain. One possible reason is that differences in the time of day may be more pronounced among cases of milder severity, which are more likely to fall below a HDRS of 8 with a 50 per cent improvement. Eastman et al. (1998) have concluded that the failure to demonstrate a consistent treatment effect across all outcome measures suggests that difference between treatment is not robust. Our estimated NNT of 7 (that is, treating 7 patients in the morning will lead to 1 extra remission compared to later in the day) is respectable, if not decisive.

3. Treatment with a light-visor was no more effective with higher than with lower intensities.

This result casts doubt on the effectiveness of the visor method of delivery of light, since the basic tenet of all light-therapy studies is that bright light should be more effective than dim light. It is unclear why visors should be less effective than light-boxes. In general, the quality of the studies is higher than in the earlier light-box studies, so poor methodology is not to blame for this negative result. All had parallel groups, most were of 2 weeks duration, and the sample sizes were greater than in the light-box studies. Direct comparisons of light-boxes vs. light-visors are few, but do not demonstrate inferiority of the light-visor. Therefore, one interpretation of this finding is that light therapy itself is ineffective, since there was no strong a priori reason to separate light given by these two modalities. The light-visor studies have superior design characteristics, and there is no credible reason why they should be less effective than light-boxes (nor is there empirical evidence in direct comparisons that they are less effective). This inconsistency must be explored further in future.

4. Non-seasonal depressive disorder

At first sight, the results of the studies in non-seasonal affective disorder appear to support a non-specific effect of light on depression. However, these studies have marked heterogeneity due to the one unusual study with only a one-day outcome assessment. When this is removed, the result is no longer significant. Thus, until further studies are available, phototherapy must be assumed to be specific to SAD.

Comment on the methodology of light-therapy trials

The decision to include only randomized controlled trials removed the most important sources of bias in previous meta-analyses and, as expected, produced a more conservative estimate of the size of the treatment effect. The decision to include only the first treatment in crossover studies removed additional bias due to order effects and was further justified by finding marked variations in the definitions of washout periods.

Randomization alone is no longer the only security required in controlled trials. Unless the randomization code is concealed from the clinical trialists (for example, by being held at a distant site), the effect size is increased by about 30 per cent (Schultz *et al.* 1995). All but one of the included studies failed to report the steps taken to ensure allocation concealment. This bias would probably occur less in crossover studies, because investigators would have expected all subjects to receive all treatments. Inclusion of only the first treatment in our analysis should therefore have reduced the allocation bias that might have been a problem in the parallel studies. In fact, in the type 1 studies, three of the four with a parallel design had odds ratios less than the overall pooled estimate. In the type 2 studies, the four with a parallel design had the lowest odds ratios. Therefore, poor allocation concealment may not have had a large influence on the results. Even if one assumes that it did operate to the degree found by Schulz *et al.* (1995), it would only have increased the NNT for SAD treatment from 4 to 5.

Another limitation of the studies is their very short treatment duration. Thus, our positive findings relate only to the first 2 to 4 weeks of treatment. Few studies report the methods used to ensure the independence of raters, for example, by asking them to guess which treatment the patients had received. Sample sizes were too small in all studies. A power calculation drawn from the effect size of the meta-analysis suggests a sample size of 106 patients per group, to allow for 20 per cent drop outs, in order to achieve an 80 per cent probability of 5 per cent significance. 'Intention to treat' analyses were seldom performed, most studies being based on those who completed treatment, especially in crossover studies.

A key question for the field has been the attempt to develop a credible 'placebo' treatment for light. Although this has added substantially to knowledge in the field, it now appears more important to correct the fundamental design flaws as described in this chapter than to pursue ever more abstruse pseudo-placebos. Many well-developed treatments in medicine and psychiatry, such as behaviour therapy, are supported by RCTs that are not placebo-controlled, and so the absence of a credible placebo should not unduly concern evidence-based practitioners.

15.3 **Antidepressants**

There are very few clinical trials on the use of antidepressants in specifically winter depression. Extrapolation may be appropriate from the effects of antidepressants on depression with atypical symptoms (non-seasonal), since the range of symptoms is similar. Many patients who attend a specialist SAD clinic have already tried a range of antidepressants in previous winters, and clinically it is therefore possible to make educated guesses about the most and least appropriate classes of drug. Most patients with winter depression actively avoid tricyclics because of their sedative properties. Monoamine oxidase inhibitors might be expected to be effective for the atypical syndrome, but few use them due to the risk of adverse reactions. In bipolar SAD, lithium may be indicated after the first few attacks of hypomania, if they are severe enough to merit intervention.

It is the class of SSRIs in which treatment trials are most available. Sertraline shows clear evidence for effectiveness in SAD from one RCT (Moscovitch *et al.* forthcoming). Fluoxetine is also widely used; there have been two studies of this drug, one with positive results and one negative. The evidence from these studies in which SAD is the specific indication, taken together with the serotonergic deficit in the pathophysiology of SAD (see the chapter by Neumeister *et al.*), make SSRIs the treatment of first choice for patients who either do not respond sufficiently to light therapy or whose schedules do not allow time for enough exposure.

There remain many questions about the use of antidepressants in SAD. For example, after a patient has responded to treatment, how long should they remain on it? Usually a major depressive episode should be treated for 4 to 6 months after recovery. If there have been a number of recent recurrences, the recommendation is to treat for 5 years. Do these apply to winter SAD? Can SSRIs prevent the onset of the next winter episode, if the patient remains on it through the summer when he or she would not normally need the treatment? If so, the treatment strategy is clear — prophylaxis is indicated for those with an established cycle. If not, then prophylaxis may do harm, since the patient will be taking treatment in summer for no reason. In addition, in order to achieve remission in the autumn, they may need to increase the dose, each year until intolerable side-effects occur. At present, there are no trials addressing this crucial point, but my own practice is to discontinue the drug after the expected date of remission, unless there are continuing symptoms. The advantages of doing so are that, if a new episode appears the following autumn, the patient can go back on the antidepressant that worked the previous winter.

What can be done if both light and SSRIs have failed to be effective? As with all treatment-resistant depression, there is very little research evidence for effectiveness of any single intervention, except the addition of lithium to an antidepressant. For example, there is no formal safety and efficacy data on the combination of light and SSRIs, but there have been many years of clinical experience and no reported adverse effects of this common strategy. Increasing the light-therapy dose to the maximum tolerated (usually limited by feasibility rather than side-effects) can sometimes be helpful. Increasing the dose of the SSRI can also be helpful.

In non-seasonal depression, there is evidence that the dual-acting antidepressants, such as tricyclics, venlafaxine, and mirtazapine, are more effective than the SSRIs. The choice between them depends on the patient's symptom profile. Particularly male patients, with the less common combination of a seasonal cycle and classical endogenous symptoms, may benefit from tricyclics or mirtazapine, since they improve sleep and increase appetite. However, the majority of patients (females with the atypical syndrome) are more likely to respond without adverse effects to venlafaxine, which also has a wide dose range and evidence for a dose response curve. It can therefore be started at a low dose at the beginning of winter and increased in line with the severity of the syndrome, reducing towards the spring as remission is expected.

15.4 Conclusion

The treatment of winter depression with light therapy using a light-box has considerable clinical and research evidence in its favour. However, there remain certain crucial questions that must be answered. One strategy would be to carry out a trial of light therapy which was pragmatic (perhaps an open comparison with an antidepressant), with a parallel-group design using concealment of randomization and blind raters over a 6 to 8 week treatment period (or even a whole winter). Recruitment should be by screening clinic attenders to reduce the treatment expectations seen in self-selected patients. Analysis should be by intention to treat with robust endpoints such as remission. The numbers entered should be about 120 per group. Although this would be a challenging study to undertake, it will have to be done if light therapy is to move into the group of widely accepted treatments in medicine.

References

Eastman, C.I., Young, M.A., Fogg, L.F., Liu, L., and Meaden, P.M. (1998) Bright light treatment of winter depression. *Arch Gen Psychiatry*, **55**:883–9.

Lee, T.M.C., Blashko, C.A., Janzen, H.L., Paterson, J.G., and Chan, C.C.H. (1997) Pathophysiological mechanism of seasonal affective disorder. *J Affect Disord*, **46**:25–38.

Lee, T.M.C., Chan, C.C.H., Paterson, J.G., Janzen, H.L., and Blashko, C.A. (1997) Spectral properties of phototherapy for seasonal affective disorder: a meta analysis. *Acta Psychiatr Scand*, **96**:117–21.

Lewy, A.J., Bauer, V.K., Cutl er, N.L., Sack, R.L., Ahmed, S., and Thomas, K.H., *et al.* (1998) Morning vs evening light treatment of patients with winter depression. *Arch Gen Psychiatry*, **55**:890–6.

Moscovitch, A., Blashko, C.A., Eagles, J.M., Darcourt, G., Thompson, C., Kasper, S., *et al.* (forthcoming) A placebo controlled trial of sertraline in the treatment of outpatients with seasonal affective disorder. *J Clin Psychopharmacology*.

Sackett, D., Richardson, W.S., Rosenberg, W., and Haynes, R.B. (1997) *Evidence based medicine.* Churchill Livingstone, New York.

Schulz, K.F., Chalmers, I.C., Hayes, R.J., and Altman, D.G. (1995) Empirical evidence of bias. *JAMA*, **273**:408–12.

Sibbald, B. and Roberts, C. (1998) *Crossover trials.* **BMJ**, 316:1719.

Tam, E.M., Lam, R.W., and Levitt, A.J. (1995) Treatment of seasonal affective disorder: a review, *Can J Psychiatry*, **40**:457–66.

Terman, M., Terman, J.S., Quitkin, F.M., McGrath, P.J., Stewart, J.W., and Rafferty, B. (1989) Light therapy for seasonal affective disorder: a review of efficacy, *Neuropsychopharmacology*, **2**:1–22.

Terman, M., Terman, J.S., and Ross, D.C. (1998) A controlled trial of timed bright light and negative air ionization for treatment of winter depression. *Arch Gen Psychiatry*, **55**:875–82.

Part two

Pathogenesis

Chapter 16

The photoperiod

Bengt F. Kjellman

16.1 Introduction

In animals, seasonal photoperiodic changes are of importance since they affect behaviour and physiology. Seasonal breeding in certain species is regulated by photoperiodic changes (Hoffmann 1981). Hibernation has some features in common with winter SAD.

Since winter SAD usually begins in the fall/autumn when the photoperiod is diminishing in time, and since the first successful treatments of patients with winter SAD were performed by extending the photoperiod (Lewy *et al.* 1982; Rosenthal *et al.* 1984, 1985; Wirz–Justice *et al.* 1986), changes in the photoperiod were initially considered to be of importance for the pathogenesis of winter SAD. However, later studies by Wehr *et al.* (1986), Hellekson *et al.* (1986), and Isaacs *et al.* (1988) showed that light may have therapeutic effects in winter SAD without photoperiodic extension.

16.2 Latitude

If the photoperiod is a part of the pathogenesis of winter SAD, the larger photoperiodic variance over the season at higher latitudes should lead to a higher prevalence of winter SAD closer to the poles.

Early studies (Potkin *et al.* 1986; Rosen *et al.* 1990) in the USA seemed to confirm this hypothesis, finding a correlation between higher prevalence of winter SAD with higher latitudes. A later study in Alaska also seemed to confirm this correlation (Booker and Hellekson 1992). On the other hand, findings from studies in Finland (Partonen *et al.* 1993), Japan (Sakamoto *et al.*1993), Iceland (Magnússon and Stefansson 1993), and Canada (Levitt and Boyle 1997) did not fit the hypothesis.

The epidemiological findings and the correlation between prevalence and latitude have recently been reviewed (Mersch *et al.* 1999; Magnússon 2000). Mersch and co-workers calculated the correlation between prevalence and latitude in North America and in Europe. Overall, including both continents, they found a non-significant correlation ($r = 0.07$, $p = 0.415$). But the correlation for North America was strong ($r = 0.70$, $p = 0.003$) and for Europe, almost significant ($r = 0.70$, $p = 0.061$). Their conclusion was that, if latitude influences prevalence, this influence is only weak. They also discussed other contributing factors like climate, which could explain the difference between North America and Europe, since places on the same latitude in Europe as in North America have a milder climate. The influence of climate and weather will be discussed in detail in the chapter by Young.

Other factors that could influence the prevalence of winter SAD include the snow in the north and genetic vulnerability. Magnússon and Axelsson (1993) found a low prevalence of winter SAD in Icelandic descendants living in the Manitoba district of Canada. Madden *et al.* (1996) calculated that 29 per cent of the variance in seasonality could be explained by genetic influence. Jang *et al.* (1997) found an even higher genetic influence on seasonality — 69 per cent for men and 45 per cent for women.

Thus, even if there are positive correlations between latitude and prevalence of winter SAD, other factors seems to contribute to a large extent.

16.3 Time of the year

A large number of studies have examined the influence of season in winter SAD and in healthy people. Rosenthal *et al.* (1984) reported a high correlation between the percentage of patients depressed at any given month and the mean monthly temperature and the length of the photoperiod. Albert *et al.* (1991) studied 10 patients with winter SAD. They found an influence both of season and weather on energy levels. In a study using SPAQ at the latitude of 60° N, strong positive effects on mood of sunny and long days and negative effects of short days were reported (Lingjærde and Reichborn–Kjennerud 1993).

A study with divergent results to most others was reported by Magnússon *et al.* (2000). They sent the Hospital Anxiety and Depression (HAD) rating scale to 1000 persons in Iceland. They could not find any seasonal variation in HAD scores. They interpreted the results as a low genetic vulnerability for seasonal influences on mood in Iceland, in line with the low prevalence of winter SAD.

In another Scandinavian study, Molin *et al.* (1996) followed 126 patients with winter SAD from September to March in Copenhagen, Denmark. The patients completed the Beck Depression Inventory (BDI) every second week and the results were correlated to the photoperiod and local weather. A significant correlation was found between the BDI scores and minutes of sunshine, global radiation (lux per day), length of daylight, and temperature. They concluded that the results were in accordance with the hypothesis that lack of light is a contributing factor for the development of winter SAD.

16.4 Natural light exposure

Of great importance is, of course, how much light exposure an individual receives during different days and different seasons. With urbanization, an increasing amount of indoor work has reduced the level of light exposure for the modern society.

Eastman (1990) had 12 patients with winter SAD recording the time spent outdoors during daylight hours during one week in winter and one in summer. There was more than twice as much sunlight exposure in summer compared to winter (3.0 vs. 1.2 hours a day). The Eastman study was replicated in Switzerland in a larger group of winter SAD patients and healthy controls (Graw *et al.* 1999). They reported that, as compared with the winter-depressive state among winter-SAD patients, mood and alertness as well as sleep improved in the summer relative to control values, but that this did not correlate with the amount of light exposure. In the summer, patients with winter SAD spent more time outdoors than controls, but in the winter there was no difference. The authors concluded that winter-SAD patients may have a greater vulnerability to the amount of light received in winter.

It is best to measure light exposure using light measurement devices. Espiritu *et al.* (1994) studied 106 volunteers, 40 to 60 years old, in San Diego at 32° N — a location with much sunshine. The median time spent in more than 1000 lux was only 58 minutes. Subjects scoring higher on the atypical SAD mood scores spent less time in bright illumination. Cole *et al.* (1995) compared the ambient illumination exposure in healthy individuals in San Diego with Rochester, Minnesota at 44° N. In Rochester, the illumination exceeded 1000 lux only 23 minutes per day during winter. The annual average of time spent outdoors in more than 1000 lux was significantly higher in San Diego than in Rochester. However, seasonal variation in outdoor illumination was far more pronounced in Rochester.

Light exposure measurements have been used in two studies on SAD. Oren *et al.* (1994) studied 13 patients with winter SAD and 13 normal subjects with light monitoring for one week in the winter. There was no difference in the light-exposure profiles, but the severity of depression was inversely related to the photoperiod among the patients, suggesting that vulnerability to short photoperiods may be related to depression in winter SAD. Guillemette *et al.* (1998) compared 11 individuals with subsyndromal SAD (S-SAD) with 8 without seasonal problems. When calculating time spent in an illumination of more than 1000 lux there was no difference between the groups, and both groups spent more time in more than 1000 lux in the summer (1.6 hours) than in winter (0.5 hours). Guillemette and co-workers concluded that S-SAD individuals may have a lower sensitivity to light.

16.5 **Effect of the photoperiod**

Since the photoperiod is identical every year, Young *et al.* (1997) postulated that the onset of symptoms in winter-SAD patients should begin earlier at higher latitudes after the equinox on 22 September. To test this hypothesis, they first used data from published reports. They found a highly significant correlation between risk of onset and latitude between 39° N and 49° N, but not at 60° N. They explained the latter finding as a 'ceiling' effect in human ability to respond to short photoperiods. This appeared to occur at a photoperiod of about 9.5 hours.

In their own study, Young and collaborators studied 190 patients with winter SAD during one year between 1988 and 1994. The week of onset was defined as the week of onset of the first symptom(s). They reported that 74 per cent of the onsets occurred from mid-September to the first week of November, with a peak in mid-October.

The three environmental factors studied were sunshine, solar radiation, and temperature. A multiple regression with the environmental variables as the independent variables and onset risk deviation as the dependent variable was statistically significant, but hours of sunshine was the only individual predictor that approached significance ($p < 0.06$). However, this correlation was highly dependent on one data point. Thus none of the environmental variables were clearly related to onset risk. The photoperiod correlated $r = 0.97$ to cover all seasonal patterns of risk and accounted for 26 per cent of the total variance in weekly risk ($r = 0.51$, $p < 0.01$). The environmental factors explained no additional variance. The conclusion was that the photoperiod, and not environmental factors, was of importance for the onset of winter SAD. The photoperiodic effect could be due to earlier sunset or later sunrise or both.

What conclusions regarding the role of the photoperiod in the pathogenesis of winter SAD can be drawn from these studies with sometimes divergent results? The photoperiod and climatic factors such as temperature, hours of sunshine, solar radiation, and so on, are highly inter-correlated. Many studies have not had the adequate design to be able to differentiate between these variables. The study of Young and collaborators is the one that best could separate the effect of the photoperiod and that of the environmental variables. This and several other studies suggest that photoperiod changes may influence the onset and clinical course of winter SAD. How strong this influence is remains to be defined.

16.6 Hypotheses

What is the mechanism behind the possible effect of the changing photoperiod on the onset and cause of winter SAD? This will be briefly discussed.

There are six major hypotheses regarding the aetiology of winter SAD and the antidepressant effect of bright-light therapy (LT). These are the melatonin, amplitude, phase-shift, entrainment, photon-count, and neurotransmitter-associated hypotheses.

Support for the melatonin hypothesis may be the finding that the β-adrenergic-blocking drug, propranolol, given in the morning to reduce melatonin levels, had a better antidepressant effect than placebo in winter-SAD patients (Schlager 1994). On the other hand, Thalén et al. (1995) found a significant decrease of melatonin amplitude during the night after 10 days of LT. However, the change was not related to the clinical outcome.

There is little support for the amplitude hypothesis in the literature but more support for the phase-shift and entrainment hypotheses.

Klerman et al. 1996 have shown that even low light intensities such as ordinary indoor artificial light could phase-shift and entrain circadian rhythms in healthy individuals. Teicher et al. (1997) studied locomotor activity levels and rhythm in 25 patients with winter SAD and 20 healthy controls. Winter-SAD patients seemed to be about 50 minutes phase delayed. The inter-daily stability was lower in winter-SAD patients, pointing at a possible entrainment deficit resulting in a phase delay. Recently, Wehr et al. (2000), in a constant regime study, found that the intrinsic duration of melatonin secretion was longer in winter than in summer in winter-SAD patients (8.8 hours vs. 8.1 hours, $p < 001$). In healthy volunteers there was no change. The difference between the groups' responses to change of season was statistically significant ($p < 0.05$). These findings support the hypothesis that responses to seasonal changes in the length of day induce winter SAD. Thalén and collaborators (1995) reported a phase advancement of about one hour on melatonin rhythm after 10 days of LT, but found no correlation between these changes and clinical outcome measured with depression ratings.

The photon-count theory has been advocated strongly in a meta-analysis showing that morning and evening LT are superior to LT at other times of the day (Lee et al. 1997).

Bouhuys et al. (1994) have pointed at the importance of cognitive sensitivity to symbolic light for the onset time of winter SAD.

There are many studies that support the neurotransmitter hypothesis, especially regarding the importance of serotonergic disturbances for the pathogenesis of winter SAD (Szádóczky et al. 1989; Stain–Malmgren et al. 1998).

16.7 Mechanisms of action

What then is the mechanism behind the possible photoperiodic influences on the pathogenesis of winter SAD?

The most plausible effect seems to be the influence of the changing photoperiod on circadian rhythms and entrainment. However, winter-SAD patients seem to have about the same real-light exposure in winter as healthy people do. So, if light and the photoperiod is of importance, winter-SAD patients should have a lowered sensitive to light exposure. Regarding the retina, there is no consistent finding of lowered sensitivity to light among winter-SAD patients in the winter. Thus, it is more probable that there is a lowered sensitivity in the circadian oscillators in the suprachiasmatic nuclei (SCN). Since the serotonergic function is vital for the function of the SCN, a serotonergic insufficiency could be the pathogenesis for the lower sensitivity of the circadian oscillator in winter-SAD patients.

References

Albert, P.S., Rosen, L.N., Alexander Jr, J.R., and Rosenthal, N.E. (1991). Effect of daily variation in weather and sleep on seasonal affective disorder. *Psychiatry Res*, **36**:51–63.

Booker, J.M. and Hellekson, C.J. (1992). Prevalence of seasonal affective disorder in Alaska. *Am J Psychiatry*, **149**:1176–82.

Bouhuys, A.L., Meesters, Y., Jansen, J.H.C., and Bloem, G.M. (1994). Relationship between cognitive sensitivity to (symbolic) light in remitted seasonal affective disorder patients and the onset time of a subsequent depressive episode. *J Affect Disord*, **31**:39–48.

Cole, R.J., Kripke, D.F., Wisbey, J., Mason, W.J., Gruen, W., Hauri, P.J, *et al.* (1995). Seasonal variation in human illumination. Exposure at two different latitudes. *J Biol Rhythms*, **10**:324–34.

Eastman, C.I. (1990). Natural summer and winter sunlight exposure patterns in seasonal affective disorder. *Physiol Behav*, **48**:611–16.

Espiritu, R.C., Kripke, D.F., Ancoli-Israel, S., Mowen, M.A., Mason, W.J., Fell, R.L., *et al.* (1994). Low illumiation experienced by San Diego adults: assocition with atypical depressive symptoms. *Biol Psychiatry*, **35**:403–7.

Graw, P, Recker, S, Sand, I., Kraüchi, K., and Wirz–Justice, A. (1999). Winter and summer outdoor light exposure in woman with and without seasonal affective disorder. *J Affect Disord*, **56**:163–9.

Guillemette, J. Hébert, M., Paquet, J., and Dumont, M. (1998). Natural bright light exposure in the summer and winter in subjects with and without complaints of seasonal mood variations. *Biol Psychiatry*, **44**:622–8.

Hellekson, C.J., Kline, J.A., and Rosenthal, N.E. (1986). Phototherapy for seasonal affective disorder in Alaska. *Am J Psychiatry*, **143**:1035–7.

Hoffmann, K. (1981). Photoperiodism in vertebrates. In *Handbook of behavioral neurobiology* (ed. J. Aschoff), pp. 449–73. Plenum Publishing Corp., New York.

Isaacs, G., Stainer, D.S., Sensky, T.E., Moor, S., and Thompson C. (1988). Phototherapy and its mechanism of action in seasonal affective disorder. *J Affect D isord*, **14**:13–19.

Jang, K.L., Lam, R.W., Livesley, W.J., and Vernon, P.A. (1997). Gender differences in the heritability of seasonal mood change. *Psychiatry Res*, **70**:145–54.

Klerman, E.B., Dijk, D.J., Kronauer, R.E., and Czeisler, C.A. (1996). Simulations of light effects on human circadian pacemaker: implications for assessment of intrinsic period. *Am J Physiol*, **270**:271–82.

Lee, T.M.C., Blashsko, C.A., Janzen, H.L, Paterson J.H., and Chan, C.C.H. (1997). Pathophysiological mechanism of seasonal affective disorder. *J Affect Disord*, **46**:25–36.

Levitt, A.J. and Boyle, M.H. (1997) Latitude and the variation in seasonal depression and seasonality of depressive symptoms. *Soc Light Treatment Biol Rhythms Abstracts*, **9**:14.

Lewy, A.J., Kern, H.A., Rosenthal, N.E., and Wehr, T.A. (1982). Bright arificial light treatment of a manic-depressive patient with a seasonal mood cycle. *Am J Psychiatry*, **139**:1496–8.

Lingjærde, O. and Reichborn–Kjennerud, T. (1993). Characteristics of winter depression in the Oslo area (60° N). *Acta Psychiatr Scand*, **88**:111–20.

Madden, P.A.F., Heath, A.C., Rosenthal, N.E., and Martin, N.G. (1996). Seasonal changes in mood and behavior. Role of genetic factors. *Arch Gen Psychiatry*, **53**:47–55.

Magnússon, A. (2000). An overview of epidemiological studies on seasonal affective disorder. *Acta Psychiatr Scand*, **101**:176–84.

Magnússon, A. and Axelsson, J. (1993). The prevalence of seasonal affective disorder is low among decendants of Icelandic emigrants in Canada. *Arch Gen Psychiatry*, **50**:947–51.

Magnússon, A. and Stefansson, J. (1993). Prevalence of seasonal affective disorders in Iceland. *Arch Gen Psychiatry*, **50**:941–6.

Magnússon, A., Axelsson, J., Karlsson, M.M., and Oskarsson, H. (2000). Lack of seasonal mood change in the Icelandic population. *Am J Psychiatry*, **157**:234–398.

Mersch, P. P.A., Middendorp, H.M., Bouhuys, A.L., Beersma., D.G.M., and van den Hoofdakker R.H. (1999). Seasonal affective disorder and latitude: a review of the literature. *J Affect Disord*, **53**:35–48.

Molin, M., Mellerup, E., Bolwig, T., Scheike, T., and Dam, H. (1996). The influence of climate on development of winter depression. *J Affect Disord*, **37**:151–5.

Oren, D.A., Moul, D.E., Schwartz, P.J., Brown, C., Yamada E.M., and Rosenthal, N.E. (1994). Exposure to ambient light in patients with seasonal affective disorder. *Am J Psychiatry*, **151**:591–3.

Partonen, T., Partinen, M., and Lönnqvist, J. (1993). Frequencies of seasonal major depressive symptoms at high latitudes. *Eur Arch Psychiatry Clin Neurosci*, **243**:189–92.

Potkin, S.G., Zetin, M., Stamenkovic, V., Kripke, D., and Bunney, Jr, W.E. (1986). Seasonal affective disorder: prevalence varies with latitude and climate. *Clin Neuropharm*, **9**(**suppl. 4**):181–3.

Rosen, L.N., Targum, S.D., Terman M., Bryant M.J., Hoffman H., Kasper, S.F., *et al*. (1990). Prevalence of seasonal affective disorder at four latitudes. *Psychiatry Res*, **31**:131–44.

Rosenthal, N.E., Sack, D.A., Gillin, C, Lewy, A.J., Goodwin, F.K., Davenport, Y., *et al*. (1984). Seasonal affective disorder. A description of the syndrome and preliminary findings with light therapy. *Arch Gen Psychiatry*, **41**:72–80.

Rosenthal, N.E, Sack, D.A., Carpenter C.J., Parry, B.L., Mendelson W.B., and Wehr, T.A. (1985). Antidepressant effects of light in seasonal affective disorder. *Am J Psychiatry*, **142**:163–70.

Sakamoto, K., Kamo, T., Nakadaira, S., Tamura, A., and Takahashi, K. (1993). A nationwide survey of seasonal affective disorder at 53 outpatient university clinics in Japan. *Acta Psychiatr Scand*, **87**:258–65.

Schlager, D.S.(1994). Early morning administration of short-acting ß blockers for treatment of winter depression. *Am J Psychiatry*, **151**:1383–5.

Stain–Malmgren, R., Kjellman, B.F., and Åberg–Wistedt A. (1998). Platelet serotonergic functions and light therapy in SAD. *Psychiatry Res*, **78**:163–72.

Szádóczky, E., Falus, A., Arató, M., Németh, A., Tezéri, G., and Moussong–Kovács, E. (1989). Phototherapy increases platelet 3H-imipramine binding in patients with winter depression. *J Affect Disord*, **16**:121–5.

Teicher, M.H., Glod, C.A., Magnus, E., Harper, D., Benson, G., Krueger, K., *et al*. (1997). Circadian rest-activity disturbances in seasonal affective disorder. *Arch Gen Psychiatry*, **54**:124–30.

Thalén, B–E., Kjellman, B.F., Mørkrid,L., and Wetterberg, L. (1995). Melatonin in light treatment of patients with seasonal and nonseasonal depression. *Acta Psychiatr Scand*, **92**:274–84.

Wehr, T.A., Jacobsen ,M., Sack, D.A., Arendt J., Tamarkin, L., and Rosenthal, N.E. (1986). Phototherapy of seasonal affective disorder. Time of day and suppression of melatonin are not critical for antidepressant effects. *Arch Gen Psychiatry*, **43**:870–5.

Wehr, T.A., Duncan Jr, W.C., Sher, L., Schwarz, P.E., Turner, E.M., Postolache, T., *et al*. (2000). SNC signal of change of season in seasonal affective disorder. *Soc Light Treatment Biol Rhythms Abstracts*, **12**:2.

Wirz–Justice, A., Buccheli, C., Graw, P., Kielholz P., Fisch H–U., and Woggon B. (1986). Light treatment of seasonal affective disorder in Switzerland. *Acta Psychiatr Scand*, **74**:193–204.

Young, M.A., Meaden, P.M., Fogg, L.F., Cherin, E.A., and Eastman, C.I. (1997). Which environmental variables are related to the onset of seasonal affective disorder? *J Abnorm Psychol*, **106**:554–62.

Chapter 17

Weather

Michael A. Young

17.1 Introduction

All sorts of things and weather
Must be taken in together,
To make up a year
And a sphere.

Ralph Waldo Emerson (1847)

Everyone talks about the weather, but nobody does anything about it.

Charles Dudley Warner (1897)

As noted by Emerson, weather is an unavoidable part of our experience. These literary observations suggest a number of empirical scientific questions about the consequences of weather. First, does everyone complain about the weather? Is a negative reaction to particular types of weather a universal, normal phenomenon or is it part a specific syndrome? Second, does nobody do anything about the weather? Or are there particular responses to the weather that either some or all humans make (albeit not to change the weather)? And third, are physiological and behavioural changes attributed to the weather truly due to the weather or to other things? Unfortunately, there is little research that addresses these issues and methodological issues make understanding the results complicated.

17.2 Reactions to weather conditions

Anecdotal reports suggest that many patients with SAD spontaneously complain about cold winter temperatures and dark cloudy days. However, I am not aware of any systematic collection or assessment of these reports. In addition, complaints about the weather are common in the general population. This raises the possibility that the weather-related complaints of SAD sufferers are no different from those of anyone else and that the weather plays no particular role in SAD. Alternatively, those with SAD may be physiologically or psychologically more sensitive to weather in general or to specific aspects of weather. This sensitivity could be a trait that plays a role in determining the onset or severity of SAD, or it may be clinical feature of the SAD syndrome.

In a study that suggests a psychological sensitivity, Bouhuys *et al.* (1994) found that SAD patients who were more sensitive to lighting conditions when judging the emotions in pictures of faces had an earlier onset of episodes of winter depression. In thinking about this issue, it is useful to distinguish between complaints about the experience of the weather (for example, it is unpleasant when it is so cold) and complaints about one's reaction to the weather (symptom complaints such as 'I feel tired when its cloudy'), although this distinction has not been previously noted.

Weather refers to atmospheric conditions such as temperature, wind, cloudiness, humidity, and barometric pressure, at a given time and place. This contrasts to climate which refers to the average or typical values of these factors. For example, if the weather were unusually warm one week in February, we would expect people's behaviour to reflect this particular weather, not the cold climatic conditions that are more typical of this time of year. Because weather changes over periods of days and weeks, studies that relate monthly or seasonal averages of weather variables to similar averages in behaviour are not adequate to provide evidence for the influence of weather. In addition, because many weather variables are highly inter-correlated (Young *et al.* 1997), it is difficult to identify which variable is truly associated with behaviour or psychopathology. While this requires a data analysis with statistical controls, the usual multiple regression techniques are not effective with *highly* inter-correlated independent variables.

Also, as noted by Peck (1990), time-series data present a number of data-analysis problems which most authors, by computing simple correlations, have not addressed. For example, Sakamoto *et al.* (1993) found that SAD prevalence at different latitudes was associated to total hours of sunshine from September through March, but not with mean December temperature (both averaged over 30 years). In another latitude study, Okawa *et al.* (1996) found that monthly SAD symptoms correlated with sunshine and temperature. However, for the reasons already noted, it is difficult to interpret these studies in terms of weather.

17.3 **Effects on symptoms**

A related issue is exposure to the weather that putatively affects symptom presentation. In a study in Iceland, Magnusson and Stefansson (1993) did not detect a difference in seasonal problems between those who worked outdoors (with presumably more exposure to the weather) and those who worked indoors. Wirz–Justice *et al.* (1992) found that people with seasonal problems spent less time outdoors than those without seasonal problems. This is logical given their depressions, but it also means that these seasonal sufferers have less exposure to the weather than those who are not seasonal. The seasonal group would have no less knowledge of the weather, which is relevant if the effect of weather is mediated by their cognitions about it.

Existing research on weather and behaviour can be divided into three types: studies of weather and SAD, studies of weather and other disorders, and studies of weather and human functioning in general. Unfortunately, only three reports could be found that directly address the issue of weather and SAD. These studies took quite different methodological approaches to the subject.

Molin *et al.* (1996) studied the symptom severity of 126 Danish winter-depression patients during September to May, prior to beginning treatment. On alternate weeks the severity of depression was assessed with the Beck Depression Inventory. A multiple regression analysis indicated that depression severity was predicted by:

1. a shorter average length of day in the week of, and the week preceding, the depression assessment, and;

2. cooler average temperatures in the period 2 to 3 weeks prior to the depression assessment.

Thus, both the length of day and the temperature had independent effects on depressive symptoms in the early, pre-treatment phase of episodes. However, it is difficult to explain why there would be a two-week delay in the effect of temperature on symptoms, especially because after two weeks the temperature is likely to have changed in unpredictable ways. Significant effects were not found for minutes of sunshine, barometric pressure, global radiation, and rainfall.

Albert *et al.* (1991) studied the effect of daily weather (minimum temperature, hours of sunshine, barometric pressure, and relative humidity) on daily the energy level and sleep duration in 10 SAD patients over 2 to 5 years. Weather effects on sleep and energy were not present after first accounting for seasonal patterns. However, seasonal patterns were present after first accounting for the effects of daily weather. Thus, weather did not account for the seasonal energy and sleep patterns in these SAD subjects. Some individual subjects did show weather effects in particular seasons; however, the particular season and the specific weather factor was highly idiosyncratic. Thus, although weather may have had some impact on these individuals, the impact was not consistent in a way that would indicate that the effects were related to SAD.

In contrast to these studies of weekly and daily variations in symptoms, Young *et al.* (1997) studied the effects of weather on the onset of episodes in 190 winter-depression patients in Chicago. The onset of *actual* episodes was determined, in contrast to most other studies which ask subjects to report when their symptoms *typically* began. Because the study was conducted over seven years, the weather in any given week of any given year could be related to the risk of onset in each week of each year. In order to control for the high covariance of weather factors, the authors examined whether higher (or lower) than average onset risk was associated with higher (or lower) than average weather conditions. No evidence was found for an impact of temperature, hours of sunshine, or global radiation on the onset of SAD episodes. Length of day was highly related to risk of onset.

These three studies hardly allow for a definitive conclusion. However, the most parsimonious interpretation of the results to date is that weather may have an impact on the self-reported symptoms of individuals with SAD, but that it does not account for the disorder itself. No research has compared SAD patients to controls to determine whether SAD patients generally, or during an episode of SAD, have an increased responsiveness to weather. It may be that they are equally as sensitive to weather as the population at large but, because their SAD brings them to the clinic in the winter, their weather-attributed symptoms are considered part of the SAD syndrome.

A number of studies and case reports have addressed weather and other affective disorders. Several studies have observed a higher admissions rate for mania in the summer months (for example, Peck 1990). This may indicate something about mania. However, because there are no studies with comparison groups with a different diagnosis, it also may indicate something about admission or other associated factors. Also, studies such as these, which examine data in each of 12 months, have only 12 data points on which to calculate correlations and thus low power to find statistical significance.

Fukuda and Yoshinaga (1993) reported a case of SAD (spring type) in which they considered 6 out of 10 episodes of onset to be related to temperature increases. However, this was based on visual interpretation of graphical data that could just as easily be interpreted as exhibiting no particular pattern. Summers and Shur (1992) reported a case of unipolar depression in which many onsets of depression followed sudden increases in solar radiation; this occurred regardless of season. Eagles (1994) reported a case of rapid cycling bipolar disorder in which mood correlated with hours of sunshine over a period of 62 days.

A literature also exists concerning the effect of weather variables on mood and behaviour in normal or unscreened samples (for example, Howarth and Hoffman 1984). Based on a literature search, this research appears not to have continued in the 1990s. These studies suggest that increased humidity tends to be related to decreased concentration and increased sleepiness. Increased temperature, or perhaps any uncomfortable temperature, has been associated with increased aggressive behaviour. Studies in this area vary tremendously in research design, the data that are collected, and the data-analysis methods used. Many conceptual and methodological issues are reviewed by Persinger (1987).

17.4 **Conclusions**

There is great methodological diversity in research regarding the role of weather in SAD. Attention to the following eight issues would benefit study design and interpretation.

1. Are data from normal or clinical samples? If clinical, what diagnoses are included and to what populations can the results be generalized? Do weather factors function differently in SAD patients than in healthy subjects?

2. Is the outcome variable the presence or absence of a diagnosis, the severity of symptoms, or more specific phenomena such as mood, behaviour, or performance/functioning? Are results relevant to normal range behaviour and/or pathology?

3. Are outcome variables measured or reported repeatedly over time or are subjects reporting their understanding of how they are affected by weather?

4. Do the design and analysis allow the separation of specific weather factors from length of day and other confounds?

5. If the study includes time-series data (for example, a long run of days or weeks) are data analysed using appropriate time-series methods? For example, if weather at time 1 is to predict symptoms at time 2, then one needs to control for symptoms at time 1.

6. Is the time scale (for example, days, weeks, months) appropriate to the expected effect of the weather factors being studied?

7. Is the time period over which data are collected appropriate to the question being asked? For example, variations in symptoms of SAD during January and February, when symptoms are more severe but relatively stable, are not likely to reflect mechanisms related to the onset of the episode.

8. Does the study indicate something about weather variables as aetiological factors or as moderators of severity?

In conclusion, more research is needed, with clearer conceptualization of the issues involved and more consistent and rigorous methodology. Existing research suggests that weather variables are not a factor in the basic aetiology of SAD. Weather may affect how individuals with SAD feel, but these effects tend to be idiosyncratic to the individual. The experiences of those with SAD may be similar to the weather complaints of non-SAD individuals, may exacerbate SAD symptoms, or may be exacerbated by SAD symptoms.

Clinically, it seems appropriate to deal with each patient individually by collecting data as in a single-subject design (Barlow and Hersen 1984) to determine if weather truly is contributing to the patient's symptoms. If so, behavioural or cognitive interventions can improve the patient's ability to cope with weather conditions. Treating the SAD itself also should be helpful either by directly reducing weather-related symptoms or by reducing the impact of weather-related symptoms, thus improving the patient's overall condition.

References

Albert, P.S., Rosen, L.N., Alexander, J.R., and Rosenthal, N.E. (1991) Effect of daily variation in weather and sleep on seasonal affective disorder. *Psychiatry Research* **36**:51–63.

Barlow, D.H. and Hersen, M. (1984) *Single case experimental designs*. Pergamon Press, New York.

Bouhuys, A.L., Meesters, Y., Jansen, J.H., and Bloem, G.M. (1994) Relationship between cognitive sensitivity to (symbolic) light in remitted seasonal affective disorder patients and the onset time of a subsequent depressive state. *Journal of Affective Disorders* **31**:39–48.

Eagles, J.M. (1994) The relationship between mood and daily hours of sunlight in rapid cycling bipolar illness. *Biological Psychiatry* **36**:422–4.

Fukuda, M. and Yoshinaga, C. (1993) Onset of depressive episodes in a woman with seasonal affective disorder of 'spring type' coincident with atmospheric temperature, but not with sunshine duration. *Japanese Journal of Psychiatry and Neurology* **47**:777–82.

Howarth, E. and Hoffman, M.S. (1984) A multidimensional approach to the relationship between mood and weather. *British Journal of Psychology* **75**:1523.

Magnusson, A. Stefansson, J.G. (1993). Prevalence of seasonal affective disorder in Iceland. *Archives of General Psychiatry* **50**:941–6.

Molin, J., Mellerup, E., Bolwig, T., Scheike, T., and Dam, H. (1996) The influence of climate on development of winter depression. *Journal of Affective Disorders* **37**:151–5.

Okawa, M., Shirakawa, S., Uchiyama, M., Oguri, M., *et al.* (1996) Seasonal variation of mood and behavior in a healthy middle-aged population. *Acta Psychiatrica Scandinavica* **94**:211–16.

Peck, D.F. (1990) Climate variables and admission for mania: a reanalysis. *Journal of Affective Disorders* **20**:249–50.

Persinger, M.A. (1987) Mental processes and disorders: a neurobehavioral perspective in human biometeorology. *Experientia* **43**:39–48.

Sakamoto, K., Kamo, T., Nakadaira, S., Tamura, A., and Takahashi, K. (1993) A nationwide survey of seasonal affective disorder at 53 outpatient university clinics in Japan. *Acta Psychiatrica Scandinavica* **87**:258–65.

Summers, L. and Shur, E. (1992) The relationship between onsets of depression and sudden drops in solar radiation. *Biological Psychiatry* **32**:1164–72.

Wirz–Justice, A., Kräuchi, K., Graw, P., Schulman, J., and Wirz, H. (1992) *Seasonality in Switzerland: an epidemiological survey. 4th annual meeting of the Society for Light Treatment and Biological Rhythms*. Bethesda, Maryland, USA.

Young, M.A., Meaden, P.M., and Fogg, L.F. (1997) Which environmental variables are causal factors in the onset of seasonal affective disorder? *Journal of Abnormal Psychology* **106**:556–62.

Chapter 18

Melatonin

David S. Schlager

18.1 **Introduction**

The role of melatonin in seasonal affective disorder (SAD) remains unresolved, informed largely by two competing hypotheses which are, in turn, based on divergent models of depression. The 'phase shift' hypothesis in SAd (Lewy *et al.*, 1987a,b) in one which models human depression as disorder of circadian entrainment (e.g., Wehr *et al.*, 1979; Ehlers *et al.*, 1988). The 'melatonin' hypothesis, on the other hand, begins with SAD's apparent, if far from certain, homology with normal mammalian seasonality and melatonin's known role in modulating suc rhythms, also recognizing growing consideration of adaptive functions served by depressive behaviours (Nesse, 2000).

Reflecting this dual theoretical pedigree, melatonin in SAD has been considered with regard to two parameters of its nocturnal secretion – timing and duration – thought to subserve separate if overlapping functions in mammalian timekeeping. Melatonin is secreted by te pineal during nighttime darkness, its secretion controlled by te circadian pacemaker in the supreciasmatic nucleus with photic input from the retina. Melatonin thus constitutes an endocrine signal of darkness such that the *timing* of nightly secretion functions to convey nightlength and, by extension, 'time of year' information to modulate annual (seasonal) rhythms.

The timing of melatonin in SAD is the focus of the 'phase shift' hypothesis (PSH, Lewy *et al.*, 1987), which grew out of findings that human melatonin can be suppressed by bright artificial light (Lewy *et al.*, 1980) and that such light has antidepresent effects in human winter-SAD (Lewy *et al.*, 1982; Rosenthal *et al.*, 1984). This hypothesis regards the timing of melatonin noctunal as a marker of circadian phase (Lewy *et al.*, 1999), albeit with important phase shifting properties of its own (Lewy *et al.*, 1998c). Ot proposes that winter SAD is caused by pothogenic exposure or sensitivity to wintertime light-dark conditions which, in turn, produces circadian phase delays of melatonin and possibly other circadian rhythms relative to the sleep-wake cycle (1988b). It further suggests that corrective wintertime phase-advances by morning artificial light or afternoon exogenous melatonin is the means by which such interventions produces an antidepressant effect (Lewy *et al.*, 2000).

Melatonin duration as SAD neuro-modulator – the 'melatonin' hypothesis – was suggested by immediate comparisons with melatonin's concurrently elucidated role in driving or entraining mammalian seasonal reproduction (e.g., Bartness and Goldman, 1989; Karsch *et al.*, 1991) autumn-seasonal weight ggain (see Wade, 1989), and torpor and hibernation (see Saarela and Reiter, 1994). Indeed, by the time light therapy came into widespread practical use as a seasonal antidepressant, commercial manipulations of livestock seasonal breeding and weight-gain cycles using light and melatonin were also underway (e.g., Chemineau *et al.*, 1988; Williams and Ward, 1988). Initial phototherapy studies in SAD failed to provide empricial support for the 'melatonin' hypothesis (MH). More recent work has revived the possibility that human melatonin serves as both a calendar and clock (Reiter, 1993), linking long-night melatonin duration with wintertime recurrence and artificiality induced short-night melatonin duration with the antidepressant effect of light treatment (Wehr, 1997).

'Patogenic' melatonin in SAD then is defined by the phase-shift and melatonin hypothesis, respectively, as secretion that is either later or longer than normal. This chapter aims to review recent findings which bear on the proposal role of melatonin in SAD. It will review relevant studies which measured melatonin in SAD, reconsider animal models of normal seasonality in neurovegetative and reproductive functions, and recent adaptationist analyses of human depression.

18.2 Melatonin correlates of mood

Empirical support for the PH in SAD has come in the form of recent human studies which diseemed within subject correlations between treatment induced melatonin phase advance and antidepressant response (Lewy *et al.*, 2000; Terman *et al.*, 2001). Recent support for the MH induces observed seasonal differences in melatonin duration in SAD patients but not controlls, in both laboratory and naturalistic settings (Wehr, 2000). Such findings represent results from a general category of testing to find correlation between melatonin timing (phase) or duration and mood state. Such melatonin correlates of mood can be divided into several categories, including melatonin comparisons between winter depressive and normal controls, comparisons, within winter depressives of their winter depressed and naturally remitted state, and within winter depressives before and after treatment. The latter melatonin change with treatment includes time-of-day of treatment studies and a small number of non-photic treatment studies aimed at manipulating melatonin. A brief review of these categories of findings as they bear on the PSH and MH is summarized in Table 1. The most common tests of the two hypotheses has come in the form of observed correlations between mood change and change in melatonin timing or duration. For the purpose of later discussion, these can be labelled as follows:

♦ **Type 1** – wintertime-depressed subjects before and after antidepressant treatment.

♦ **Type 2** – wintertime-depressed subjects compared with wintertime euthymic controls.

♦ **Type 3** – seasonal depressives in their wintertime depressed compared to summertime remitted states.

As summarized in Table 18.1, support for the PSH has come most strongly from type 1 studies (Lewy *et al.* 1998a, 2000; Terman *et al.*, 2001) which showed significant phase advance of dim light melatonin onset (DLMO) as a correlate of antidepressant response. Type 2 and 3 studies have been sometimes (Lewy *et al.* 1987*b*, 1988*a*), but not always, supportive of the PSH (Checkley *et al.* 1993; Levendosky *et al.* 1991).

The MH is supported most strongly by type 2 and 3 studies, which observed significantly longer duration of nocturnal melatonin in winter compared to summer, but only in SAD patients, not normal controls (Wehr *et al.* 2000). There have been no type 1 study tests of the MH.

Table 18.1 Findings which bear on the phase-shift and/or melatonin hypotheses

	Phase-shift hypothesis (Melatonin phase delayed)	Melatonin hypothesis (Melatonin longer than normal)
Melatonin in winter depressives before and after treatment (type 1)	Phase advanced after treatment (Lewy *et al.* 1998, 2000; Terman *et al.*, 2001)	No data
Melatonin in winter depressives vs. euthymic controls (type 2)	Depressives delayed cf. to controls (e.g. Lewy *et al.* 1988a) No difference between depressives and controls (e.g. Checkley *et al.* 1993)	Winter–summer differences significant in seasonal depressives but not euthymic controls (Wehr *et al.* 2000)
Melatonin in seasonal depressives in winter cf. to summer (type 3)	Minimal data	Longer in winter depressed cf. to summer euthymic state (Wehr *et al.* 2000)
Time of day of light efficacy	Morning more effective than evening light (Lewy *et al.* 1998a; Terman *et al.* 1989, 1998)	Evening more effective than control (Terman *et al.* 1998)
Non-photic antidepressant treatment	Afternoon exogenous melatonin superior to placebo (Lewy *et al.* 1998b, 2000)	Early-morning beta-adrenergic blockers vs. placebo (Schlager 1994; Schlager *et al.* 1996)
Relevant animal studies	Equivocal (for review, see Rosenwasser 1992)	Seasonal reproduction (Bartness & Goldman 1989) Thermoregulation (Saarela & Reiter 1994) Annual weight rhythms (Wade 1989)

Two comments are relevant to type 1 study design and results. First, those studies which observed a phase advance of DLMOI during light treatment to correlate with antidepressant response cannot, without analysing whole-night melatonin profiles, rule out a correlation between antidepressant response and shortened melatonin duration produced by morning light-induced phase advance of melatonin offset even greater than observed phase advance of melatonin onset. Such a response would be predicted by Wehr's (1997) finding that seasonal variation in duration is correlated largely with morning offset and might thus be shortened by morning light regardless of any concurrent phase advance of DLMO As one example, Terman *et al.*, (2001) demonstrated a correlation between magnitude of DLMO phase-advance and clinical response, but measured whole night melatonin in only a small subgroup and did not formally discuss any potential duration changes produced by apparent phase advance of melatonin offset concurrently produced.

This prediction is also generally consistent with recent observations that phase advance of DLMO beyond a certain magnitude no longer correlates with an antidepressant response (for example, Lewy 1998a) theoretically because such patients represent a true phase advance without concomitant decreased duration of melatonin.

A second point is that the data from a sizeable number of whole-night melatonin profiles of winter-depressed patients, before and after light treatment, that have been collected by researchers in type 1 studies in recent years are probably amenable to reanalysis for melatonin duration as a co-correlate/pr edictor of antidepressant response.

18.3 Melatonin manipulations

A more direct test of melatonin's role in winter SAD is one which controls for light-dark exposure and its other circadian effects while experimentally manipulating melatonin itself. This type of study has taken two forms: suppression of endogenous melatonin by means other than light exposure and administration of exogenous melatonin.

Non-photic suppression of melatonin was conceived and originally studied by Rosenthal and colleagues, who administered a beta-adrenergic blocker, atenolol, previously shown to suppress pineal melatonin secretion (Rosenthal *et al.* 1988), to winter depressives. Their study showed no overall superiority of atenolol to placebo, but highlighted some brisk individual responses to intervention.

This author conducted two follow-up studies administering a shorter-acting beta-blocker, propranolol, in the early morning, in order to more closely mimic the melatonin suppressive effects of natural summertime and artificial wintertime early morning light in winter SAD. The first study, an open trial followed by a double-blind placebo-discontinuation phase, showed significantly greater tendency to relapse in improved subjects who were switched to placebo compared to those who continued on propranolol at 6.00 a.m. (Schlager 1994).

The second study, of 17 women and 5 men with DSM-IV recurrent major depression with seasonal pattern (SAD), attempted to replicate the finding of antidepressant effect of early-morning propranolol administration while directly measuring the melatonin suppressive effects of such treatment (Schlager *et al.* 1996). To enter, subjects scored at least 12 on the 21-item Hamilton Rating Scale for Depression (HRSD) or at least 9 on the HRSD and at least 18 on the 29-item Structured Interview Guide for the Hamilton-SAD version (SIGH-SAD). Subjects were randomized to receive either placebo or 30 mg of propranolol at 6.00 a.m. for 5 days, after which, the dose for subjects feeling no better (or worse) was doubled to 2 pills (of placebo or 60 mg of propranolol). Final assessment was after 14 days of treatment.

As shown in Table 18.2, significant differences between drug and placebo were observed in decreases of depression severity scores on both the SIGH-SAD (mean decrease = 16.2 and

Table 18.2 Baseline and post-treatment depression ratings by treatment condition

Depression score	Propranolol (n = 12) Mean (SD)	Placebo (n = 11) Mean (SD)	Drug–placebo differences Repeated measures ANOVA (df = 1.21)
Hamilton (21-item)			
Baseline	14.8 (3.3)	16.9 (5.9)	$F = 9.7$, $p < 0.01$
Post-treatment	6.3 (6.0)	14.6 (6.6)	
8 atypical items			
Baseline	14.5 (5.3)	15.2 (5.3)	$F = 2.5$, $p =$ NS
Post-treatment	6.7 (5.6)	10.5 (3.9)	
SIGH-SAD (29-item)			
Baseline	29.3 (5.1)	32.1 (5.7)	$F = 7.4$, $p < 0.05$
Post-treatment	13.1 (11.3)	25.2 (7.8)	

6.9, respectively; repeated measures ANOVA F = 7.4, df = 1,21; p < 0.05) and HRSD (mean decrease = 8.5 and 2.3, F = 9.7, p < 0.01). Mean propranolol dose was 46 mg. No subjects receiving active medication reported significant adverse effects.

The data support earlier findings (Schlager 1994) that this treatment is effective for winter depression. Such treatment, if effective, has advantages over conventional light treatment in terms of cost and convenience.

As for the test of melatonin suppression as the mediator for an antidepressant response, measurement of urinary melatonin metabolite 6-sulfatoxymelatonin (aMTs) in winter depressives, before and after treatment with either propranolol or placebo, was analysed to determine whether aMTs reduction was greater among those randomized to active drug compared to placebo and whether there was correlation between treatment-associated reductions in aMTs and depression severity ratings.

Urine was collected by each subject on the day prior to starting the pills and again at the end of the treatment trial. On each of the two occasions, urine collected was that produced and voided between 7.00 a.m. and 12.00 noon. Total aMTs (mg) in each collection represents the product of urine volume (ml) and assayed aMTs concentration (ng/ml).

Nineteen subjects completed both the treatment trial and urine collections. Among those taking propranolol, mean daily dose was 42 mg. Significant differences in decreases of depression severity scores was observed between drug and placebo groups on both the SIGH-SAD (mean decrease = 15.4 and 6.8, respectively; repeated measures ANOVA F = 5.4, df = 1,17; p < 0.05) and Hamilton Rating Scale for Depression (mean decrease = 8.1 and 2.2, F = 6.8, p < 0.02). Treatment-associated decrease in total morning aMTs was not significantly greater among subjects randomized to active drug (mean change = −0.415 mg) compared to those on placebo (mean change = +0.369; repeated measures ANOVA F = 1.04, df = 1,18; p = 0.32), nor was there any significant correlation between clinical improvement and aMTs reduction in the morning urine collection.

The findings provide no support for the notion of melatonin suppression as a mediator for the antidepressant effect of beta-blockers in SAD. At the same time, the argument against such an association is limited, in the current data, by failure to observe significant melatonin suppression among active-drug compared to placebo subjects. Such a failure suggests an active-drug condition inadequately dosed or inappropriately timed to test the question. Another, neither unlikely nor mutually exclusive, possibility is that the study as designed requires a larger 'n' to detect melatonin suppression of only the peri-dawn tail of nocturnal secretion or any correlation between suppression and clinical response (Schlager et al. 1997).

Lewy's recent study using exogenous afternoon melatonin represents another and more definitive test of the two hypotheses. This study is based on earlier evidence of a human phase- response curve to exogenous melatonin (Lewy et al. 1998c) demonstrating that morning or evening administration of melatonin should produce a circadian phase shift in an opposite direction to that produced by bright light administered at the same times. Thus, late afternoon or evening melatonin would be expected to produce a circadian phase advance while theoretically lengthening the physiologic melatonin signal or at least avoiding the potential shortening of melatonin duration induced by evening light treatment.

The treatment study compared administration of approximately 0.3 mg of melatonin, over 6 to 8 hours, just after morning wake-up time to the same 0.3 mg dose, over 6 to 8 hours, beginning 7 hours after wake-up — essentially a morning vs. evening design. All 81 subjects took capsules every 2 hours throughout their waking day in a placebo-controlled parallel design. The study measured DLMO and SIGH-SAD before and after 3 weeks of treatment, finding a statistically significant correlation between decrease in depression ratings and phase advance of melatonin onset, though only among those patients exhibiting phase advance of less than 1.5 hours. Whole-night melatonin profiles were not reported.

18.4 Animal models — defect or adaptation

Conceptually, the PSH and MH diverge in considering SAD as a physiologic defect or an evolved seasonal adaptation, respectively. The PSH regards depression as a seasonal caused by a physiologic defect in the timekeeping machinery, which dysrhythmia produces morbidity without advantage or defence. The MH, by contrast, represents the same depression as a synchronization of behavioural and ecological cycles, an evolved adaptation (or at least a vestige thereof), preserved despite attenuated cycles of lightdark signals and akin to animal seasonal adaptations to seasonal environmental challenges.

Having framed it this way, and before considering animal data which bear on the question, it should be said, that even evolved adaptations can present in altered or 'pathologic' forms under conditions of attenuated time cues, dissociation between seasonal light and temperature cues, or countless other deviations from the uniform laboratory conditions 'that are simply unattainable in human experimentation' (Zucker 1989). In spite of this and other limitations, relevant animal models of seasonal behavioural rhythms and growing consideration of human depression as an evolved defence provide collateral support for recent evidence that seasonal changes in human melatonin duration may modulate the photoperiodic control of SAD (Wehr 1991, 1997; Wehr et al. 1993, 2000).

The phase-shift or circadian disturbance hypotheses of depression have focused attention on circadian entrainment, postulating pathogenic light sensitivity (for example, Nathan et al. 1999; Terman and Terman 1999) or light exposure (for example, Eastman 1990; Oren et al. 1994; Cole et al. 1995; Guillemette et al. 1998; Hebert et al. 1998) to explain phase-angle abnormalities. Animal models used to test these hypotheses have been hampered by uncertain face validity and by uncertainty over the direction of cause and effect in circadian abnormalities and depression (for review, see Rosenwasser 1992).

On the MH side, discovery of SAD raised immediate and obvious comparisons with melatonin's role in photoperiodic control of mammalian models of seasonality. At the same time, early questions about the relevance to SAD of animal models of seasonality were raised, citing dissimilarities between human SAD and mammalian torpor (Mrosovsky 1989) and absence of strict seasonal breeding rhythms among healthy humans or SAD patients. Furthermore, melatonin has not been shown to play a definitive role in regulation of any human rhythm, though effects on circadian entrainment (Lewy and Sack 1997), reproductive function (Luboshitsky 1999), and sleep have been suggested.

While neither thermoregulation nor reproduction models seem to have much face validity for human mood seasonality, animal models of annual weight rhythms may be more relevant (Wade 1989). Autumnal weight gain is a common seasonal pattern in animals and humans. In humans, it has been detected in general population samples (for example, VanStavaren et al. 1986), suggesting that the magnitude of weight change in winter SAD may represent an extreme on a population continuum, much as might other symptoms of this clinical disorder. In animal models like the hamster, weight increases are greater in females than in males and the weight gain can occur in the absence of increased caloric intake, indicating a role for decreased activity and/or changing macronutrient composition of preferred food. The weight gain in hamsters can be induced by exposure to either short photoperiods or 'long-night' melatonin infusion, indicating coexisting melatonin-dependent and melatonin-independent pathways (Wade 1989).

Finally, it is of interest that weight gain in response to melatonin is graded in hamsters, with 'lower-dose' short-day melatonin infusions producing a significant but lesser weight gain than 'higher-dose' long-night melatonin, and the former without the latter's concomitant reproductive quiescence (Bartness and Wade 1984). This finding, and other examples of dissociation of seasonal traits under exotic environmental circumstances (for example, Joy and Mrosovsky 1982), may be relevant to humans. Recent findings suggest that in individuals where seasonal differences in melatonin are significant, such differences are still less robust in modern naturalistic environments than they are in the same individuals under experimentally produced 'pre-industrial' light–dark conditions (Wehr 1997). This gradation of response to photoperiodic time cues may underlie some of the variation in human mood severity and phenomenology.

Another problem is that seasonal depression, inarguably a disorder, with subjective suffering and functional impairment, seems an unlikely adaptation. This question has been considered by recent work suggesting that symptoms and illness in general (Williams and Nesse 1991), and depression in particular (Nesse 2000), might well represent evolved adaptive behaviour. The relevant general concept is that of an evolved defence, in which disorders can represent adaptations which, though painful and even costly to the organism in themselves, are less costly than the failure to respond to the threat against which they defend. Examples of such evolved defences include cough, morning sickness in early pregnancy (to avoid consuming teratogens during morphogenesis), and forms of anxiety from simple phobia to panic (for example Klein 1993).

Considering depression as a defence requires characterizing specific behaviours, the functions they perform, and the situations in which they are evoked, discerning a fit between the three that seems too complex and efficient to be the product of chance (Williams 1962). Many functions and evocative situations have been proposed for negative affective states — all of them behavioral states:

> ... shaped to help organisms cope with unpropitious circumstances useful because they inhibit dangerous or wasteful actions ... Decreased motivation and activity would obviously be useful mainly in situations in which action would be futile or dangerous. Organisms carefully regulate when and where they exert effort; foraging theory offers robust predictions for one such type of effort. (Nesse 2000)

Winter depression's autumnal weight gain, decreased activity, and general disengagement are superficially similar to certain animal models of preparation for and survival of the energetic challenges of winter. And as in humans, some such models do not exhibit annual reproductive rhythms (for example, rats or cattle).

Beyond any specific match between behaviour and environment, several more global clues which suggest that depression is an adaptation (Nesse 2000) are applicable to SAD. These include the observation that defences, but not defects, are regulated by cues (that is, seasonal light–dark change) associated with situations in which they are useful (Mrosovsky 1989); a general, if imperfect correlation between observed prevalence or severity of the defence (winter depression) and the magnitude of the situation which triggers it (that is, cold and dark) (Oren *et al.* 1994; Mersch *et al.* 1999); the high prevalence among persons of reproductive age; and a continuum of severity within populations that makes distinguishing pathologic from non-pathologic difficult (Nesse 2000).

Signal detection in certain defences, like some types of anxiety, is designed with hair-trigger responses which, though responsible for much normal suffering, are selectively maintained by the dire penalty (that is, death) incurred by a single missed threat. An analogy for this concept is the household smoke alarm, whose annoying sensitivity to 'burnt toast' is actively maintained to ensure an early alert in the rare case of actual fire. As applied to SAD, this concept suggests that the adaptiveness of winter depression may have less to do with surviving the predictable component of wintertime energetic stress than the variable component. Temperature and food supply varies not only between summer and winter but also, substantially, from winter to winter. To defend against extreme energetic challenge of an especially harsh winter, sensitivity to a reliable, if inexact, predictive trigger — the photoperiod — could have been conceivably maintained by selection until very recently, even if the energy-conserving responses were often costly and unnecessary but rarely life-saving.

Another question is raised by the observation that mammalian seasonal adaptations, when present, are generally highly prevalent within long-lived, temperate-zone living populations (Bronson 1989) — clearly not the case for human SAD. The prevalence of a human wintertime, depressive adaptation has probably been lowered for several reasons consistent with the adaptationist notion. Least likely is that the trait is no longer subject to selective pressures of earlier, and energetically harder times, and thus no longer adaptive and is in the process of downward genetic drift. More likely is that modern artificial light and dark exposure are responsible for loss of seasonal (for example, melatonin) variation in some persons in whom such variation can be evoked under experimentally produced 'pre-industrial' conditions (Wehr 1997). Second, winter depression, like depression in general, is largely a syndrome of reproductive-age persons and the relative proportion of this demographic group in the general population has, in recent times, decreased in proportion to improvements in infant mortality and average life expectancy, lowering the relative prevalence compared to that of mammalian adaptations.

Finally, population heterogeneity of a trait does not, in itself, rule out an adaptive function. Rather, polymorphisms of phenotype and genotype are common and a growing body of evidence suggests that natural selection plays an active role in maintaining such polymorphisms (see Hudson 1996). Even in classical one-locus, over-dominant, random-mating genetic models, natural selection leads only to maximization of mean fitness, such that the fitness of any particular individual need not reach the maximum level of the population (Rose and Lauder 1996b).

Probably the most familiar example of adaptive polymorphism, and one which formally embraces the concept of disease as adaptation, is that of the heterozygous advantage. In this model, a mutation which confers net reproductive advantage will increase in frequency even if it causes vulnerability to disease. The classic example is sickle-cell anaemia — a single-locus genetic polymorphism in which the recessive allele for haemoglobin S produces enough benefit by protecting heterozygous carriers against malaria in endemic environments that its gene frequency is maintained despite the dire consequences to homozygous individuals (Allison 1954).

The heterozygous advantage argument has been applied to various conditions with known deleterious effects on reproduction but stable gene frequencies within populations (for example, Huxely 1964; Srinivasan and Padmavati 1997). In SAD, the observed population continuum in vulnerability to wintertime symptoms may include some form of heterozygous advantage, with 'milder' forms balancing the adverse consequences to more severely affected individuals.

The purpose of all this adaptationist speculation is not to suggest that Darwinian paradigms provide any direct bearing on a role for melatonin duration in SAD or against a phase-angle abnormality in the aetiology of depression. On the other hand, recognizing the adaptive potential of depressive behaviour in observed form, demographic groups, and prevalence is relevant to proposing a role for melatonin as an effector of photoperiodic time measurement in human seasonality. Together, they support at least reconsideration of melatonin's role in SAD as more physiologic than pathophysiologic and as a role homologous to that in animal wintertime adaptations.

18.5 Conclusions

Two main melatonin findings support the role of circadian phase-angle abnormality (the PSH) in SAD. The first is the observed phase advance of DLMO with antidepressant morning light in winter depressives. The limitations of this type of finding is that it has not been consistently observed and that it does not, without concurrent measurement of melatonin offset, rule out decreased duration as a consequence and active ingredient of morning light. A second, and more compelling, recent finding is that exogenous melatonin administered in the afternoon, but not the morning, produced antidepressant effects and DLMO phase advances in SAD. This finding, if replicated, would represent very strong support for the PSH because the control condition — an empty capsule — is a valid placebo and because the active treatment, if it phase advances melatonin, would not, like morning light, be as likely to shorten melatonin as advance it. Still, direct melatonin measurements remain to be reported in this type of experiment.

The main support for the MH comes from several sources. Ultimately it derives from the validity of a few well-studied animal models of photoperiodic time measurement in which melatonin duration has proved to be the effector signal by which the SCN regulates seasonal change. Further support is provided by naturalistic studies which show that SAD patients, but not controls, show significant lengthening of melatonin duration in winter compared to summer. The hypothesis is consistent with findings that evening light is more effective than placebo and that morning light is more effective than evening light, the latter predicted by observations that seasonal variation in melatonin duration correlates more strongly with morning melatonin offset than with evening (DLMO) onset. The major limitation of the MH is that no study, to my knowledge, has measured melatonin duration before and after light treatment in SAD.

Future research will no doubt attempt such measures of duration as a correlate of antidepressant response. Also relevant would be a reanalysis, if not a meta-analysis, of available whole-night melatonin profiles in light treatment studies to determine whether melatonin duration correlates with clinical change.

SAD, to the extent that it has captured the fancy of anyone other than those affected by its symptoms, has from the moment of its recent discovery promised two things — a human behaviour and disorder with relevant animal models; and an environmental trigger which, whether or not still relevant to fitness, is easier to manipulate than other environmental risk factors for depression.

Acknowledgements

Supported in part by NIMH grant MH5389301.

References

Allison, A.C (1954) Protection afforded by the sickle-cell trait against subtertian malarial infection. *British Medical Journal*, 1:290–292.

Bartness, T.J., Wade, G.N. (1984) Photoperiodic control of body weight and energy metabolism in Syrian hamters (Mesocricetus auratus): role of pineal gland, melatonin, gonads, and diet. *Endocrinology. 114*:492–498.

Bartness, T.J. and Goldman, B.D. (1989) Mammalian pineal melatonin: a clock for all seasons. *Experientia*, 45:939–45.

Bronson, F.H. (1989) *Mammalian reproductive biology*, p. 133. .University of Chicago, Chicago.

Checkley, S.A., Murphy, D.G.M., Abbas, M., Marks, M., Winton, F., Palazidou, E., *et al.* (1993) Melatonin rhythms in seasonal affective disorder. *British Journal of Psychiatry*, 163:332–7.

Chemineau, P., Pelletier, J., Guerin, Y., Colas, G., Ravault, J.P., Toure, G., *et al.* (1988) Photoperiodic and melatonin treatments for the control of seasonal reproduction in sheep and goats. *Reproduction and Nutritional Development*, 28(2B):409–22.

Cole, R.J., Kripke, D.F., Wisbey, J., Mason, W.J., Gruen, W., Hauri, P.J., *et al.* (1995) Seasonal variation in human illumination exposure at two different latitudes. *Journal of Biological Rhythms*, 10:324–34.

Eastman, C.I. (1990) Natural summer and winter sunlight exposure patterns in seasonal affective disorder. *Physiology and Behavior*, 48:611–16.

Eastman, C.I., Young, M.A., Fogg, L.F., Liu, L., and Meaden, P.M. (1998) Bright light treatment of winter depression: a placebo-controlled trial. *Archives of General Psychiatry*, 55:883–9.

Ehlers, C.L., Frank, E., and Kupfer, D.J. (1988) Social zeitgebers and biological rhythms: a unified approach to understanding the etiology of depression. *Archives of General Psychiatry*, 45: 948–52.

Guillemette, J., Hébert, M., Paquet, J., and Dumont, M. (1998) Natural bright light exposure in the summer and winter in subjects with and without complaints of seasonal mood variations. *Biological Psychiatry*, 44:622–8.

Healy, D. (1987) Rhythm and blues: neurochemical, neuropharmacological and neuropsychological implications of a hypothesis of circadian rhythm dysfunction in the affective disorders. *Psychoph armacology*, 93:271–85.

Hébert, M., Dumont, M., and Paquet, J. (1998) Seasonal and diurnal patterns of human illumination under natural conditions. *Chronobiology International*, 15:59–70.

Hudson, R.R. (1996) Molecular population genetics of adaptation. In *Adaptation* (ed. M.R. Rose and G.V. Launder), pp. 291–309. Academic Press, San Diego.

Huxley, Sir J.S., Myr, E., Osmond H., *et al.* (1964) Schizoprenia as a genetic morphism. *Nature* 204:220–225, 1964.

Joy, J.E. and Mrosovsky, N. (1982) Circannual cycles of molt in ground squirrels. *Canadian Journal of Zoology*, 60:3227–31.

Karsch, F.J., Woodfill, C.J.I., Malpaux, B., Robinson, J.E., and Wayne, N.L. (1991) Melatonin and mammalian photoperiodism: synchronization of annual reproductive cycles. In *The suprachiasmatic nucleus* (ed. D.C. Klein, R.Y. Moore, and S.M. Reppert), pp. 217–32. Oxford University Press, New York.

Klein, D.F. (1993) False suffocation alarms, spontaneous panics, and related conditions. *Archives of General Psychiatry*, 50:306–17.

Levendosky, A.A., Joseph–Vanderpool, J.R., Hardin, T., Sorek, E., and Rosenthal, N.E. (1991) Core body temperature in patients with seasonal affective disorder and normal controls in summer and winter. *Biological Psychiatry*, 29:524–34.

Lewy, A.J., Wehr, T.A., Goodwin, F.K., Newsome, D.A., and Markey, S.P. (1980) Light suppresses melatonin suppression in humans. *Science*, 210:1267–9.

Lewy, A.J., Kern, H.J., Rosenthal, N.E., *et al.* (1982) Bright artificial light treatment of a manic-depressive with a seasonal mood cycle. *American Journal of Psychiatry*, 139:1496–8.

Lewy, A.J., Sack, R.L., Miller, S., and Hoban, T.M. (1987a) Antidepressant and circadian phase-shifting effects of light. *Science*, 235:352–4.

Lewy, A.J., Sack, R.L., Singer C.M., and White, D.M.. (1987*b*) The phase-shift hypothesis for bright light's therapeutic mechanism of action: theoretical considerations and experimental evidence. *Pscyhopharmacology Bulletin*, **23**:349–53.

Lewy, A.J., Sack, R.L., Singer, C.M., White, D.M., and Hoban, T.M. (1988*b*) Winter depression and the phase shift hypothesis for bright light's therapeutic effect. *Journal of Biological Rhythms*, **3**:121–34.

Lewy, A.J. and Sack, R.L. (1997) Exogenous melatonin's phase-shifting effects on the endogenous melatonin profile in sighted humans: a brief review and critique of the literature. *Journal of Biological Rhythms*, **12**:588–94.

Lewy, A.J., Bauer, V.K., Cutler, N.L., Sack, R.L., Ahmed, S., Thomas, K.H., *et al.* (1998*a*) Morning vs evening light treatment of patients with winter depression. *Archives of General Psychiatry*, **55**:890–96.

Lewy, A.J., Bauer, V.K., Cutler, N.L., and Sack, R.L. (1998*b*) Melatonin treatment of winter depression: a pilot study. *Psychiatry Research*, **77**:57–61.

Lewy, A.J., Bauer, V.K., Ahmed, S., Thomas, K.H., Cutler, N.L., Singer, C.M., *et al.* (1998*c*) The human phase response curve (PRC) to melatonin is out of phase with the PRC to light. *Chronobiology International*, **15**:71–83.

Lewy, A.J., Cutler, N.L., and Sack, R.L. (1999) The endogenous melatonin profile as a marker for circadian phase position. *Journal of Biological Rhythms*, **14**:227–36.

Lewy, A.J., Bauer, V.K., Bish, H.A., Evces, C.E., Hasler, B.P., Emens, J.S., *et al.* (2000) Antidepressant response correlates with the phase advance in winter depression. *Society for Light Treatment and Biological Rhythms Abstracts*, **12**:22.

Luboshitsky, R. and Lavie, P. (1999) Melatonin and sex hormone relationships — a review. *Journal of Pediatric Endocrinology and Metabolism*, **12**:355–62.

Mersch, P.P., Middendorp, H.P., Bouhuys, A.L., Beersma, D.G.M., and van den Hoofdakker, R.H. (1999) Seasonal affective disorder and latitude: a review of the literature. *Journal of Affective Disorders*, **53**:35–48.

Mrosovsky, N. (1989) Seasonal affective disorder, hibernation and annual cycles in animals: chipmunks in the sky. In *Seasonal affective disorder and phototherapy* (ed. N.E. Rosenthal and M. Blehar), pp. 127–48. Guilford Press, New York.

Nathan, P.J., Burrows, G.D., and Norman, T.R. (1999) Melatonin sensitivity to dim white light in affective disorders. *Neuropsychopharmacology*, **21**:408–13.

Nesse, R.M.(2000) Is depression an adaptation. *Archives of General Psychiatry*, **57**:14–20.

Oren, D.A., Moul, D.E., Schwartz, P.J., Brown, C., Yamada, E.M., and Rosenthal, N.E. (1994) Exposure to ambient light in patients with winter seasonal affective disorder. *American Journal of Psychiatry* **15**:591–3.

Reiter, R.J. (1993) The melatonin rhythm: both a clock and a calendar. *Experientia*, **49**:654–64.

Rose. M.R, Launder, G.V. (1996*b*) Post-spandrel adaptationism. In *Adaptation* (ed. M.R. Rose and G.V. Launder), pp. 1–10 Academic Press, San Diego.

Rosenthal, N.E., Sack, D.A., Gillin, J.C., Lewy, A.J., Goodwin, F.K., Davenport, Y., *et al.* (1984) Seasonal affective disorder. A description of the syndrome and preliminary findings with light therapy. *Archives of General Psychiatry*, **41**:72–80.

Rosenthal, N.E., Jacobsen, F.M., Sack, D.A., Arendt, J, James, S.P., Parry, B.L., *et al.* (1988). Atenolol in seasonal affective disorder: a test of the melatonin hypothesis. *American Journal of Psychiatry*, **145**:52–6.

Rosenwasser, A.M. (1992) Circadian rhythms and depression. *Light Therapy and Biological Rhythms*, **4**:35–9.

Saarela, S. and Reiter, R.J. (1994) Function of melatonin in thermoregulatory processes. *Life Sciences*, **54**:295–311.

Schlager D. (1994) Early morning administration of short-acting beta-adrenergic blockers for treatment of winter depression. *American Journal of Psychiatry*, **151**:1383–5.

Schlager, D., Norman, C., and Brown, G. (1996) Early-morning short-acting beta-adrenergic blockers for treatment of winter depression: a replication. *Society for Light Treatment and Biological Rhythms Abstracts*, **8**:15.

Schlager, D., Norman, C., and Brown, G. (1997) Early-morning short-acting beta-adrenergic blockers for treatment of winter depression: a replication and a test of the melatonin hypoth esis. *American Psychiatric Association Annual Meeting Abstract*.

Souêtre, E., Pringuey, D., Salvati, E., and Robert, P. (1985) Circadian rhythms and depression. *Annals of Medical Psychology (Paris)*, **143**:845–70.

Srinivasan, T.N., Padmavati, R. (1997) Fertility and schizophrenia: evidence for increased fertility in the relatives of schizophrenic patients. *Acta Psychiatrica Scandinavica*, **96**:260–4.

Terman, J.S., Terman, M. (1999) Photopic and scotopic light detection in patients with seasonal affective disorder and control subjects. *Biological Psychiatry* **46**:1642–8.

Terman, J.S., Terman, M., Lo, E.C. Cooper, T.B. (2001) Circadian time of morning light administration and therapeutic response in winter depression. *Archives of General Psychiatry*, **58**:69–75.

Terman, M,. Terman, J.S., Quitkin, F.M., McGrath, P.J., Stewart, J.W., and Rafferty, B. (1989) Light therapy for seasonal affective disorder: a review of efficacy. *Neuropsychopharmacology*, **2**:1–22.

Terman, M., Terman, J.S., and Ross, D.C. (1998) A controlled trial of timed bright light and negative air ionization for treatment of winter depression. *Archives of General Psychiatry*, **55**:875–82.

VanStaveren, W.A., Deurenberg, P., Burema, J., DeGroot, L.C.P.G.M., and Hautvast, J.G.A.J. (1986) Seasonal variation in food intake, pattern of physical activity and change in body weight in a group of young adult Dutch women consuming self-selected diets. *International Journal of Obesity*, **10**:133–45.

Wade, G.N. (1989) Seasonal variations in body weight and metabolism in hamsters. In *Seasonal affective disorder and phototherapy* (ed. N.E. Rosenthal and M. Blehar), pp. 105–26. Guilford Press, New York.

Wehr, T.A.. (1991) The duration of human melatonin secretion and sleep respond to changes in daylength (photoperiod). *Journal of Clinical Endocrinology and Metabolism*, **73**:1276–80.

Wehr, T.A. (1997) Melatonin and seasonal rhythms. *Journal of Biological Rhythms*, **12**:517–26.

Wehr, T.A. (1998) Effect of seasonal changes in daylength on human neuroendocrine function. *Hormone Research* **49**:118–24.

Wehr, T.A., Wirz-Justice, A, Goodwin, F.K., Duncan, W., and Gillin, J.C. (1979) Phase advance of circadian sleep-wake cycles as an antidepressant. *Science*, **206**:710–13.

Wehr, T.A., Jacobsen, F.M., Sack, D.A., Arendt, J., Tamarkin, L., and Rosenthal, N.E. (1986) Phototherapy of seasonal affective disorder: time of day and suppression of melatonin are not critical for antidepressant effects. *Archives of General Psychiatry*, **43**:870–75.

Wehr, T.A., Moul, D.E. Barbato, G., Giesen, H.A., Seidel, J.A., Barker, C., *et al.* (1993) Conservation of photoperiod-responsive mechanisms in humans. *American Journal of Physiology*, **265**:R846–57.

Wehr, T.A., Duncan Jr, W.C., Sher, L., Schwartz, P.E., Turner, E.M., Postolache, T., *et al.* (2000) SCN signal of change of season in seasonal affective disorder. *Society of Light Treatment and Biological Rhythms Abstracts*, **12**:2.

Williams, G.C. (1966) *Adaptation and natural selection: a critique of some current evolutionary thought.* Princeton University Press, Princeton.

Williams, H. and Ward, S. (1988) Melatonin and light treatment of ewes for autumn lambing. *Reproduction and Nutritional Development*, **28(2B)**:423–9.

Williams, G.C. and Nesse, R.M. (1991) The dawn of Darwinian medicine. *Quarterly Review of Biology*, **66**:1–22.

Zucker, I. (1989). Seasonal affective disorders: animal models non fingo. In *Seasonal affective disorder and phototherapy* (ed. N.E. Rosenthal and M. Blehar), pp. 149–64. Guilford Press, New York.

Chapter 19

Sleep

Jianhua Shen and Colin M. Shapiro

19.1 Insomnia associated with depression

Sleep disturbances are a common complaint in mood disorders (Reynolds 1987). SAD patients whose depressed mood recurs regularly in the winter season report hypersomnia more often (Rosenthal *et al.* 1984; Thompson *et al.* 1988) than the classical insomnia associated with depression. It is of particular interest to consider sleep in SAD for several reasons. First, the high sensitivity and specificity of sleep architecture changes in depression make it one of the (if not *the*) most important biological markers in psychiatry. Second, if there is a specific pattern in one form of depression then an understanding of this condition will be important in itself but will also potentially add to the knowledge of this field in general. Third, there is the opportunity to study the subjective and objective sleep congruence in this population.

Rosenthal and Wehr (1987) reported that hypersomnia was present in over 80 per cent of SAD subjects. Consistent with this, another large-sample study by Anderson *et al.* (1994) found that among the responses of 293 SAD patients on a symptom questionnaire, 235 (80 per cent) reported increased sleep in the winter compared with the summer, 30 (10 per cent) reported decreased sleep, 14 (5 per cent) complained of both, and the remaining 5 per cent did not report sleep-length differences. Ten of these patients kept daily sleep logs for one year. They recorded more mean total hours of sleep per 24 hours in the autumn (7.7 ± 0.6 hours) and winter (7.5 ± 0.7 hours), than in the spring (7.2 ± 0.7 hours) and summer (7.0 ± 0.6 hours). In particular, self-recorded sleep lengths in October, November, and December were significantly longer than in May. The SAD patient who reported the most marked seasonal change slept an average of 5.8 hours on weekdays in May to 11.3 hours on weekends in October. When weekdays are calculated separately from weekends, the mean maximum seasonal differences recorded were 2.3 hours for weekdays and 2.7 hours for weekends. Despite the increased length of sleep, these patients did not feel rested, and daytime drowsiness was a frequent phenomenon. Although these patients reported more frequent daytime naps in the autumn and winter, they did not report dozing off at inappropriate times or experiencing irresistible sleep onset.

We investigated 115 SAD patients with the Seasonal Patterns Assessment Questionnaire (SPAQ), a widely-used instrument that elicits the six key features of SAD. From data collected, we estimated each participant's total hours of sleep over a 24-hour period across the four seasons. Individuals with SAD reported the highest hours of sleep during winter (9.9 ± 2.28) and the fewest hours in summer (7.4 ± 1.22) with intermediate sleep duration for autumn (8.6 ± 1.76) and spring (8.4 ± 1.27) (Shapiro *et al.* 1994).

Complaints of hypersomnia in SAD appear to reflect a combination of earlier sleep onset, difficulty wakening, a low capacity to be awake at unusual times, and a lower quality of night-time sleep (Putilov *et al.* 1994). In the study by Rosenthal *et al.* (1984), all but 1 of the 29 patients (97 per cent) reported sleeping longer when depressed, with 79 per cent going to sleep earlier and 77 per cent waking up later.

19.2 Hypersomnolence may not be unique to SAD

Although SAD patients reported increased sleep during the winter season, hypersomnolence may not be a specific feature of SAD. Rosen *et al.* (1990) reported increased amounts of nocturnal sleep during autumn and winter in SAD patients, but similar changes were also found in the general population. The extent of winter/autumn oversleeping recorded by SAD patients did not differ dramatically from that reported by the general population. In a study (Anderson *et al.* 1994) among 1571 individuals from the general population, winter sleep increases of 2 hours a day relative to summer were reported by nearly half. As a whole, adults from the general population reported sleeping more in the winter (7.8 hours) than in the autumn (7.4 hours), spring (7.3 hours), or summer (7.1 hours). Females reported more sleep per night than males (females 7.5 hours, males 7.3 hours), but both genders described significantly different sleep length across each of the four seasons. Wirz-Justice *et al.* (1984) have also reported seasonal variations in sleep length among healthy individuals who tend to sleep less in May and June and more in October and November.

Electroencephalographic (EEG) data collected by Brunner *et al.* (1996) did not support the assumption of an involvement of sleep mechanisms in the pathogenesis of winter depression. Sleep diary data collected by Wirz–Justice *et al.* (1989) showed that sleep duration is generally not altered after successful light treatment (LT). When measured on a daily basis, sleep duration of SAD patients in Switzerland does not differ significantly between summer and winter (Brunner *et al.* 1993; Kräuchi *et al.* 1993). Furthermore, daily estimates of sleep duration and timing do not correlate with therapeutic response (Wirz–Justice and Anderson 1990) and have no predictive value for the success of LT (Kräuchi *et al.* 1993). Thus, most polysomnographic sleep data, as well as some data on prospective daily ratings of sleep duration, question the validity of hypersomnia as a intrinsic feature of SAD, unless patients are specifically selected for this characteristic (Brunner *et al.* 1996).

The Multiple Sleep Latency Test (MSLT) in patients with SAD has also failed to show evidence for increased sleep propensity during the day (Putilov *et al.* 1995). The MSLT is a formal polysomnographic test described by Carskadon and Dement (1977) in which patients are required to lie in a darkened room for 20 minutes at 2-hourly intervals during the day, for 4 or 5 tests. The time to fall asleep is taken as an indicator of daytime sleepiness.

In our study (Shapiro *et al.* 1994), sleep time differed significantly as indicated by a one-factor (season) analysis of variance. When entered simultaneously into a multiple regression equation, the entire set of items of the SPAQ accounted for a significant proportion of variance in depressive symptoms. However, examination of the individual beta weights for each of the SPAQ items indicated that only social activity levels were significantly related to depressive symptoms. Even when changes in sleep duration were included in the multiple regression analysis, neither this variable nor the other five SPAQ items were significantly related to the severity of depressive symptoms. Although the Hamilton scale item concerning hypersomnia indicated a significant reduction from pre- (1.3 ± 1.23) to post-treatment (0.7 ± 0.93), this was not corroborated by sleep-diary data collected just prior to and just after treatment: total hours of daily sleep did not change significantly (pre-treatment, 7.5 ± 0.86 versus post-treatment, 7.4 ± 0.68). Comparison of mean pre-treatment daily hours of sleep did not differ significantly across individuals whose SPAQ responses ranged from 'none' to 'extremely marked' seasonal variation in sleep duration. Similar results were obtained when we examined post-treatment sleep-diary information. Total diary sleep hours, as assessed by the sleep diary, were significantly shorter than self-report of sleep duration in the same season on the SPAQ.

When the SAD patients were asked to provide global retrospective descriptions, summarizing sleep over an extended period, there was a pattern of response that concurs with the widely-publicized description of SAD. However, the more detailed prospective sleep-diary information failed to corroborate this pattern. Interrelations among the seven individual items comprising the SPAQ also failed to support the hypothesized centrality of sleep change in SAD. When all of the seven items were regressed on Hamilton depression scores, only the item corresponding to social activity related significantly to the severity of depressive symptoms. This finding is consistent with extensive literature regarding the behavioural component of affective disorders. The failure to detect a relation of similar magnitude between depressive symptom severity and sleep behaviour as reported on the SPAQ also challenges the assumption that hypersomnia is the central feature of SAD.

19.3 **Polysomnographic findings**

Many authors (for example, Reynolds *et al.* 1986; Wehr *et al.* 1988; Reynolds 1987; Benca *et al.* 1992) have reported polysomnographic features of non-seasonal endogenous depressions. The sleep abnormalities of non-seasonal depressions primarily include shortened REM latency; increased REM sleep in the first third of the night; increased REM density; decreased delta sleep; reversal of the amount of slow wave sleep (SWS) in the first and second sleep cycles; early morning awakening; increased sleep latency; and increased nocturnal awakenings. These features are described in a patient-oriented book (Kennedy *et al.* 1998).

Sleep in SAD patients was found to have little resemblance to sleep in non-seasonal endogenous depression. A number of studies have investigated sleep structures and sleep EEGs in depressed SAD patients (Rosenthal *et al.* 1989; Endo 1993; Partonen *et al.* 1993; Anderson *et al.* 1994; Kohsaka *et al.* 1994; Brunner *et al.* 1996). In a winter-SAD study (Anderson *et al.* 1994), the polysomnographic data were compared with those from the same individuals in summer and those patients after LT, and with age- and gender-matched healthy controls. In this study, the sleep changes of SAD patients were decreased delta sleep and decreased sleep efficiency. The total sleep time of SAD patients was significantly longer in winter (6.8 ± 1.5 hours) than in summer (5.8 ± 0.6 hours). In summer, the sleep length of the SAD patients (5.8 ± 0.6 hours) was shorter than that of the controls (6.6 ± 0.7 hours). Analysis of delta sleep revealed that the patients demonstrated a significantly lower percentage of delta sleep in winter than in summer. Among healthy controls, there was no difference between winter and summer in duration of delta sleep.

However, another study (Brunner *et al.* 1996) revealed that SAD patients had better sleep than the controls. These patients showed higher sleep efficiency, longer total sleep time, and more stage 2 sleep during the entire sleep episode. SAD patients also were less wakeful during the first 4 hours of sleep, whereas REM sleep and slow wave sleep parameters did not differ between the SAD patients and healthy controls.

Table 19.1 Polysomnographic features of depression*

Sleep continuity disorders	Slow wave sleep (SWS or deep sleep)	REM sleep abnormalities deficits
Increased sleep latency	Decreased overall	Decreased REM latency
Increased wakefulness	Reversal in amounts of SWS in the	Increased overall
Sleep fragmentation	1st and 2nd sleep cycles	Increased 1st REM period
Decreased sleep efficiency		Increased REM Density
Increased early morning wake time		

* Reprinted with permission from *Defeating depression* by S.H. Kennedy, S.V. Parikh, and C.M. Shapiro (1998)

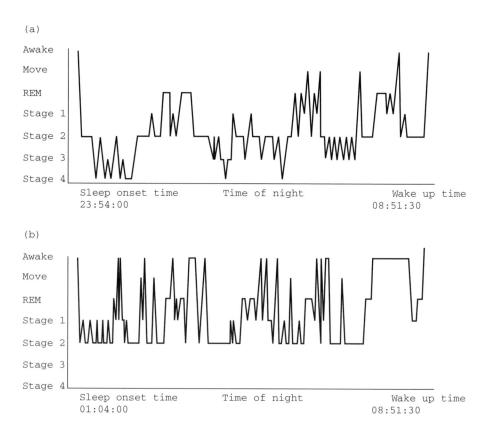

Fig. 19.1 (a) The sleep hypnogram of a healthy, normal person. Note that there is a great deal of stage 3 and 4 sleep early in the night and that the first REM or dream period occurs at about 90 minutes after sleep onset. (b) The hypnogram of a symptomatic depressed person. Note that there are many awakenings during the night, no deep sleep in this example, and very early REM sleep. (Reprinted with permission from *Defeating depression* by S.H. Kennedy, S.V. Parikh, and C.M. Shapiro, 1998.).

Taken together, there is no strong evidence that polysomnographic measures of SAD patients differ from those of healthy controls. In agreement with this notion, none of the sleep EEG studies in SAD (Rosenthal *et al.* 1989; Endo 1993; Partonen *et al.* 1993; Kohsaka *et al.* 1994) has found the pattern of sleep EEG changes that characterizes endogenous melancholic depression.

19.4 **Effects of light treatment on sleep**

After light treatment (LT), significant subjective and polysomnographic sleep improvement was observed in both SAD patients and control subjects. Increases of sleep efficiency and delta sleep were the major findings. Other findings included decreased REM density, increased amount and percentage of REM sleep, increased or decreased total sleep time, as well as reduced stage 1 sleep. The exposure to bright light resulted in a significant decrease in subjective sleepiness early in the evening in the patients, but not in the control subjects (Partonen *et al.* 1996). These findings were interpreted as a normalization of decreased sleep efficiency in depressed SAD patients (Brunner *et al.* 1996).

The most frequently reported finding after LT in SAD is increased sleep efficiency. Increased sleep maintenance has been reported after evening LT in healthy elderly subjects (Campbell *et al.* 1993) as well. Anderson *et al.* (1994) found that sleep efficiency was significantly enhanced following a week of bright-light treatment compared with the efficiency following room-light exposures. Only one LT study has been reported with healthy subjects administered bright light in the afternoon when no phase shifts of circadian rhythms are expected (Carrier and Dumont 1995), and it was concluded that good sleep in young subjects cannot be further improved by LT. Changes in sleep parameters could not demonstrate that LT *per se*, independent of circadian, clinical, behavioural, and/or methodological contributions, alters sleep stages (Brunner *et al.* 1996).

A curtailment of sleep, possibly related to activation and rebound activities, was documented in the sleep diaries of a group of SAD patients. They reported a reduction of their daily sleep duration by an average of 73 minutes during LT. In contrast, the controls reported an insignificant increase in their average daily sleep duration (Brunner *et al.* 1996). However, these findings are different from ours. Based on sleep-diary report, the sleep duration of our 115 SAD patients following LT was similar to the pre-treatment amount (Shapiro *et al.* 1994). Sleep-diary recordings of depressed SAD patients in Switzerland also indicated that their average winter sleep duration (6.9–7.4 hours per day) was not significantly different from that following successful LT or in summer (Wirz–Justice *et al.* 1984).

Increased SWS was found by Anderson *et al.* (1994) using combined morning and evening LT, but not by Brunner *et al.* (1996) using midday light. Using morning LT alone, an increase of SWS in the first 3 hours of the night has been reported in one study (Endo 1993), whereas in another no modifications of sleep stage parameters were found (Partonen *et al.* 1993).

Regarding the effects of LT on power spectra, Brunner *et al.* (1996) found that the absolute values of power density did not differ between SAD patients and controls in any frequency bin. The spectral changes were similar for both patient and control groups. In all cases, the recovery nights had increased EEG activity in the low delta band. A slight attenuation of EEG activity was present in the spindle frequencies. The decrease reached significance in the 12.25–14.0 Hz range for the SAD patients. As evaluated by paired comparisons, SAD patients had significantly increased EEG activity in the 0.75–6.0 Hz range for the baseline night, whereas the changes in the recovery night did not reach significance in any frequency bin.

SAD patients and controls differed significantly in their response to LT in the 1.75–4.0 Hz and 4.75–6.0 Hz band.

It is clear that there are some variations among the reports regarding the effect of LT. This may be due to differences in the light exposure regimen, such as the duration and the total number of days.

19.5 Effects of total sleep deprivation on sleep of SAD patients

The effect of sleep deprivation on the EEG is not dependent on the level of physical activity. Total sleep deprivation (TSD) resulted in increases in total sleep time, sleep efficiency, slow wave sleep, and total minutes of REM sleep during the recovery night, and it reduced sleep latency, the amount of wakefulness, and stage 1 sleep (Brunner *et al.* 1996). In a study evaluating sleep deprivation in SAD patients and normal controls, several other changes were found in both groups. In particular, REM latency of the SAD patients was markedly reduced. This phenomenon was also found after sleep deprivation in elderly men and women (Reynolds *et al.* 1986), but not in healthy young men (Borbély *et al.* 1981; Dijk *et al.* 1993).

Since a delayed onset of REM sleep is often seen in disrupted sleep, TSD may reduce REM sleep latency by consolidating sleep in the middle-aged and elderly. In female SAD patients, power spectra of non-REM sleep were changed by TSD. The power spectra changes were nearly identical to those found in healthy young men (Borbély *et al.* 1981; Dijk *et al.* 1990, 1993). Increased EEG activity in all frequencies below 11 Hz was accompanied by slightly attenuated values in the spindle frequencies (12.25–14.0 Hz). The increase of power density in the low delta frequencies is comparable or even larger than that reported after TSD in healthy young men (Borbély *et al.* 1981; Dijk *et al.* 1993).

19.6 Possible pathophysiological mechanisms

The relationship between sleep and circadian phase has spawned several explanations. It has been suggested that in healthy subjects the duration of a sleep episode partly depends on the circadian phase. Sleep episodes tend to end during the rising phase of the circadian temperature rhythm (Zulley *et al.* 1981, Gillberg and Åkerstedt 1982). The daytime regulation of the core temperature by serotonin 1A receptors appears normal in SAD. The magnitude of serotonin 1A receptor-activated hypothermia is controlled in the central nervous system by a thermostat whose operation appears to be modulated by both melatonin and the minimum core temperature (Schwartz *et al.* 1998). However, endogenous circadian rhythms are separable from sleep (Czeisler *et al.* 1987). At times, the temperature rhythm and sleep will become 'internally desynchronized'; the temperature rhythm will maintain a period of about 24.5 hours whereas the sleep–wake cycle period will be clearly different (for example, 19 hours or 35 hours). Variables that are associated with the circadian process include temperature, cortisol, thyroid-stimulating hormone (TSH), melatonin, and REM sleep (Czeisler *et al.* 1987).

Hypotheses about the pathophysiology of SAD have focused on abnormalities in circadian pacemaker function, such as a phase delay (Lewy *et al.* 1985, 1987), diminished amplitude of circadian rhythms during winter (Czeisler *et al.* 1987, 1989), or abnormal response to the photoperiod (Rosenthal *et al.* 1984). Accordingly, the therapeutic effects of bright light have been attributed to its ability to normalize aberrant circadian rhythms. Since the circadian pacemaker is a major determinant of sleep propensity, sleep timing, and sleep structure

(Zulley *et al.* 1981), light-induced modifications of the pacemaker may also have repercussions on sleep.

Lewy *et al.* (1985) hypothesized that most SAD patients have a phase delay in their endogenous circadian rhythm relative to sleep and that the antidepressant effect of light may be mediated by the phase-advancing effect of morning light. In winter depressives, compared to non-depressed controls, they found the circadian rhythm of melatonin to be phase-delayed relative to sleep. Terman *et al.* (1988) have also found phase-delayed melatonin rhythms in SAD. Properly timed bright light caused a significant phase advance (Lewy *et al.* 1987; Sack *et al.* 1990), and it can also increase the amplitude of the temperature rhythm. Thus, Czeisler *et al.* (1987) have proposed a hypothesis that the endogenous circadian amplitude is low in SAD and that bright-light therapy increases the amplitude to normal levels.

Avery *et al.* (1997) assessed circadian temperature, cortisol, and TSH rhythms during a constant routine research in female hypersomnic SAD patients and controls before and after morning bright-light treatment. After sleep was standardized for 6 days, the subjects were sleep-deprived and at bed rest for 27 hours while rectal temperature, cortisol, and TSH levels were assessed. The minimum of the fitted rectal temperature rhythm was phase-delayed in the SAD group compared to the controls (5.42 a.m. versus 3.16 a.m.). With bright-light treatment, the minimum advanced from 5.42 a.m. to 3.36 a.m. The minimum of the cortisol rhythm was phase-delayed in the SAD group compared to the control group — 12.11 a.m. versus 11.03 p.m. With bright-light treatment, the minimum advanced from 12.11 a.m. to 11.38 p.m. The peak phase of the TSH rhythm was not significantly phase-delayed in SAD subjects compared to controls, though the trend appeared to be toward a phase delay. After bright-light therapy, the TSH peak phase did not change significantly in the SAD subjects; the trend was a phase advance. These results suggest that circadian rhythms are phase-delayed relative to sleep in SAD patients and that morning bright light phase-advances those rhythms.

In a study of ambulatory monitoring of rectal temperature, Rosenthal *et al.* (1990) found that the temperature amplitude of SAD subjects was similar to that of controls. Although there was no systematic shift in phase with the photoperiod extension, temperature minima were advanced in 6 of 10 SAD patients and delayed in 4 of 10. It was suggested that those SAD patients who advanced their rhythms with LT tended to experience more hypersomnia at baseline, a greater increase in temperature amplitude with light treatment, and a better antidepressant response. Those whose temperature rhythms were phase-delayed with bright light tended to have early morning awakening, reduced amplitude increase, and inferior antidepressant response.

In SAD patients, LT lowered core temperature during sleep in proportion to its antidepressant efficacy (Schwartz *et al.* 1998). When the SAD patients and controls were re-studied in the summer, the amplitudes were not different, but the overall mean temperature across the 24-hour period was lower for both groups (Levendosky *et al.* 1991). In contrast to endogenous melancholic depressed in-patients, who usually have high nocturnal temperatures and low temperature amplitude (Avery *et al.* 1997), SAD patients rarely show these abnormalities either in an ambulatory study (Rosenthal *et al.* 1990) or in constant-routine studies.

The circadian rhythms of cortisol obtained without a constant routine were found to be similar in SAD patients compared to controls both in phase and amplitude; the rhythms did not change with successful bright light (Joseph–Vanderpool *et al.* 1991). Since sleep has a suppressing effect on cortisol (Weitzman *et al.* 1983), those cortisol data do not reflect the unmasked endogenous circadian rhythm of cortisol. SAD patients had normal cortisol and adrenocorticotropic hormone (ACTH) levels, but their responses to corticotropin-releasing hormone (CRH) were delayed and significantly reduced (Joseph–Vanderpool *et al.* 1991; Partonen 1995). With bright-light therapy, the responses of cortisol and ACTH to CRH significantly increased. James *et al.* (1986) found that only 2 of 20 SAD subjects showed dexamethasone non-suppression.

Joffe (1991) and Bauer *at al.* (1993) found that single time-point assessment of thyroid function is normal in SAD patients and does not change significantly after successful LT. Raitiere (1992) found that 17 (35 per cent) of 49 SAD patients had elevated TSH compatible with mild primary hypothyroidism, and that this proportion was significantly greater than that seen in non-seasonal depressed patients. Circadian profiles without a constant routine have shown no differences between SAD patients and controls, but with bright-light treatment the nocturnal TSH values decreased significantly; however, sleep suppresses TSH secretion and masks the endogenous rhythm. It has been shown that responsiveness of TSH to thyrotropin-releasing hormone stimulation is reduced in SAD subjects (Coiro *et al.* 1994).

Overall, the data generally support the hypothesis that the circadian rhythms obtained under constant routine conditions are phase-delayed in SAD subjects compared to controls and that morning bright-light treatments phase-advance those circadian rhythms (see also the chapter by Boivin). However, there are some discrepancies among the reports. The cortisol data offer some support for the low circadian amplitude hypothesis. These data suggest that the phase-delay hypothesis and the low circadian amplitude hypothesis are not mutually exclusive.

19.7 **Conclusion**

This review suggests that an impairment of circadian rhythm is part of the pathogenesis of SAD and that there is a pattern of delayed sleep phase in such patients. The relationships between circadian rhythms and their modifiers in the treatment of SAD patients require further study.

References

Anderson, J.L., Rosen, L.N., Mendelson, W.B., Jacobsen, F.M., Skwerer, E.G., Joseph–Vanderpool, J.R., *et al.* (1994) Sleep in full/winter seasonal affective disorder: effects of light and changing seasons. *J Psychosomatic Res* **38**:323–37.

Avery, D.H., Dahl, K., Savage, M.V., Brengelmann, G.L., Larsen, L.H., Kenny, M.A., *et al.* (1997) Circadian temperature and cortisol rhythms during a constant routine are phase-delayed in hypersomnic winter depression. *Biol Psychiatry* **41**:1109–23.

Bauer, M.S., Kurtz, J., Winokur, A., Phillips, J., Rubin, L., and Marcus, J. (1993) Thyroid function before and after four-week light treatment in winter depressives and controls. *Psychoneuroendocrinology* **18**:437–43.

Benca, R.M., Obermeyer, W.H., Thisted, R.A., and Gillin, J.C. (1992) Sleep and psychiatric disorders. A meta-analysis. *Arch Gen Psychiatry* **49**:651–8.

Borbély, A.A., Baumann, F., Brandeis, D., Strauch, I., and Lehmann, D. (1981) Sleep deprivation: effect on sleep stages and EEG power density in man. *Electroenceph Clin Neurophysiol* **51**: 483–93.

Brunner, D.P., Kräuchi, K., Leonhardt, G., Graw, P., and Wirz–Justice, A. (1993) Sleep parameters in SAD: effects on midday light, season, and sleep deprivation. *Sleep Res* **22**:396.

Brunner, D.P., Kräuchi, K., Dijk, D-J., Leonhardt, G., Haug, H-J., and Wirz–Justice, A. (1996) Sleep electroencephalogram in seasonal affective disorder and in control women: effects of midday light treatment and sleep deprivation. *Biol Psychiatry* **40**:485–96.

Campbell, S.S., Dawson, D., and Anderson, M.W. (1993) Alleviation of sleep maintenance insomnia with timed exposure to bright light. *J Am Geriatr Soc* **41**:829–36.

Carrier, J. and Dumont, M. (1995) Sleep propensity and sleep architecture after bright light exposure at three different times of day. *J Sleep Res* **4**:202–11.

Carskadon, M.A. and Dement, W.C. (1977) Sleep tendency: an objective measure of sleep loss. *Sleep Res* **6**:200

Coiro, V., Colp, R., Marchesi, C., *et al.* (1994) Lack of seasonal variation in abnormal TSH secretion in patients with seasonal affective disorder. *Biol Psychiatry* **35**:36–41.

Czeisler, C.A., Kronauer, R.E., Mooney, J.J., Anderson, J.L., and Allan, J.S. (1987) Biologic rhythm disorders, depression, and phototherapy: a new hypothesis. *Psych Clin N Amer* **10**:687–709.

Czeisler, C.A., Kronauer, R.E., Allan, J.S., Duffy, J.F., Jewett, M.E., Brown, E.N., *et al.* (1989) Bright light induction of strong (type 0) resetting of the human circadian pacemaker. *Science* **244**:1328–33.

Dijk, D.J., Brunner, D.P., and Borbély, A.A. (1990) Time course of EEG power density during long sleep in humans. *Am J Physiol* **258**:R650–61.

Dijk, D.J., Hayes, B., and Czeisler, C.A. (1993) Dynamics of electroencephalographic sleep spindles and wave activity in men: effect of sleep deprivation. *Brain Res* **626**:190–9.

Endo, T. (1993) Morning bright light effects on circadian rhythms and sleep structure of SAD. *Jikeikai Med J* **40**:295–307.

Gillberg, M. and Åkerstedt, T. (1982) Body temperature and sleep at different times of day. *Sleep* **5**:378–88.

James, S., Wehr, T., Sack, D., Parry, B., Rogers, S., and Rosenthal N.E. (1986) The dexamethasone suppression test in seasonal affective disorder. *Compr Psychiatry* **27**:224–6.

Joffe, R. (1991) Thyroid function and phototherapy in seasonal affective disorder. *Am J Psychiatry* **148**:393.

Joseph–Vandepool, J.R., Rosenthal, N.E., Chrousos, G.P., *et al.* (1991) Abnormal pituitary-adrenal responses to corticotropin-releasing hormone in patients with seasonal affective disorder: Clinical and pathophysiological implications. *J Clin Endocrinol Metab* **72**:1382–7.

Kennedy, S.H., Parikh, S.V., and Shapiro, C.M. (1998) Defeating depression. Joli Joco Publications, Inc., Thornhill, USA.

Kohsaka, M., Honma, H., Fukuda, N., Kobayashi, R., and Honma, K. (1994) Does bright light change sleep structures in seasonal affective disorder? *Soc Light Therapy Biol Rhythms Abstracts* **6**:32.

Kräuchi, K., Wirz–Justice, A., and Graw, P. (1993) High intake of sweets late in the day predicts a rapid and persistent response to light therapy in winter depression. *Psychiatry Res* **46**:107–17.

Levendosky, A.A., Joseph-Vanderpool, J.R., Hardin, T., Sorek, E., and Rosenthal, N.E. (1991) Core body temperature in patients with seasonal affective disorder and normal controls in summer and winter. *Biol Psychiatry* **29**:524–34.

Lewy, A.J., Sack, R.L., and Singer, C.M. (1985) Treating phase-typed chronobiologic sleep and mood disorders using appropriately timed bright artificial light. *Psychopharmacol Bull* **21**:368–72.

Lewy, A.J., Sack, R.L., Miller, L.S., and Hoban, T.M. (1987) Antidepressant and circadian phase-shifting effects of light. *Science* **235**:352–4.

Partonen, T. (1995) A mechanism of action underlying the antidepressant effect of light. *Medical Hypotheses* **45**:33–4.

Partonen, T., Appelberg, B., and Partinen, M. (1993) Effects of light treatment on sleep structure in seasonal affective disorder. *Eur Arch Psychiatry Clin Neurosci* **242**:310–13.

Partonen, T., Vakkuri, O., Lamberg–Allardt, C., and Lönnqvist, J. (1996) Effects of bright light on sleepiness, melatonin, and 25-hydroxyvitamin D (3) in winter seasonal affective disorder. *Biol Psychiatry* **39**:865–72.

Putilov, A.A., Booker, J.M., Danilenko, K.V., and Zolotarev, D.Y. (1994) The relation of sleep-wake patterns to seasonal depressive behavior. *Arctic Medical Res* **53**:130–6.

Putilov, A.A., Danilenko, K.V., Palchikov, V.E., and Schergin, S.M. (1995) The multiple sleep latency test in seasonal affective disorder: no evidence for increased sleep propensity. *Soc Light Treatment Biol Rhythms Abstracts* **7**:30.

Raitiere, M.N. (1992) Clinical evidence for thyroid dysfunction in patients with seasonal affective disorder. *Psychoneuroendocrinology* **17**:23141.

Reynolds III, C.F., Kupfer, D.J., Hoch, C.C., Stack, J.A., Houck, P.R., and Berman, S.R. (1986) Sleep deprivation in healthy elderly men and women: effects on mood and on sleep during recovery. *Sleep* **9**:492–501.

Reynolds III, C.F. (1987) Sleep and affective disorders: a minireview. *Psych Clin N Am* **10**:583–91.

Rosen, L.N., Targum, S.D., Terman, M., Bryant, M.J., Hoffman, H., Kasper, S.F., *et al.* (1990) Prevalence of seasonal affective disorder at four latitudes. *Psychiatry Res* **31**:131–44.

Rosenthal, N.E., Sack, D.A., Gillin, J.C., Lewy, A.J., Goodwin, F.K., Davenport, Y., *et al.* (1984) Seasonal affective disorder: a description of the syndrome and preliminary findings with light therapy. *Arch Gen Psychiatry* **41**:72–80.

Rosenthal, N.E. and Wehr, T.A. (1987) Seasonal affective disorder. *Psychiatr Ann* **17**:670–4.

Rosenthal, N.E., Skwerer, R.G., Levendosky, B.A., Joseph–Vanderpool, J.R., Jacobsen, F.M., Duncan, C.C., *et al.* (1989) Sleep architecture in seasonal affective disorder: the effects of light therapy and changing seasons. *Sleep Res* **18**:440.

Rosenthal, N.E., Levendosky, A.A., Skwerer, R.G., *et al.* (1990) Effects of light treatment on core body temperature in seasonal affective disorder. *Biol Psychiatry* **27**:39–50.

Sack, R.L., Lewy, A.J., White, D.M., Singer, C.M., Fireman, M.V., and Van Diver, R. (1990) Morning versus evening light treatment for winter depression: evidence that the therapeutic effects of light are mediated by circadian phase shifting. *Arch Gen Psychiatry* **47**:343–51.

Schwartz, P.J., Rosenthal, N.E., and Wehr, T.A. (1998) Serotonin 1A receptors, melatonin, and the proportional control thermostat in patients with winter depression. *Arch Gen Psychiatry* **55**: 897–903.

Shapiro, C.M., Devins, G.M., Feldman, B., and Levitt, A.J. (1994) Is hypersomnolence a feature of seasonal affective disorder? *J Psychosom Res* **38**(Suppl. 1):49–54.

Terman, M., Terman, J.S., Quitkin, F.M., *et al.* (1988) Response of the melatonin cycle to phototherapy for seasonal affective disorder. *J Neural Transm* **72**:147–65.

Thompson, C., Stinson, D., Fernandez, M., Fine, J., and Isaacs, G. (1988) A comparison of normal, bipolar and seasonal affective disorder subjects using the Seasonal Pattern Assessment Questionnaire. *J Aff Dis* **14**:257–64.

Wehr, T.A., Rosenthal, N.E., and Sack, D.A. (1988) Environmental and behavioral influences on affective illness. *Acta Psychiat Scand* **Suppl 341** (77):44–52.

Weitzman, E., Zimmerman, J.C., Czeisler, C.A., and Ronda, J. (1983) Cortisol secretion is inhibited during sleep in normal man. *J Clin Endocrinol Metabol* **56**:352–8.

Wirz–Justice, A., Wever, R.A., and Aschoff, J. (1984) Seasonality in freeruning circadian rhythms in man. *Naturwissenschaften* **71**:316–19.

Wirz–Justice, A., Graw, P., Kräuchi, K., Brunner, M., and Pöldinger, W. (1989) Light and season modify sleep rating and carbohydrate intake in SAD. *Sleep Res* **18**:157.

Wirz–Justice, A. and Anderson, J. (1990) Morning light exposure for the treatment of winter depression: the one true light therapy? *Psychopharmacology* **26**:511–20.

Zulley, J., Wever, R., and Aschoff, J. (1981) The dependence of onset and duration of sleep on the circadian rhythm of rectal temperature. *Pflügers Arch* **391**:312–18.

Chapter 20

Carbohydrate intake

Kurt Kräuchi and Anna Wirz–Justice

20.1 Introduction

Psychiatrists have long made analogies between hibernation and depression, because of the apparently withdrawn state and its periodicity (Giedke 1987; Lange 1928). And indeed, the resurgence of interest in such analogies has been stimulated by the diagnosis of recurrent winter depression. Designated SAD, these patients experience regular depressive episodes in autumn or winter with remission in spring and summer (Rosenthal *et al.* 1984). The depressive state is characterized by hypersomnia and fatigue, and changes in eating style are prominent (Rosenthal *et al.* 1984). Most patients with SAD report increased appetite and 'carbohydrate (CHO) craving', higher food intake, and weight gain during their winter depression. Therefore, studying SAD could help to reveal the often assumed association between CHO intake, CHO metabolism, and mood in a seasonal time course. This chapter summarizes studies dealing with the link between mood, CHO intake, and metabolic functions.

20.2 Is seasonality in food selection and metabolism a normal phenomenon?

In healthy subjects, seasonal rhythms in psychological, physiological, and behavioural dimensions have been widely documented, as have those neurochemical and hormonal measures considered relevant for affective illness (for review, see Aschoff 1981; Lacoste and Wirz–Justice 1989). Early studies documented seasonal rhythms of total caloric intake in adults and even in children (Debry *et al.* 1975; Sargent 1954). This has been confirmed in a more recent study showing increased total caloric intake, especially of CHO, in the autumn (De Castro 1991). Seasonal variation of other macronutrients and specific foods (for example, fibres, dairy products) have also been reported, but with inconsistent results (reviewed in Kräuchi and Wirz–Justice 1992).

Whether these discrepancies are a result of different methods for measuring food intake, or from a real reduction in amplitude of seasonal rhythms over the last decades, as seen in many other variables (Aschoff 1981), is unclear. In a representative telephone survey in Switzerland we found that sweet- and starch-rich CHO foods are more often selected during autumn to spring than in summer, whereas protein-rich foods did not exhibit a seasonal pattern (unpublished results).

20.3 **CHO intake related to depression**

The symptoms just described are atypical for major depression. Most patients with major affective disorder have sleep loss, diminished appetite and food intake, an inability to taste and to enjoy food, and loss of body weight (for example, Amsterdam *et al.* 1987; Davidson and Turnbull 1986; Paykel 1977). Only about 15 per cent report increased appetite and body weight (for example, Davidson and Turnbull 1986; Paykel 1977). A direct comparison of major affective disorders with or without a seasonal periodicity has shown that 67 per cent and 23 per cent, respectively, exhibited CHO craving (Garvey *et al.* 1988). In a group of untreated, severely depressed patients, a decrease in appetite and food intake was found but, with a relative excess of CHO and a preference for sweets (Kazes *et al.* 1994). It has been claimed that increased CHO consumption (primarily in the form of sucrose) in depressed subjects is consistent with the often described characteristic of CHO craving, and may relate to the development or maintenance of depression (Christensen and Somers 1996).

In early childhood, sweets initially serve as one of the attractive sensory experiences (Steiner 1979). Oral sweet solutions induce rapid and sustained calming in crying newborns and increase mouthing and hand–mouth contact (Barr *et al.* 1999). But also adults give the highest 'hedonic ratings' to substances which are sweet, particularly if they are combined with high fat content (Drewnowski and Greenwood 1983). Thus, during the depressive state regressive behaviours are activated which were positively experienced in early childhood — that is, behaviours learned in early years as a way of solving emotional problems via food (Steiner 1979). All these studies suggest that an excess in CHO intake is not restricted to a seasonal disturbance such as SAD, it can be more generally related to depressive mood.

20.4 **Seasonal rhythms of food selection and metabolism in SAD**

Food intake and body weight changes in SAD have previously been studied by retrospective self-estimation using a single application of the Seasonal Pattern Assessment Questionnaire (SPAQ) (Kasper *et al.* 1989; Kräuchi and Wirz–Justice 1992; Rosenthal *et al.* 1987), or under semi-natural laboratory conditions (Wurtman and Wurtman 1989). We have replicated the selective nutrient choice of depressed SAD patients in a series of independent ambulatory studies (reviewed in Kräuchi and Wirz–Justice 1992). The highest CHO intake occurred in the afternoon and evening. Successful light therapy selectively suppressed CHO intake. Additionally, those patients with the highest consumption of sweets in the second half of the day responded best to light treatment (Kräuchi *et al.* 1993).

SAD patients have not only appetite and weight disturbances, but also dysfunctional eating attitudes which are not, however, as extreme as those of bulimia (Berman *et al.* 1993). A significant correlation between seasonal body weight changes and body dissatisfaction was interpreted as discomfort with body shape during winter when weight had increased (Berman *et al.* 1993).

The Dutch Eating Behaviour Questionnaire (DEBQ) has provided new insight with respect to 'eating style'. SAD patients showed higher values in 'emotional' and 'external' eating than controls (Kräuchi *et al.* 1997). In contrast to patients with bulimia and anorexia nervosa, who are high 'restraint' eaters, SAD patients were not. Additional items revealed that SAD patients selectively ate sweets under emotionally difficult conditions (when depressed, anxious, or lonely) (Kräuchi *et al.* 1997). Furthermore, seasonal body weight change was highest in those subjects with high 'emotional' and 'restraint' eating, together with a high body mass index (Kräuchi *et al.* 1997). This result is in accord with the concept of disinhibition of dietary restraint in extreme emotional situations (for example, the depressive state).

There is a sparse literature noting an association between depression and altered glucose regulation. For example, the prevalence for depression among patients with diabetes mellitus is higher than in the general population and conversely, affective disorders are significantly associated with poorer glucose control and increased reporting of diabetic symptoms (Eaton *et al.* 1996; Mueller *et al.* 1969).

We investigated the link between mood, glucose, and metabolism in a combined set-up which included a glucose tolerance test and hedonic ratings of sucrose solutions (alliesthesia test, Cabanac 1971). The alliesthesia test is based on the perception of an external stimulus (for example, a sweet taste) as either pleasant or unpleasant, depending on signals from inside the body (for example, glucose homeostasis). SAD patients perceived high sucrose concentrations as more pleasant when they were depressed than when they were euthymic after light therapy or in summer (Kräuchi *et al.* 1999). Seasonal alterations in taste detection and recognition threshold have also been reported in SAD (Arbisi *et al.* 1996).

The change in hedonic ratings is reflected in changes in metabolic functions: in the glucose tolerance test, SAD patients have impaired insulin sensitivity only during the winter depressive phase, which is normalized after 1 week of bright-light therapy and spontaneously in summer (Kräuchi *et al.* 1999). The more rapid post-glucose glycaemia may impair glycaemic control in depressed SAD patients. However, in all individuals the baseline and 2-hour post-prandial plasma levels of glucose and insulin were within the non-diabetic range. Allen *et al.* (1992) have reported that insulin sensitivity improved after light therapy in a patient with both SAD and insulin-dependent diabetes mellitus. Taken together, these results suggest that a real 'metabolic demand' for glucose could underlie the characteristic CHO craving in SAD patients during their winter depression. Their increased CHO consumption can be therefore considered as an attempt at self-medication, perhaps via monoaminergic mechanisms with specific neuroanatomical substrate (for a detailed discussion, see Kräuchi *et al.* 1993).

In spite of the established, clinically significant, abnormal CHO regulation in SAD, the pathophysiology of this disturbance and the mechanism of its responsiveness to light remains unknown.

References

Allen, N.H.P., Kerr, D., Smythe, P.J., Martin, N., Osola, K., and Thompson, C. (1992). Insulin sensitivity after phototherapy for seasonal affective disorder. *Lancet*, **339**:1065–6.

Amsterdam, J.D., Settle, G., Doty, R.L., and Abelman, E.A.W. (1987). Taste and smell perception in depression. *Biological Psychiatry*, **22**:1477–81.

Arbisi, P.A., Levine, A.S., Nerenberg, J., and Wolf, J. (1996). Seasonal alteration in taste detection and recognition threshold in seasonal affective disorder: the proximate source of carbohydrate craving. *Psychiatry Research*, **59**:171–82.

Aschoff, J. (1981). Annual rhythms in man. In *Handbook of behavioral neurobiology, Vol. 4* (ed. J. Aschoff), pp. 475–87. Plenum Publishing Corp., New York.

Barr, R.G., Pantel, M.S., Young, S., Wright, J.H., Hendricks, L.A., and Gravel R. (1999). The response of crying newborns to sucrose: is it a 'sweetness' effect? *Physiology and Behavior*, **66**:409–17.

Berman, K., Lam, R.W., and Goldner, E.M. (1993). Eating attitudes in seasonal affective disorder and bulimia. *Journal of Affective Disorders*, **29**:219–25.

Cabanac, M. (1971). Physiological role of pleasure. *Science*, **173**:1103–7.

Christensen, L. and Somers, S. (1996). Comparison of nutrient intake among depressed and nondepressed individuals. *International Journal of Eating Disorders*, **20**:105–9.

Davidson, J. and Turnbull, C.D. (1986). Diagnostic significance of vegetative symptoms in depression. *British Journal of Psychiatry*, **148**:442–6.

De Castro, J.M. (1991). Seasonal rhythms of human nutrient intake and meal pattern. *Physiology and Behavior*, **50**:243–8.

Debry, G., Bleyer, R., and Reinberg, A. (1975). Circadian, circannual and other rhythms in spontaneous nutrient and caloric intake of healthy four-year olds. *Diabète & Metabolisme (Paris)*, **1**:91–9.

Drewnowski, A. and Greenwood, M.R.C. (1983). Cream and sugar: human preferences for high-fat foods. *Physiology and Behavior*, **30**:629–33.

Eaton, W.W., Armenian, H., Gallo, J., Pratt, L., and Ford, D.E. (1996). Depression and the risk for the onset of type II diabetes: a prospective population-based study. *Diabetes Care*, **19**:1097–102.

Garvey, M.J., Wesner, R., and Godes, M. (1988). Comparison of seasonal and non-seasonal affective disorders. *American Journal of Psychiatry*, **145**:100–2.

Giedke, H. (1987). Schlaf, Winterschlaf und Depression. In *Schlaf-Wach-Funktionen* (ed. H. Hippius, E. Rüther, and M. Schmauss), pp. 55–76. Springer Verlag, Berlin.

Kasper, S., Wehr, T.A., Bartko, J.J., Gaist, P.A., and Rosenthal, N.E. (1989). Epidemiological findings of seasonal changes in mood and behavior: a telephone survey of Montgomery County, Maryland. *Archives of General Psychiatry*, **46**:823–33.

Kazes, M., Danion, J.M., Grange, D. *et al.* (1994). Eating behaviour and depression before and after antidepressant treatment: a prospective, naturalistic study. *Journal of Affective Disorders*, **30**:193–207.

Kräuchi, K. and Wirz–Justice, A. (1992). Seasonal patterns of nutrient intake in relation to mood. In *The biology of feast and famine: relevance to eating disorders* (ed. G.H. Anderson and S.H. Kennedy), pp. 157–82. Academic Press, Orlando.

Kräuchi, K., Wirz–Justice, A., and Graw, P. (1993). High sweets intake late in the day predicts a rapid and persistent response to light therapy in winter depression. *Psychiatry Research*, **46**:107–17.

Kräuchi, K., Reich, S., Wirz–Justice, A. (1997). Eating style in seasonal affective disorder: who will gain weight in winter? *Comprehensive Psychiatry*, **38**:80–7.

Kräuchi, K., Keller, U., Leonhardt, G., Brunner, D.P., and van der Velde H.H-J (1999). Accelerated post-glucose glycaemia and altered alliesthesia-test in seasonal affective disorder. *Journal of Affective Disorders*, **53**:23–6.

Lacoste, V. and Wirz–Justice, A. (1989). Seasonal variation in normal subjects: an update of variables current in depression research. In *Seasonal affective disorder and phototherapy* (ed. N.E. Rosenthal and M. Blehar), pp. 167–229. Guilford Press, New York.

Lange, J. (1928). Die endogenen und reaktiven Gemütserkrankungen und die manisch-depressive Konstitution. In *Handbuch der Geisteskrankheiten* (ed. O. Bumke). Springer Verlag, Berlin.

Mueller, P.S., Heninger, G.R., and McDonald, R.K. (1969). Intravenous glucose tolerance test in depression. *Archives of General Psychiatry*, **21**:470–7.

Paykel, E.S. (1977). Depression and appetite. *Journal of Psychosomatic Research*, **21**:401–7.

Rosenthal, N.E., Sack, D.A., Gillin, J.C., *et al.* (1984). Seasonal affective disorder: a description of the syndrome and preliminary findings with light therapy. *Archives of General Psychiatry*, **41**:72–80.

Rosenthal, N.E., Genhart, M., Jacobsen, F.M., Skwerer, R.G., and Wehr T.A. (1987). Disturbances of appetite and weight regulation in seasonal affective disorder. *Annals of the New York Academy of Science*, **499**:216–30.

Sargent, F. (1954). Season and the metabolism of fat and carbohydrate: a study of vestigial. *Meteorological Monographs*, **2**:68–80.

Steiner, J.E. (1979). Human facial expressions in response to taste and smell stimulation. *Advances in Child Development and Behavior*, **13**:257–95.

Wurtman, R.J. and Wurtman, J.J. (1989). Carbohydrates and depression. *Scientific American*, **260**:68–75.

Chapter 21

Monoamines

Alexander Neumeister, Anastasios Konstantinidis,
Nicole Praschak–Rieder, Matthäus Willeit, Eva Hilger,
Jürgen Stastny, and Siegfried Kasper

21.1 Introduction

SAD (winter pattern) is a condition characterized by regularly occurring depressions in autumn and winter, alternating with non-depressed periods in spring and summer (Rosenthal *et al.* 1984). Light therapy is recognized as an effective treatment for this condition and is routinely prescribed (Neumeister *et al.* 1999*b*). Extensive research during the last two decades has focused on the pathogenesis of SAD and the mechanisms of action of light therapy. However, we still do not fully understand the aetiology of SAD and such mechanisms.

Several biological abnormalities have been found in patients with SAD compared with healthy controls. Such differences include alterations in hormonal profiles, biochemical challenges, immune responses, and visual evoked phenomena. Some of these parameters are known to change following successful light treatment.

Neurotransmitters have been postulated as playing a key role in the pathogenesis of SAD and also in the mechanisms of action of light therapy. Two neurotransmitter systems have been the main focus of interest during the past decade — serotonin (5-HT) and catecholamines — and evidence has been gathered for the role of each of these. However, it seems likely that the two transmitter systems interact and play important roles, either in different anatomic areas or neurobiologic systems of the brain. This chapter introduces the monoamine hypothesis of SAD and light therapy and demonstrates how this hypothesis can influence the practice and research of SAD in the future.

21.1 Seasonality and brain serotonin function

There is considerable evidence in the literature that there exists a seasonal variation in several phenomena, such as mood, feeding behaviour, and suicide, and that these phenomena may be related to changes in central and peripheral 5-HT function (Maes *et al.* 1995). As will be discussed, changes in 5-HT function have been postulated to be involved also in the pathogenesis of SAD. Thus it appears to be of interest whether possible seasonal fluctuations in 5-HT function exist only in SAD patients or whether these fluctuations are physiological.

In healthy subjects and non-psychiatric patients several studies have described seasonal variations in central and peripheral 5-HT function. Studies in humans involve either static (for example, biochemical levels in body fluids or blood elements) or dynamic (for example, neuroendocrine responses to pharmacological challenges) measurements. Several lines of evidence based on static measures support the hypothesis of seasonal fluctuations of 5-HT function in humans:

1. Hypothalamic 5-HT concentrations in human post-mortem brain specimens are decreased in winter after values peak in autumn (Carlsson *et al.* 1980).

2. Levels of plasma tryptophan, the precursor of 5-HT, show a bimodal seasonal pattern (Maes *et al.* 1995).

3. Platelet 5-HT uptake and ^{3}[H]-imipramine binding show a seasonal pattern, albeit with some differences in seasonal peaks and troughs (Whitaker *et al.* 1984; Tang and Morris 1985; Arora and Meltzer 1988; deMet *et al.* 1989).

4. Levels of 5-HT and its metabolites in cerebrospinal fluid show seasonal fluctuations, varying with latitude and population studied (Asberg *et al.* 1980; Brewerton *et al.* 1988).

5. Serum melatonin concentrations demonstrate summer and winter peaks in healthy males (Arendt *et al.* 1977).

6. Recently, Neumeister *et al.* (2000*b*) reported a significantly reduced *in vivo* availability of hypothalamic 5-HT transporter sites in winter, compared with summer, in healthy female subjects (Fig. 21.1).

There are only a few reports in the literature on seasonal variations in 5-HT function using dynamic measures. JosephVanderpool *et al.* (1993) reported a seasonal variation in behavioural responses to the administration of *meta*-chlorophenylpiperazine (m-CPP) in patients with SAD with higher 'activation/euphoria' scores in SAD patients during winter compared with summer or after successful light therapy. More recently, Cappiello *et al.*

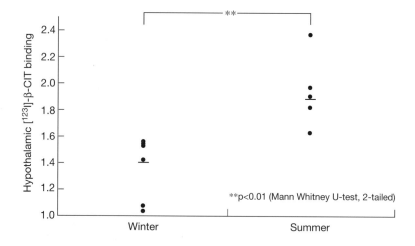

Fig. 21.1 Hypothalamic serotonin transporter availability in healthy female subjects as measured with [^{123}I]-ß-CIT during summer (n = 5) and during winter (n = 6).

(1996) demonstrated a seasonal variation in neuroendocrine (prolactin) response to intravenous tryptophan administration in unipolar, non-melancholic depressed patients. Interestingly, seasonality was more pronounced in female than in male patients. No such seasonal variability was found in bipolar, melancholic, or psychotic patients or in healthy controls.

Conclusively, substantial evidence is published in the literature arguing for a seasonal variation of central and peripheral 5-HT function in patients suffering from depression and also in healthy controls. Thus, we can hypothesize that seasonality of brain 5-HT function is physiological and may represent a predisposing factor for non-seasonal depression and in particular for seasonal depressions. However, it has to be said that the variability in the specific seasonal peaks and nadirs reported by different researchers reflects the use of different study designs, methodologies, sample sizes, and measures of 5-HT function. Consequently, further studies are needed to clarify the role of seasonal variations in central and peripheral 5-HT function in the regulation of human behaviour and in the pathogenesis of affective disorders, and in particular of SAD.

21.3 The serotonin hypothesis of SAD

Several lines of evidence suggest that brain 5-HT systems are intimately involved in the pathogenesis of SAD. Originally, Coppen (1967) nominated this neurotransmitter to play a key role in the pathogenesis of depressive disorders in general. Interestingly, even in their first clinical trial on the effects of light therapy in SAD, Rosenthal *et al.* (1984) raised the assumption that brain 5-HT systems may be involved in the pathogenesis of SAD. This was based on the observation that SAD patients have a characteristic psychopathological profile with a predominance of atypical symptoms (for example, hyperphagia and carbohydrate craving). Many of the neurovegetative functions, which seem to be disturbed in SAD, have been shown to have an important relationship to brain 5-HT systems.

21.3.1 Psychopathology of SAD and serotonin

Abnormalities in eating behaviour and food preference have been observed in patients with SAD (Rosenthal *et al.* 1984). Hyperphagia and carbohydrate craving are typical symptoms of SAD and have also been described in patients suffering from atypical depression (Paykel 1977). These patients differ from the anorectic depressive patients by being more often female and more mildly depressed. Moreover, these atypical depressed patients show a more pronounced reduction in sexual interest. These clinical features are also observed in patients with SAD. Interestingly, in SAD patients, hyperphagia often becomes worse with increasing severity of depression.

Several studies suggest that carbohydrates may play a crucial role in SAD: carbohydrate intake increases when the patients are symptomatically depressed, but not after successful light therapy or during summer (Kräuchi and Wirz–Justice 1992). It is noteworthy that a high intake of carbohydrates in the second half of the day is a positive predictor of light-therapy response (Kräuchi *et al.* 1993). Moreover, it has been shown that the sweet taste detection threshold is higher in SAD patients during winter, before and after light therapy, than during summer or compared with healthy controls (Arbisi *et al.* 1996). SAD patients have been shown to demonstrate a significant increase in their well-being after intake of carbohydrates (Rosenthal *et al.* 1989; Kräuchi *et al.* 1998). It has been postulated (Wurtman *et al.* 1981) that carbohydrate craving may reflect a functional 5-HT deficiency and that carbohydrate craving in SAD patients during autumn and winter represents a behavioural–biochemical feedback loop for raising the availability of 5-HT (Fernstrom 1977).

An interesting relationship has been found between bulimia nervosa and seasonality. Several groups have reported pronounced autumn/winter changes of mood and eating behaviour in bulimia nervosa patients (Lam *et al.* 1994; Levitan *et al.* 1994). These changes seem to be specific to bulimia nervosa and were not found in other eating disorders such as anorexia nervosa. Interestingly, a significant correlation between frequency of binge eating/purging and the daily photoperiod was reported in patients with bulimia nervosa (Blouin *et al.* 1992). Moreover, patients with bulimia nervosa exhibit higher seasonality scores than non-clinical samples (Brewerton *et al.* 1994; Hardin *et al.* 1991; Lam *et al.* 1991). Conversely, as already noted, SAD patients have been shown to have dysfunctional eating symptoms and attitudes similar to, although not as severe as, patients with eating disorders (Rosenthal *et al.* 1987; Berman *et al.* 1993).

Another characteristic symptom of SAD is hypersomnia. It has been speculated (Kupfer *et al.* 1972) that hypersomnic and hyposomnic depressed patients constitute two biologically distinct groups. 5-HT has been implicated in regulation of sleep (Jouvet 1969). Several investigators have studied the relationship between diet and sleep and have shown that changes in diet may induce changes in total sleep time, delta sleep, and REM sleep. It can be hypothesized that some of the changes in sleep observed in SAD patients during winter, when depressed, may be related to changes in diet and weight, and that serotonergic mechanisms may be involved.

21.3.2 Serotonergic challenge studies in SAD

One recognized strategy for clarifying the specific role of serotonergic systems in the aetiology of SAD and the mechanism of action of light therapy is to evaluate the effects of serotonergic probes with different pharmacological actions in both patients and controls. Serotonergic neurons send collaterals to limbic and neuroendocrine areas of the brain. Thus, it is reasonable to measure specifically those hormonal responses to serotonergic challenges which are believed to be controlled by serotonergic transmission. Such hormonal responses may also be used as a measure of serotonergic involvement in emotional disorders.

In SAD, different pharmacological probes have been used to evaluate possible disturbances in serotonergic transmission. There is preliminary evidence of abnormal hormonal responses to non-selective serotonergic agents and also to pre-synaptic or post-synaptic serotonergic agents in SAD.

Serotonin receptor challenge studies in SAD

Administration of the non-selective 5-HT agonist 5-hydroxytryptophan (Jacobsen *et al.* 1987) to a small group of symptomatic depressed patients with SAD and a group of age- and gender-matched healthy controls resulted in a decrease of prolactin levels and an increase of cortisol levels. No significant differences were found between patients and controls. The robust increase of serum cortisol levels in SAD patients, similar to the increase of cortisol in the control group, contrasts with findings in non-seasonal depressed patients who have shown an exaggerated cortisol response after administration of 5-hydroxytryptophan (Meltzer *et al.* 1984). The latter finding was interpreted as evidence of serotonergic supersensitivity in depression.

The failure to induce differences in prolactin and cortisol secretion after administration of 5-hydroxytryptophan between SAD patients and control subjects may indicate that both groups, patients and controls, are similar in their serotonergic function. Alternatively, it can be hypothesized that serotonergic transmission is normalized after administration of 5-hydroxytryptophan in SAD patients. This assumption is supported by studies demonstrating tryptophan to be effective in the treatment of SAD, either administered alone (McGrath *et al.* 1990; Ghadirian *et al.* 1998) or in combination with light therapy (Lam *et al.* 1997). Abnormal hormonal (prolactin) responses were also found after administration of the serotonergic agent d,l-fenfluramine (a compound that both releases 5-HT and blocks its reuptake), supporting the importance of serotonergic mechanisms in the pathogenesis of SAD (O'Rourke *et al.* 1987).

A widely used and potentially informative probe of central serotonergic function is m-CPP. The substance has affinity for a number of different 5-HT receptors, most important 5-HT-2c, but it binds also to 5-HT-1a, 5-HT-2, and moderately to a_2-noradrenergic receptors and to the human 5-HT transporter (Kahn and Wetzler 1991; Murphy *et al.* 1991). Interpretation of findings from earlier studies (Jacobsen *et al.* 1994; Joseph–Vanderpool *et al.* 1993) are problematic because of certain experimental design issues, such as the lack of a placebo control condition, lack of randomized order of presentation to light therapy, and failure to control for menstrual status in female subjects.

More recent studies (Schwartz *et al.* 1997; Levitan *et al.* 1998) addressed the aforementioned limitations and the results provide further evidence for the importance of serotonergic mechanisms in SAD: m-CPP was shown to reduce sadness in depressed patients with SAD; no behavioural effects were observed in healthy controls. Interestingly, normal subjective responses to m-CPP were found in patients with SAD after light therapy or during summer, when the patients are naturally remitted. This suggests that activation or euphoria, induced by m-CPP, may be a state marker of SAD. Hormonal responses (prolactin, corticotropin, cortisol) to m-CPP were blunted in SAD patients compared with controls. Also, m-CPP-induced noradrenaline responses in patients with SAD were blunted in comparison with controls. The blunted responsiveness of the hypothalamic-pituitary-adrenal axis and the sympathetic nervous system seem to represent trait markers of SAD, since they were observed across both light-treatment conditions.

To further explore serotonergic mechanisms in SAD, Yatham *et al.* (1997) administered sumatriptan to patients with SAD and health controls, before and after light therapy, and measured growth hormone response. Sumatriptan binds with highest affinity to 5-HT-1D receptors followed by 5-HT-1A receptors but has no affinity to other serotonergic, adrenergic, dopaminergic, or muscarinic receptors. The authors report that growth hormone response was blunted in symptomatic depressed SAD patients before light therapy compared with controls. This blunted response was not seen after successful light therapy. This finding suggests that 5-HT-1D receptors are subsensitive in SAD, when patiens are depressed, but not after light therapy. Thus, the noted 5-HT-1D receptor subsensitivity appears to be a state marker and not a trait marker. However, since sumatriptan also binds to 5-HT-1A receptors it was concluded by the authors that a role for 5-HT-1A receptors in the sumatriptan-mediated growth hormone response cannot be totally excluded. This is unlikely though since, in a different study, Schwartz and co-workers (1999) provided evidence that 5-HT-1A receptor subsensitivity is a trait marker and not a state marker.

Taken together, 5-HT receptor challenge studies have yielded further insight into serotonergic mechanisms in SAD and light therapy. Receptor subsensitivity has been shown for different receptors, either as a state marker or as a trait marker. 5-HT receptor challenge studies in SAD provide substantial evidence for altered activity at or downstream to central

5-HT receptors. However, the relative lack of specificity of the used substances leaves the question unanswered as to which particular 5-HT receptor systems might be dysfunctional in SAD. Future studies should use, depending upon availability, more specific 5-HT agonists and antagonists. This will certainly be helpful to better understand how serotonergic mechanisms and which structures within 5-HT systems are involved in the pathogenesis of SAD. However, the available data are compatible with the hypothesis that certain central nervous systems are dysfunctional in serotonergic transmission during winter depression and that they are influenced by light therapy.

Tryptophan depletion studies

Acute tryptophan depletion is a novel research strategy to study the behavioural effects of reduced serotonergic function in the brain. In humans, 5-HT activity has been manipulated by controlling the availability of its precursor, tryptophan (Neumeister et al. 1997a, b, c). Changes in brain tryptophan associated with feeding are relevant to 5-HT-mediated function, because in the brain, 5-HT synthesis depends on availability of tryptophan. The aim of tryptophan depletion is to lower 5-HT levels in the brain by lowering 5-HT synthesis via depletion of its precursor tryptophan.

In animal studies the efficacy of the method has been shown repeatedly by assessing brain 5-HT and 5-hydroxyindoleacetic levels (Young et al. 1989; Schaechter and Wurtman 1990). In humans, oral administration of 50–100 g of an amino acid composition without tryptophan leads to a robust reduction in plasma tryptophan (Young et al. 1985). This is believed to cause a significant reduction in brain 5-HT activity. A positron emission tomography study of humans showed that tryptophan depletion causes a marked lowering of brain 5-HT synthesis, supporting such an assumption (Nishizawa et al. 1997).

In order to be considered an adequate challenge test for serotonergic mechanisms, the tryptophan depletion method has to be reversible and specific. Animal experimental studies and studies in humans show that peak effects of tryptophan depletion are observed between 5 and 7 hours after ingestion of the amino acid beverage, and that 24 hours after ingestion of the beverage plasma tryptophan levels have returned to baseline again. Moreover, it was shown that the decline in plasma tryptophan is proportional to the dose of amino acids. However, animal studies suggest that the peripheral biochemical correlates of tryptophan depletion do not necessary reflect the degree of central impairment of serotonergic transmission (Stancampiano et al. 1997). Animal studies (Young et al. 1989) and a recent study in humans (Neumeister et al. 1998b) show the specificity of the tryptophan depletion paradigm for serotonergic mechanisms, since other neurotransmitters, such as tyrosine or catecholamines remained unaffected by tryptophan depletion. Thus, if the effects of tryptophan depletion are linked to neurotransmission in the brain, it is most likely that serotonergic mechanisms are affected.

It has to be considered that the tryptophan-depleting beverage includes substantial amounts of the other large neutral amino acids competing with tryptophan at the same carrier system across the blood–brain barrier. Lowering plasma tryptophan levels and increasing levels of the competing large neutral amino acids may induce changes in the metabolism of insulin and glucagon (Maes et al. 1990a, b) that may affect tryptophan uptake into the brain or has possibly behavioural and metabolic effects of its own (Baldessarini 1984).

Studies of tryptophan depletion in healthy subjects have shown inconsistent results. Healthy male subjects with their baseline ratings of depression in the upper normal range exhibit a transient worsening of their mood during tryptophan depletion (Young *et al.* 1985; Smith *et al.* 1987). In contrast, healthy male subjects who were euthymic at baseline and who were rigorously screened for any psychiatric or somatic illness remained unaffected by tryptophan depletion (Abbott *et al.* 1992; Danjou *et al.* 1990). Healthy controls with a multigenerational family history for major affective disorders reported a greater reduction in mood induced by tryptophan depletion than healthy controls without a positive family history (Benkelfat *et al.* 1994). The effects of tryptophan depletion in healthy female subjects is inconsistent since one study (Zimmerman *et al.* 1993), but not another (Oldman *et al.* 1994), reports a reduction in mood after tryptophan depletion.

In patients with non-seasonal depression, tryptophan depletion has been found to reverse the therapeutic effects of serotonergic, but not noradrenergic, antidepressants (Delgado *et al.* 1991), whereas no effects of tryptophan depletion were observed in fluoxetine-treated healthy subjects (Barr *et al.* 1997).

Regarding SAD, tryptophan-depletion studies have been performed in symptomatic depressed patients before light therapy (Neumeister *et al.* 1997*c*), and also in SAD patients during light therapy-induced remission (Lam *et al.* 1996; Neumeister *et al.* 1997*a*; Neumeister *et al.* 1998*b*). SAD patients were also studied during summer, when they were fully remitted and off therapy (Neumeister *et al.* 1998*a*, *b*; Lam *et al.* 2000). In untreated, symptomatic depressed patients with SAD no exacerbation of the depressive syndrome was induced by tryptophan depletion. This is in sharp contrast to the transient depressive relapse which was induced by tryptophan depletion in patients who were in stable, light therapy-induced remission and who were on light therapy. Such studies support the hypothesis that the antidepressant effects of light are mediated via serotonergic systems.

As already noted, SAD patients were studied also during summer when they were fully remitted and off therapy. These studies yielded inconsistent results. Neumeister *et al.* reported a transient depressive relapse induced by tryptophan depletion, whereas Lam and colleagues did not. The inconsistencies between the noted studies cannot be explained by different patient populations, since in both very homogenous groups of SAD patients were studied, similar in their clinical and demographic characteristics. One possible explanation for the noted discrepancy could be that the time from recovery of the last depressive episode differed between the two studies. It is noteworthy that during summer the depressive relapse occurred earlier and was more short-lived than during winter.

In a small study, Neumeister and colleagues (1999*a*) showed that those patients who had experienced a depressive relapse during tryptophan depletion in summer remained at high risk to develop a further depressive episode in the following winter. In contrast, those patients who remained well during tryptophan depletion in summer did not develop a depressive episode the following winter. These preliminary findings may be of importance when replicated in a larger sample of SAD patients because tryptophan depletion may help to define those patients who may benefit from long-term antidepressant treatment, either pharmacological or non-pharmacological.

Taken together, the tryptophan depletion studies which were performed by our group, including different sets of SAD patients in different clinical states (Fig. 21.2), provide substantial evidence that 5-HT plays a key role in the pathogenesis of SAD. In addition, this neurotransmitter seems to be involved in the mechanism of action of light therapy. Interestingly, in a small study we found an association between genotypes of the 5-HT transporter and changes in depression scores after tryptophan depletion (Lenzinger *et al.* 1999).

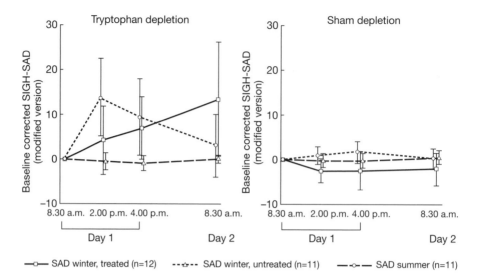

Fig. 21.2 Behavioural responses as measured with the Structured Interview Guide for the Hamilton Depression Rating Scale, Seasonal Affective Disorder Version (SIGH-SAD) to tryptophan depletion and sham depletion in patients with SAD. Patients underwent tryptophan depletion during winter prior to light therapy and after light therapy-induced remission, as well as during summer, when they were fully remitted and off therapy. Transient depressive relapses occurred after light therapy and during summer, no exacerbation of the depressive syndrome was found after tryptophan depletion when SAD patients were symptomatic depressed before starting light therapy.

Patients with SAD remain vulnerable to alterations in central 5-HT function. Thus, it can be hypothesized that the suspected serotonergic dysregulation in SAD is a trait marker and not a state marker, and that light therapy compensates for the underlying deficit. It is worth noting that no direct relationship was found between the severity of the depressive syndrome and tryptophan availability. This argues against a direct role of 5-HT in the regulation of mood in SAD. In addition, the tryptophan depletion studies do not preclude the possibility that neurobiological systems other than serotonergic may be implicated in the pathogenesis of SAD.

21.3.3 Serotonergic compounds in SAD

The hypothesis that a dysregulation within brain serotonergic systems may be one aetiological factor in SAD is also supported by the beneficial effects of serotonergic agents in the treatment of SAD. Different serotonergic compounds, such as sertraline (Blashko 1995), fluoxetine (Lam *et al.* 1995), and d,l-fenfluramine (O'Rourke *et al.* 1989) have been shown to be effective in controlled trials of SAD. More recently, the dual antidepressant, mirtazapine, has also proved efficacy in SAD (Heßelmann *et al.* 1999).

A more detailed description of the pharmacological treatment of SAD as an alternative to light therapy is given in the chapter by Kasper *et al.* Altogether, the antidepressant efficacy of serotonergic agent is further, albeit indirect, evidence for the importance of serotonergic mechanisms in SAD.

21.3.5 Single photon emission computed tomography (SPECT) studies of central serotonin transporters

In order to study whether alterations in the availability of monoamine transporters are found also in patients with SAD when depressed, Willeit and colleagues (2000) employed the SPECT ligand $[^{123}I]$-2b-carbomethoxy-3b-(4-iodophenyl)tropane ($[^{123}I]$ß-CIT) to visualize binding to the serotonin transporter (SERT) site in the human thalamus/hypothalamus midbrain area *in vivo*. The cocaine analogue $[^{123}I]$ß-CIT has been used previously to image SERT and dopamine transporter (DAT) binding sites in the human brain with SPECT. Attention needs to be paid to the fact that $[^{123}I]$ß-CIT is not a specific ligand for the SERT. Although $[^{123}I]$ß-CIT binds with high affinity for both SERTs and DATs it has been shown that striatal activity is almost exclusively associated with the DAT, while hypothalamus and midbrain activity is almost exclusively associated with the SERT (Laruelle *et al.* 1993). Thus, this apparent regional selectivity allows an assessment of SERT binding *in vivo*. The cerebellum contains negligible SERT and DAT concentrations (Bäckström and Marcusson

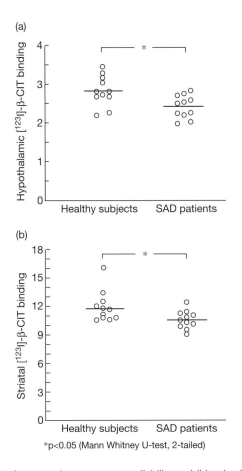

*p<0.05 (Mann Whitney U-test, 2-tailed)

Fig. 21.3 (a) Hypothalamic serotonin transporter availability and (b) striatal dopamine transporter availability in symptomatic depressed patients with SAD and healthy controls, as measured with $[^{123}I]$-ß-CIT.

1990; Cortes *et al.* 1988; Laruelle *et al.* 1988) and is thus useful as a reference region. Preliminary evidence suggests that specific [^{123}I]ß-CIT binding to SERT may be influenced by synaptic 5-HT concentrations (Jones *et al.* 1998).

SAD patients were found to have a reduced thalamic/hypothalamic availability of SERT binding sites compared with a group of age- and gender-matched healthy controls (Fig. 21.3a). This study ensured that each pair of patient and healthy control was studied within two weeks. This may be important since recently significant differences in SERT density were found in healthy female controls between summer and winter (Neumeister *et al.* 2000*b*). *The finding of a reduced availability of SERT binding sites in depressed patients with SAD is of particular interest for the pathogenesis of SAD since hypothalamic serotonergic function varies seasonally (Carlsson et al. 1980; Neumeister et al. 2000b).*

Future studies should address the question of whether the noted reduction in SERT availability during winter represents a state marker or a trait marker by studying patients before and after light therapy, and during summer when they are naturally remitted.

21.4 **The catecholamine hypothesis of SAD**

A review of the literature on the biological variables that may play a role in the pathogenesis of SAD and the mechanisms of action of light therapy revealed that during the past years serotonergic mechanisms received much more attention than catecholaminergic mechanisms. However, several lines of evidence suggest that beside 5-HT transmission, catecholaminergic transmission also may be involved in the pathophysiology of SAD and the mechanisms of action of light therapy. For example, one study showed resting plasma noradrenaline levels to be inversely correlated with the level of depression in untreated SAD patients (Rudorfer *et al.* 1993). In a study of the role of noradrenaline in the mechanism of light therapy, light therapy decreased the urinary output of noradrenaline and its metabolites (Anderson *et al.* 1992). However, plasma concentrations of 3-methoxy-4-hydroxyphenylethylenglycol (MHPG), a major metabolite of noradrenaline, did not distinguish depressed SAD patients from either light-treated SAD patients or from controls (Rudorfer *et al.* 1993). Also, cerebrospinal fluid levels did not differentiate patients from healthy controls in relation to either MHPG or the 5-HT metabolite 5-hydroxyindoleacetic acid (5-HIAA) (Rudorfer *et al.* 1993).

More, albeit indirect, evidence for the involvement of noradrenaline in the pathogenesis of SAD can be inferred from a recent open study showing the efficacy of the selective noradrenaline reuptake inhibitor, reboxetine, in the treatment of SAD (Hilger *et al.* 1999). It is worth noting that reboxetine was particularly effective for atypical symptoms of SAD.

To investigate dopaminergic mechanisms in SAD, three dependent measures were used: prolactin secretion, spontaneous eye blink rate, and temperature regulation. Dopamine via tuberoinfundibular projections to the median eminence is the primary substance involved in the tonic inhibition of prolactin secretion (Gudelsky 1981). Moreover, brain dopaminergic systems appear to modulate the rate of spontaneous eye blinking (Karson 1983) and seem also to be involved in the control of body core temperature (Lee *et al.* 1985). Studies report increased, (Jacobsen *et al.* 1987), but also decreased (Depue *et al.* 1990; Oren *et al.* 1996), basal prolactin levels in SAD patients compared with controls. One study (Depue *et al.* 1990), but not another (Barbato *et al.* 1993), showed that SAD patients have an increased eye blink rate. Initial findings of an abnormal thermoregulatory response to a thermal challenge in SAD patients compared with controls (Arbisi *et al.* 1989) were not replicated. Also, the combination of levodopa plus carbidopa was not superior to placebo in the treatment of SAD (Oren *et al.* 1994).

A recent brain imaging study (Neumeister *et al.* 2000*a*) yielded new insights into dopaminergic mechanisms in SAD. The authors studied the dopamine transporter (DAT) availability in untreated, symptomatic depressed patients with SAD and healthy controls. Patients with SAD and age- and gender-matched healthy controls were invited to participate in a [^{123}I]ß-CIT SPECT study to assess striatal density of DATs. The cerebellum was used as a reference region. The authors reported reductions in the availability of striatal DAT binding sites in untreated symptomatic depressed SAD patients compared with healthy controls (see Fig. 21.3b). It remains unclear whether these reductions represent a primary defect or an attempt to overcome a state of possible lowered dopamine availability in the synaptic cleft during a depressive episode of SAD.

More evidence for the involvement of catecholaminergic mechanisms in the pathogenesis of SAD and the mechanisms of action of light therapy comes from a monoamine depletion study using tryptophan depletion and catecholamine depletion paradigms to explore the relative contribution of these transmitter systems (Neumeister *et al.* 1998*b*). This study is important not only to the study of SAD, but also to non-seasonal depression, since it is the first to assess both tryptophan depletion and catecholamine depletion in the same patient.

Tryptophan depletion was induced by a 24-hour low tryptophan diet followed by the administration of a tryptophan-free amino acid beverage; catecholamine depletion was induced by administration of the tyrosine hydroxylase inhibitor, alpha-methyl-para-tyrosine (AMPT). Diphenhydramine was used as an active placebo during sham depletion. The effects of these interventions were evaluated with measures of depression, plasma tryptophan levels, and plasma catecholamine metabolites. As expected, tryptophan depletion significantly decreased plasma total and free tryptophan levels. Catecholamine depletion significantly decreased plasma MHPG and homovanillic acid (HVA) levels.

The primary finding of this investigation was that both tryptophan depletion and catecholamine depletion, but not sham depletion, reversed the therapeutic effects of light therapy (Fig. 21.4). Diphenhyhdramine proved to be a plausible control, since it produced a degree of drowsiness and fatigue similar to that of AMPT but did not lead to an increase of depressive mood in these patients. Interestingly, the individual item analysis showed no differences in the evoked depressive syndromes between tryptophan depletion and catecholamine depletion (Fig. 21.5). Taken together, the noted study suggests that light

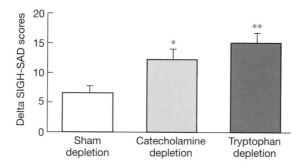

Fig. 21.4 Tryptophan and catecholamine depletion caused significantly higher delta scores than sham depletion (**p<0.01 and *p<0.05 respectively, paired t-test, 2-tailed), and no difference was found between the maximum effects of tryptophan and catecholamine depletion.

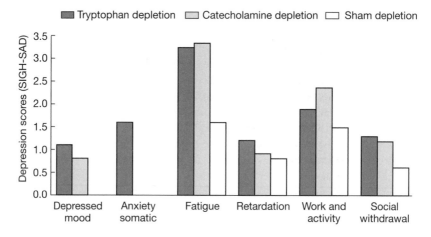

Fig. 21.5 Individual item analysis showed no differences in the evoked depressive syndrome between tryptophan depletion and catecholamine depletion.

therapy does not work exclusively via serotonergic pathways and that catecholaminergic pathways may be specifically implicated as well.

In summary, studies of catecholamine systems in SAD have been less consistent in implicating abnormalities of these neurotransmitter systems than has been the case with brain 5-HT systems. However, brain 5-HT and catecholamine systems are known to influence each other. Disturbed interactions between serotonergic and catecholaminergic systems have been reported in SAD (Schwartz *et al.* 1997). To date, it is unclear whether light therapy works by restoring disturbed interactions between these two systems to normal or by directly affecting those systems separately.

21.5 **Conclusions**

The literature on the role of brain monoaminergic systems in the pathogenesis of SAD and the mechanisms of action of light therapy shows consistently that both transmitter systems, serotonergic and catecholaminergic, seem to play a key role in this disorder and its treatment modalities. As shown, there exists substantial evidence that disturbances in monoaminergic functioning are a trait marker in SAD and that antidepressant treatments, such as light therapy or pharmacological treatments, may well compensate for this deficit.

References

Abbott, F.V., Etienne, P., Franklin, K.B.J., Morgan, M.J., Sewitch, M.J., and Young, S.N. (1992). Acute tryptophan depletion blocks morphine analgesia in the cold-pressor test in humans. *Psychopharmacology* **108**:60–6.

Anderson, J.L., Vasile, R.G., Mooney, J.J., Bloomingdale, K.L., Samson, J.A., and Schildkraut, J.J. (1992). Changes in noradrenaline output following light therapy for fall/winter seasonal depression. *Biological Psychiatry* **32**:700–4.

Arbisi, P.A., Depue, R.A., Spoont, M.R., Leon, A., and Ainsworth, B.(1989). Thermoregulatory response to thermal challenge in seasonal affective disorder: a preliminary report. *Psychiatry Research* **28**:323–34.

Arbisi, P.A., Levine, A.S., Nerenberg, J., and Wolf, J. (1996). Seasonal alteration in taste detection and recognition threshold in seasonal affective disorder: the proximate source of carbohydrate craving. *Psychiatry Research* **59**:171–82.

Arendt, J., Wirz-Justice, A., and Bradtke, J. (1977). Circadian, diurnal and circannual rhythms of serum melatonin and platelet serotonin in man. *Chronobiologia* **4**:96–7.

Arora, R.C. and Meltzer, H.Y. (1988). Seasonal variation of imipramine binding in the blood platelets of normal controls and depressed patients. *Biological Psychiatry* **23**:217–26.

Asberg, M., Bertilsson, L., Rydin, E., Schalling, D., Thorén, P., and Träskman–Bendz, L. (1980). Monoamine metabolites in cerebrospinal fluid in relation to depressive illness, suicidal behaviour and personality. In *Recent advances in neuropharmacology* (ed. B. Angrist, G.D. Burrows, and M. Lader), pp. 257–71. Pergamon, Oxford.

Bäckström, I.T. and Marcusson, J.O. (1990). High- and low-affinity 3H-desipramine-binding sites in human postmortem brain tissue. *Neuropsychobiology* **23**(2):68–73.

Baldessarini, R.J. (1984). Treatment of depression by altering monoamine metabolism: precursors and metabolic inhibitors. *Psychopharmacological Bulletin* **20**:224–39.

Barbato, G., Moul, D.E., Schwartz, P., Rosenthal, N.E., and Oren, D.A. (1993). Spontaneous eye blink rate in winter seasonal affective disorder. *Psychiatry Research* **47**(1):79–85

Barr, L.C., Heninger, G.R., Goodman, W., Charney, D.S., and Price, L.H.,(1997). Effects of fluoxetin administration on mood response to tryptophan depletion in healthy subjects. *Biological Psychiatry* **41**:949–54.

Benkelfat, C., Ellenbogen, M.A., Dean, P., Palmour, R.M., and Young, S.N. (1994). Mood-lowering effect of tryptophan depletion. Enhanced susceptibility in young men at genetic risk for major affective disorders. *Archives of General Psychiatry* **51**:687–97.

Berman, K., Lam, R.W., and Goldner, E.M. (1993). Eating attitudes in seasonal affective disorder and bulimia nervosa. *Journal of Affective Disorders* **29**(4):219–25.

Blashko, C.A.(1995). A double-blind, placebo-controlled study of sertraline in the treatment of outpatients with seasonal affective disorders. *European Neuropsychopharmacology* **5**:258.

Blouin, A., Blouin, J., Aubin, P., Carter, J., Goldstein, C., Boyer, H., *et al.* (1992). Seasonal patterns of bulimia nervosa. *American Journal of Psychiatry* **149**(1):73–81.

Brewerton, T.D., Berrettini, W., Nurnberger, J., and Linnoila, M. (1988). An analysis of seasonal fluctuations of CSF monoamines and neuropeptides in normal controls: findings with 5-HIAA and HVA. *Psychiatry Research* **23**:257–65.

Brewerton, T.D., Krahn, D.D., Hardin, T.A., Wehr, T.A., and Rosenthal, N.E. (1994). Findings from the seasonal pattern assessment questionnaire in patients with eating disorders and control subjects: effects of diagnosis and location. *Psychiatry Research* **52**:71–84.

Cappiello, A., Malison, R.T., McDougle, C.J., Vegso, S.J., Charney, D.S., Heninger, G.R., *et al.* (1996). Seasonal variation in neuroendocrine and mood responses to IV L-tryptophan in depressed patients and healthy subjects. *Neuropsychopharmacology* **15**(5):475–83.

Carlsson, A., Svennerholm, L., and Winblad, B.(1980). Seasonal and circadian monoamine variations in human brains examined post mortem. *Acta Psychiatrica Scandinavica* **61** (**Suppl. 280**):75–83.

Coppen, A. (1967). The biochemistry of affective disorders. *British Journal of Psychiatry* **113**(504):1237–64.

Cortes, R., Soriano, E., Pazos, A., Probst, A., and Palacios, J.M. (1988). Autoradiography of antidepressant binding sites in the human brain: localization using [3H]imipramine and [3H]paroxetine. *Neuroscience* **27**(2):473–96.

Danjou, P., Hamon, M., Lacomblez, L., Warot, D., *et al.* (1990). Psychomotor, subjective and neuroendicrine effects of acute tryptophan depletion in the healthy volunteer. *Psychiatric Psychobiology* **5**:31–8.

Delgado, P.L., Price, L.H., Miller, H.L., Salomon, R.M., Licinio, J., Krystal, J.H., *et al.* (1991). Rapid serotonin depletion as a provocative challenge test for patients with major depression; relevance to antidepressant action and the neurobiology of depression. *Psychopharmacological Bulletin* **27**:321–30.

DeMet, E.M., Chicz–DeMet, A., and Fleischmann, J. (1989). Seasonal rhythm of platelet 3H-imipramine binding in normal controls. *Biological Psychiatry* **26**:489–95.

Depue, R.A., Krauss, S., Ianoco, W.G., Leon, A., Muir, R., and Allen, J. (1990). Seasonal independence of low prolactin concentration and high spontaneous eye blink rates in unipolar and bipolar II seasonal affective disorder. *Archives of General Psychiatry* **47**:356–64.

Fernstrom, J.D. (1977). Effects of the diet on brain neurotransmitters. *Metabolism* **26(2)**:207–23.

Ghadirian, A.M., Murphy, B.E., and Gendron, M.J. (1998). Efficacy of light versus tryptophan therapy in seasonal affective disorder. *Journal of Affective Disorders* **50(1)**:23–7.

Gudelsky, G.A.(1981). Tuberoinfundibular dopamine neurons and the regulation of prolactin secretion. *Psychoneuroendocrinology* **6(1)**:3–16.

Hardin, T.A., Wehr, T.A., Brewerton, T.D., Kasper, S., Berrettini, W., Rabkin, J., et al. (1991). Evaluation of seasonality in six clinical populations and two normal populations. *Journal of Psychiatric Research* **25**:75–87.

Hesselmann, B., Habeler, A., Praschak–Rieder, N., Willeit, M., Neumeister, A., and Kasper, S. (1999). Mirtazapine in seasonal affective disorder (SAD): a preliminary report. *Human Psychopharmacology Clinical and Experimental* **14(1)**:59–62.

Hilger, E, Willeit, M, Praschak–Rieder, N., Neumeister, A., Stastny, J., Thierry, N., et al. (1999) Selective noradrenaline reuptake inhibitor reboxetine leads to rapid remission of atypical symptoms in patients with SAD. *Society for Light Treatment and Biological Rhythms Abstracts* **11**:19.

Jacobsen, F.M., Sack, D.A., Wehr, T.A., Rogers, S., and Rosenthal, N.E. (1987). Neuroendocrine response to 5-hydroxytryptophan in seasonal affective disorder. *Archives of General Psychiatry* **44**:1086–91.

Jacobsen, F.M., Mueller, E.A., Rosenthal, N.E., Rogers, S., Hill, J.L., and Murphy, D.L. (1994). Behavioural responses to intravenous meta-chlorophenylpiperazine in patients with seasonal affective disorder and control subjects before and after phototherapy. *Psychiatry Research* **52**:181–97.

Jones, D.W., Gorey, G.J., Zajicek, K., Das, B., Urbina, R.A., and Lee, K.S. (1998). Depletion-restoration studies reveal the impact of endogenous dopamine and serotonin on [^{123}I]-ß-CIT-SPECT imaging in primate brain. *Journal of Nuclear Medicine* **39(5)**:42(abstract).

Joseph–Vanderpool, J.R., Jacobsen, F.M., Murphy, D.L., Hill, J.L., and Rosenthal, N.E. (1993). Seasonal variation in behavioral responses to m-CPP in patients with seasonal affective disorder and controls. *Biological Psychiatry* **33**:496–504.

Jouvet, M.(1969). Biogenic amines and the states of sleep. *Science* **163**:32–41.

Kahn, R.S. and Wetzler, S. (1991). M-Chlorophenylpiperazine as a probe of serotonin function. *Biological Psychiatry* **30**:1139–66.

Karson, C.N.(1983). Spontaneous eye-blink rates and dopaminergic systems. *Brain* **106**:643–53.

Kräuchi, K. and Wirz–Justice, A.(1992). Seasonal patterns of nutrient intake in relation to mood. In *The biology of feast and famine: relevance to eating disorders* (ed. G.H. Anderson and S.H. Kennedy), pp. 157–82. Academic Press, Orlando, FL.

Kräuchi, K., Wirz–Justice, A., and Graw, P.(1993). High intake of sweets late in the day predicts a rapid and persistent response to light therapy in winter depression. *Psychiatry Research* **46(2)**:10717.

Kräuchi, K., Keller, U., Leonhardt, G., Brunner, D.P., van der Velde, P., Haug, H-J., et al. (1998). Accelerated post-glucose glycaemia and altered alliesthesia-test in seasonal affective disorder. *Journal of Affective Disorders* **53(1)**:23–6.

Kupfer, D.J. et al. (1972). Hypersomnia in manic-depressive disease: a preliminary report. *Diseases of the Nervous System* **33(11)**:720–4.

Lam, R.W., Solyom, L., and Tompkins, A. (1991). Seasonal mood symptoms in bulimia nervosa and seasonal affective disorder. *Comprehensive Psychiatry* **32**:552–8.

Lam, R.W., Gorman, C., Michalon, M., Steiner, M., and Levitt, A.J. (1994). A multicentre placebo-controlled study of fluoxetine in seasonal affective disorder. In *Program and abstracts of the annual meeting of the Society for Light Treatment and Biological Rhythms, June 1994*, p. 5. Bethesda, Md.

Lam, R.W., Gorman, C.P., Michalon, M., Steiner, M., Levitt, A.J., Corral, M.R., et al. (1995). A multi-centre, placebo-controlled study of fluoxetine in seasonal affective disorder. *American Journal of Psychiatry* **152**:1765–70.

Lam, R.W., Zis, A.P., Grewal, A., Delgado, P.L., Charney, D.S., and Krystal, J.H.(1996). Effects of tryptophan depletion in patients with seasonal affective disorder in remission after light therapy. *Archives of General Psychiatry* **53**:41–4.

Lam, R.W., Levitan, R.D., Tam, E.M., Yatham, L.N., Lamoureux, S., and Zis, A.P. (1997). L-tryptophan augmentation of light-therapy in patients with seasonal affective disorder. *Canadian Journal of Psychiatry* **42**(3):303–6.

Lam, R.W., Bowering, T.A., Tam, E.M., Grewal, A., Yatham, L.N., Shiah, I.S., *et al.* (2000). Effects of rapid tryptophan depletion in patients with seasonal affective disorder in natural summer remission. *Psychological Medicine* **30**(1):79–87.

Laruelle, M., Vanisberg, M.A., and Maloteaux, J.M. (1988). Regional and subcellular localization in human brain of [3H]paroxetine binding, a marker of serotonin uptake sites. *Biological Psychiatry* **24**(3):299–309.

Laruelle, M., Baldwin, R.M., Malison, R.T., Zea–Ponce, Y., Zoghbi, S.S., al Tikriti, M.S., *et al.* (1993). SPECT imaging of dopamine and serotonin transporters with [123I]beta-CIT: pharmacological characterization of brain uptake in nonhuman primates. *Synapse* **13**(4):295–309.

Lee, T.F., Mora, F., and Myers, R.D.(1985). Dopamine and thermoregulation: an evaluation with special reference to dopaminergic pathways. *Neuroscience and Biobehavioral Reviews* **9**(4):589–98.

Lenzinger, E., Neumeister, A., Praschak–Rieder, N., Fuchs, K., Gerhard, E., Willeit, M., *et al.* (1999). Behavioral effects of tryptophan depletion in seasonal affective disorder associated with the serotonin transporter gene? *Psychiatry Research* **85**(3):241–6.

Levitan, R.D., Kaplan, A.S., Levitt, A.J., and Joffe, R.T. (1994). Seasonal fluctuations in mood and eating behavior in bulimia nervosa. *International Journal of Eating Disorders* **16**(3):295–9.

Levitan, R.D., Kaplan, A.S., Brown, G.M., Vaccarino, F.J., Kennedy, S.H., Levitt, A.J., *et al.* (1998). Hormonal and subjective responses to intravenous m–chlorophenylpiperazine in women with seasonal affective disorder. *Archives of General Psychiatry* **55**:244–9.

Maes, M., Jacobs, M.P., Suy, E., Minner, B., Leclercq, C., Christiaens, F., *et al.* (1990*a*). Suppressant effects of dexamethasone on the availability of plasma L-tryptophan and tyrosine in healthy controls and in depressed patients. *Acta Psychiatrica Scandinavica* **81**: 19–23.

Maes, M., Maes, L., and Suy, E. (1990*b*). Symptom profiles of biological markers in depression: a multivariate study. *Psychoneuroendocrinology* **15**:29–37.

Maes, M., Scharpé, S., Verkerk, R., D'Hondt, P., Peeters, D., Cosyns, P., *et al.* (1995). Seasonal variation in plasma L-tryptophan availability in healthy volunteers. *Archives of General Psychiatry* **52**:937–46.

McGrath, R.E., Buckwald, B., and Resnick, E.V. (1990). The effect of l-tryptophan on seasonal affective disorder. *Journal of Clinical Psychiatry* **51**:162–3.

Meltzer, H.Y., Lowy, M., Robertson, A., Goodnick, P., and Perline, R. (1984). Effect of 5-hydroxytryptophan on serum cortisol levels in major affective disorders. *Archives of General Psychiatry* **41**:366–97.

Murphy, D.L., Lesch, K.P., Aulakh, C.S., and Pigott, T.A. (1991). Serotonin-selective arylpiperazines with neuroendocrine, behavioral, temperature and cardiovascular effects in humans. *Pharmacology Review* **43**:527–52.

Neumeister, A., Praschak–Rieder, N., Heßelmann, B., Rao, M-L., Glück, J., and Kasper, S. (1997*a*) Effects of tryptophan depletion on drug-free patients with seasonal affective disorder during a stable response to bright light therapy. *Archives of General Psychiatry* **54**:133–8.

Neumeister, A., Praschak–Rieder, N., Heßelmann, B., Tauscher, J., and Kasper, S. (1997*b*) Der Tryptophandepletionstest-Grundlagen und klinische Relevanz. *Der Nervenarzt* **68**:556–62.

Neumeister, A., Praschak–Rieder, N., Heßelmann, B., Vitouch, O., Rauh, M., Barocka, A., *et al.* (1997*c*) Rapid tryptophan depletion in drug-free depressed patients with seasonal affective disorder. *American Journal of Psychiatry* **154**:1153–5.

Neumeister, A., Praschak–Rieder, N., Heßelmann, B., Vitouch, O., Rauh, M., Barocka, A., *et al.* (1998*a*) Effects of tryptophan depletion in fully remitted patients with seasonal affective disorder during summer. *Psychological Medicine* **28**:257–64.

Neumeister, A., Turner, E.H., Matthews, J.R., Postolache, T.T., Barnett, R.L., Rauh, M., *et al.* (1998*b*) Effects of tryptophan depletion vs catecholamine depletion in patients with seasonal affective disorder in remission with light therapy. *Archives of General Psychiatry* **55**:524–30.

Neumeister, A., Habeler, A., Praschak–Rieder, N., Willeit, M., and Kasper, S. (1999*a*) Tryptophan depletion: a predictor of future depressive episodes in SAD? *International Clinical Psychopharmacology* **14**(5):313–15.

Neumeister, A., Stastny, J., Praschak–Rieder, N., Willeit,M., and Kasper, S. (1999b) Light treatment in depression (SAD, s-SAD & non-SAD). In *Biologic effects of light 1998. Proceedings of a symposium, Basel, Switzerland, November 13, 1998* (ed. M.F. Holick and E.G. Jung), pp. 409–16. Kluwer Academic Press, Netherlands.

Neumeister, A., Willeit, M., Praschak–Rieder, N., Asenbaum, S., Stastny, J., Hilger, E., *et al.* (2000a) Dopamine transporter availability in symptomatic depressed patients with seasonal affective disorder and healthy controls. *Psychological Medicine* (in press)

Neumeister, A., Pirker, W., Willeit, M., Praschak–Rieder, N., Asenbaum, S., Brücke, T., *et al.* (2000b) Seasonal variation of availability of serotonin transporter binding sites in healthy female subjects as measured by [^{123}I]-2β-carbomethoxy-3β-(4-iodophenyl)tropane and single photon emission computed tomography. *Biological Psychiatry* **47**:158–60.

Nishizawa, S., Benkelfat, C., Young, S.N., Leyton, M., Mzengeza, S., deMontigny, C., *et al.* (1997). Differences between males and females in rates of serotonin synthesis in human brain. *Proceedings of the National Academy of Sciences* **94**:5308–13.

Oldman, A.D., Walsch, A.E.S, Salkovski, P., Laver, D.A., and Cowen, P.J. (1994). Effect of acute tryptophan depletion on mood and appetite in healthy female volunteers. *Journal of Psychopharmacology* **8**:8–13.

Oren, D.A., Moul, D.E., Schwartz, P., Wehr, T.A., and Rosenthal, N.E. (1994). A controlled trial of levodopa plus carbidopa in the treatment of winter seasonal affective disorder: a test of the dopamine hypothesis. *Journal of Clinical Psychopharmacology* **14**:196–200.

Oren, D.A., Levendosky, A.A., Kasper, S., Duncan, C.C., and Rosenthal, N.E. (1996). Circadian profiles of cortisol, prolactin, and thyrotropin in seasonal affective disorder. *Biological Psychiatry* **39**:157–70.

O'Rourke, D., Wurtman, J.J., Brzezinski, A., Nader, T.A., and Chew, B.(1987). Serotonin implicated in etiology of seasonal affective disorder. *Psychopharmacology Bulletin* **23(3)**:358–9.

O'Rourke, D., Wurtman, J.J., Wurtman, R.J., Chebli, R., and Gleason, R. (1989). Treatment of seasonal depression with d-fenfluramine. *Journal of Clinical Psychiatry* **50**:343–7.

Paykel, E.S. (1977). Depression and appetite. *Journal of Psychosomatic Research* **21(5)**:401–7.

Rosenthal, N.E., Sack, D.A., Gillin, J.C., Lewy, A.J., Goodwin, F.K., Davenport, Y., *et al.* (1984). Seasonal affective disorder: a description of the syndrome and preliminary findings with light therapy. *Archives of General Psychiatry* **41**:72–80.

Rosenthal, N.E., Genhart, M., Jacobsen, F.M., Skwerer, R.G., and Wehr, T.A.(1987). Disturbances of appetite and weight regulation in seasonal affective disorder. *Annals of the New York Academy of Sciences* **499**:216–30.

Rosenthal, N.E., Genhart, M.J., Caballero, B., Jacobsen, F.M., Skwerer, R.G., Coursey, R.D., *et al.* (1989). Psychobiological effects of carbohydrate- and protein-rich meals in patients with seasonal affective disorder and normal controls. *Biological Psychiatry* **25**:1029–40.

Rudorfer, M., Skwerer, R., and Rosenthal, N. (1993). Biogenic amines in seasonal affective disorder: effects of light therapy. *Biological Psychiatry* **46**:19–28.

Schaechter, J.D. and Wurtman, R.J. (1990). Serotonin release varies with brain tryptophan levels. *Brain Research* **532(1–2)**:203–10.

Schwartz, P.J., Murphy, D.L., Wehr, T.A., Garcia–Borreguero, D., Oren, D.A., Moul, D.E., *et al.* (1997). Effects of meta-chlorophenylpiperazine infusions in patients with seasonal affective disorder and healthy control subjects. *Archives of General Psychiatry* **54**:375–85.

Schwartz, P.J., Turner, E.H., Garcia–Borreguero, D., Sedway, J., Vetticad, R.G., Wehr, T.A., *et al.* (1999). Serotonin hypothesis of winter depression: behavioral and neuroendocrine effects of the 5-HT (1A) receptor partial agonist ipsapirone in patients with seasonal affective disorder and healthy control subjects. *Psychiatry Research* **86(1)**:9–28.

Smith, S.E., Pihl, R.O., Young, S.N., and Ervin, F.R. (1987). A test of possible cognitive and environmental influences on the mood lowering effect of tryptophan depletion in normal males. *Psychopharmacology* **91**:451–7.

Stancampiano, R., Melis, F., Sarais, L., Cocco, S., Cugusi, C., and Fadda, F. (1997). Acute administration of a tryptophan-free amino acid mixture decreases 5-HT release in rat hippocampus in vivo. *American Journal of Physiology* **272**:R991–4.

Tang, S.W. and Morris, J.M. (1985).Variation in human platelets 3H-imipramine binding. *Psychiatry Research* **16**:141–6.

Whitaker, P.M., Warsh, J.J., Stancer, H.C., Persade, E., and Vint, C.K. (1984). Seasonal variation in platelet 3H-imipramine binding: comparable values in control and depressed populations. *Psychiatry Research* **11**:127–31.

Willeit, M., Praschak–Rieder, N., Neumeister, A., Pirker, W., Asenbaum, S., Vitouch, O., *et al.* (2000). [^{123}I]-ß-CIT SPECT imaging shows reduced brain serotonin transporter availability in drug-free depressed patients with seasonal affective disorder. *Biological Psychiatry* **47**:482–9.

Wurtman, R.J., Hefti, F., and Melamed, E. (1981). Precursor control of neurotransmitter synthesis. *Pharmacological Review* **32**:315–35.

Yatham, L.N., Lam, R.W., and Zis, A.P. (1997). Growth hormone response to sumatriptan (5-HT1D agonist) challenge in seasonal affective disorder: effects of light therapy. *Biological Psychiatry* **42**:24–9.

Young, S.N., Smith, S.E., Pihl, R.O., and Ervin, F.R. (1985). Tryptophan depletion causes a rapid lowering of mood in normal males. *Psychopharmacology* **87**:173–7.

Young, S.N., Ervin, F.R., Pihl, R.O., and Finn, P. (1989). Biochemical aspects of tryptophan depletion in primates. *Psychopharmacology* **98**:508–11.

Zimmerman, R.C., McDougle, C.J., Schumacher, M., Olcese, J., Mason, J.W., Heninger, G.R., *et al.* (1993). Effects of acute tryptophan depletion on nocturnal melatonin secretion in humans. *Journal of Clinical Endocrinology and Metabolism* **76**:1106–64.

Chapter 22

Photobiology

Megan R. Leahy and Dan A. Oren

22.1 Introduction

Surprisingly little is known of the physical basis of the effect of light treatment on SAD. Although there remains the possibility that some as yet unidentified, purely psychological process might explain the effects of light treatments in the disorder, with a wide range of excellent studies having minimized the possibility that light treatment works on the basis of a placebo effect, it is reasonable to infer that some physicochemical process mediates this process of a light signal being converted into a behavioural effect. According to what is now termed the 'first law of photochemistry' — as formulated by Theodor Grotthus (1785–1822) and John William Draper (1811–82) — for light to produce a chemical reaction, it must first be absorbed by or act upon a molecule (Fleming 1971; Stradins 1971). But we still do not know the photoreceptor molecule or molecules that are critical to the antidepressant response in SAD.

22.2 Identifying the photoreceptor(s)

Knowledge of the photoreceptor molecule(s) and cells that mediate light in SAD would also, conceivably, be of immense value to understanding the pathogenesis of a common psychiatric syndrome, and perhaps open a proverbial 'window' into the brain. Until the photoreceptor has been identified, the method of measuring the light used for therapeutic purposes will remain arbitrary. The commonly used unit of measure for light with respect to light therapy is the 'lux'. Lux is a psychophysical measurement of how bright the eye perceives light; it is not a count of photons and energy or another direct physical quantity. This creates a problem, however. Since lux is a measurement of perception, 10 000 lux of red light carries less energy and more photons than similarly bright 10 000 lux of green light or 10 000 lux of white light. Lux may not be the ideal quantity for comparison of measurements within and between studies because of this inconsistency. Knowledge of the relevant photoreceptor(s) would allow construction of a purely physical scale to measure light's antidepressant effects.

Using commonly accepted principles of photobiology, several research groups have been working to identify the photoreceptor(s) involved with the therapeutic effects of light. According to such principles, the first step is to define an 'action spectrum', which measures the relative response of the relevant outcome to different stimulus wavelengths. The second step is to define 'absorption spectra' for candidate photoreceptor molecules. Such spectra identify those wavelengths that the molecule absorbs and reflects. Each molecule has a characteristic absorption spectrum that is dependent upon the atomic structure of its photopigments. (For example, see the absorption spectrum of rhodopsin, Fig. 22.1). As first studied in plant photobiology, when an action spectrum for a process matches an absorption spectrum for a candidate photoreceptor, by virtue of parsimony, the candidate photoreceptor is presumed to be a real photoreceptor (Galston 1994).

For historical reasons and relying on presumed parsimony, researchers have hypothesized that the known visual photoreceptor rhodopsin-based molecules were primary receptors for circadian and neuroendocrine regulation, and presumably therefore for winter depression treatment as well (Brainard *et al.* 1984; Bronstein *et al.* 1987; Podolin *et al.* 1987; Thiele and Meissl 1987). That peak sensitivity of the circadian and neuroendocrine system has been found to be in the blue–green portion of the visible spectrum is consistent with the rhodopsin model.

22.3 Investigating the electromagnetic spectrum for efficacy of light therapy

Several studies have been conducted concerning different colours of light and their efficacy in treating SAD. Three specific studies compared red, blue, and green portions of the spectrum with white light. The first study, a comparison of one week of red, blue, or white light therapy, with equal photon densities equivalent to that commonly used with white light treatment for SAD, demonstrated white to be superior to blue or red light (Brainard *et al.* 1990). The second study compared green and red light at the same photon densities. Here, green light had a significantly better therapeutic effect than red light (Oren *et al.* 1991). In a third study, white and green light proved helpful for symptoms (Stewart *et al.* 1991). Since green light included the primary absorption wavelengths for rhodopsin and appeared to include the wavelengths of light most effective in humans in suppressing melatonin (Brainard *et al.* 1985) — which many surmised was somehow related to the antidepressant response — rhodopsin-based molecules remained strong potential candidates as antidepressant photoreceptors.

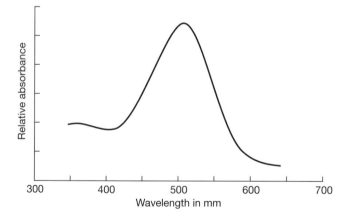

Fig. 22.1 Absorption spectrum for rhodopsin. (Adapted from Wolken 1975.)

The use of the ultraviolet (UV) portion of the spectrum in light therapy has been debated and studied. Although UV wavelengths might have antidepressant effects, they are not required for the treatment response, and are contraindicated because of possible risks of stimulating skin cancers or ocular cataracts (Lam *et al.* 1991; Oren *et al.* 1990; Oren *et al.* 1991).

Limited research has been published on the use of infrared light in the treatment of SAD. One study has raised the possibility that infrared light is effective in preventing the onset of winter depression but does not suggest that infrared light is superior to white light (Meesters *et al.* 1999).

22.4 **Non-visual photoreceptors**

Following the 1984 report of Takahashi *et al.* showing that hamster circadian rhythm photoreceptors exhibited properties that were unusual for rhodopsin (the capacity for integration of time and intensity and a high threshold for bleaching), serious consideration has been given to the possibility that other molecules might be at work. Several other studies have since supported this proposition. In 1995, Czeisler *et al.* reported that exposing the eyes to 6000 lux of white light could suppress melatonin production in some humans with complete visual blindness.

The assumption that light therapy operates through the visual system has been the prominent assumption driving research on light therapy for depression, largely supported by Wehr *et al.* (1987) who demonstrated a superior response to ocular over extraocular light for winter depression. When Oren *et al.* (1993) looked for clear evidence of visual dysfunction in the disorder — which might support the visual system as a pathway of direct effectiveness in light therapy — none could be found. These data supported the idea of a non-visual ocular photoreceptive process.

Drawing upon an evolutionary argument, Oren (1996) therefore proposed that blood-borne pigments in the eye (haemoglobin, bilirubin) mediate circadian and antidepressant regulation via 'humoral phototransduction', with the eye as the site of most efficient exposure of blood to light. Campbell and Murphy (1998) subsequently reported that delivering a single, 3-hour bright-light pulse of 13 000 lux to the back of the knees of human volunteers permits systematic resetting of the circadian rhythms of body temperature and melatonin. This finding, which still requires independent confirmation, might also be explained by humoral phototransduction. Other groups, however, have argued that human melatonin is not suppressed by extraocular light (Lockley *et al.* 1998; Jean–Louis *et al.* 2000) and that hamster circadian rhythms do not shift in response to extraocular light (Yamazaki *et al.* 1999).

Recent work in genetic knock-out rodents by Lucas *et al.* (1999) and Freedman *et al.* (1999) clearly established that some novel, non-visual system must mediate the circadian rhythm system in rodents, and presumably humans. Recently, Provencio *et al.* (2000) reported the identification of a new human opsin, melanopsin, which has been found in the cells of the mammalian inner retina, the presumed site of melatonin-suppressing photoreceptors. They have suggested that melanopsin may be a circadian photoreceptor.

Solving this photoreceptor mystery must remain an important goal for psychiatry.

References

Brainard, G.C., Richardson, B.A., King, T.S., and Reiter, R.J. (1984). The influence of different light spectra on the suppression of pineal melatonin content in the Syrian hamster. *Brain Research*, **294**:333–9.

Brainard, G.C., Lewy, A.J., Menaker, M., Fredrickson, R.H., Miller, L.S., Weleber, R.G., *et al.* (1985). Effect of light wavelength on the suppression of nocturnal plasma melatonin in normal volunteers. *Annals of the New York Academy of Sciences*, **453**:376–8.

Brainard, G.C., Sherry, D., Skwerer, R.G., Waxler, M., Kelly, K., and Rosenthal, N.E. (1990). Effects of different wavelengths in seasonal affective disorder. *Journal of Affective Disorders*, **20**:209–16.

Bronstein, D.M., Jacobs, G.H., Haak, K.A., Neitz, J., and Lytle, L.D. (1987). Action spectrum of the retinal mechanism mediating nocturnal light-induced suppression of rat pineal gland *N*-acetyltransferase. *Brain Research*, **406**:352–6.

Campbell, S.S. and Murphy, P.J. (1998). Extraocular circadian phototransduction in humans. *Science*, **279**:396.

Czeisler, C.A., Shanahan, T.L., Klerman, E.B., Martens, H., Brotman, D.J., Emens, J.S., *et al.* (1995). Suppression of melatonin secretion in some blind patients by exposure to bright light. *New England Journal of Medicine*, **332**:6–11.

Fleming, D. (1971). John William Draper. In *Dictionary of scientific biography* (ed. C.C. Gillispie), Vol. IV., pp. 181–3. Scribner's, New York.

Freedman, M.S., Lucas, R.J., Soni, B., Schantz, Mv., Muñoz, M., David–Gray, Z., *et al.* (1999). Regulation of mammalian circadian behavior by non-rod, non-cone, ocular photoreceptors. *Science*, **284**:502–4.

Galston, A.W. (1994). *Life processes of plants*. Scientific American Library, New York.

Jean–Louis, G., Kripke, D.F., Cole, R.J., and Elliott, J.A. (2000). No melatonin suppression by illumination of popliteal fossae or eyelids. *Journal of Biological Rhythms*, **15**:265–9.

Lam, R.W., Buchanan, A., Clark, C.M., and Remick, R.A. (1991). Ultraviolet versus non-ultraviolet light therapy for seasonal affective disorder. *Journal of Clinical Psychiatry*, **52**:213–16.

Lockley, S.W., Skene, D.J., Thapan, K., English, J., Ribeiro, D., Haimov, I., *et al.* (1998). Extraocular light exposure does not suppress plasma melatonin in humans. *Journal of Clinical Endocrinology and Metabolism*, **83**:3369–72.

Lucas, R.J., Freedman, M.S., Muñoz, M., Garcia–Fernández, J-M., and Foster, R.G. (1999). Regulation of the mammalian pineal by non-rod, non-cone, ocular photoreceptors. *Science*, **284**:505–7.

Meesters, Y., Beersma, D.G.M., Bouhuys, A.L., and van den Hoofdakker, R.H. (1999). Prophylactic treatment of seasonal affective disorder (SAD) by using light visors: bright white or infrared light? *Biological Psychiatry*, **46**:239–46.

Oren, D.A. (1996). Humoral phototransduction: blood is a messenger. *Neuroscientist*, **2**:207–10.

Oren, D.A., Rosenthal, F.S., Rosenthal, N.E., Waxler, M., and Wehr, T.A. (1990). Exposure to ultraviolet B radiation during phototherapy. *American Journal of Psychiatry*, **147**:675–6.

Oren, D.A., Brainard, G.C., Johnston, S.H., Joseph–Vanderpool, J.R., Sorek, E., and Rosenthal, N.E. (1991). Treatment of seasonal affective disorder with green light and red light. *American Journal of Psychiatry*, **148**:509–11.

Oren, D.A., Moul, D.E., Schwartz, P.J., Alexander, J.R., Yamada, E.M., and Rosenthal, N.E. (1993). An investigation of ophthalmic function in winter seasonal affective disorder. *Depression*, **1**:29–37.

Podolin, P.C., Rollag, M.D., and Brainard, G.C. (1987). The suppression of nocturnal pineal melatonin in the Syrian hamster: dose-response curves at 500 nm and 360 nm. *Endocrinology*, **121**:266–70.

Provencio, I., Rodriguez, I.R., Jiang, G., Pär Hayes, W., Moreira, E.F., and Rollag, M.D. (2000). A novel human opsin in the inner retina. *Journal of Neuroscience*, **20**:600–5.

Stewart, K.T., Gaddy, J.R., Byrne, B., Miller, S., and Brainard, G.C. (1991). Effects of green or white light for treatment of seasonal depression. *Psychiatry Research*, **38**:261–70.

Stradins, J.P. (1971). Theodor (Christian Johann Dietrich) von Grotthuss. In *Dictionary of scientific biography* (ed. C.C. Gillispie), Vol. V, pp. 558–9, Scribner's, New York.

Takahashi, J.S., DeCoursey, P.J., Bauman, L., and Menaker, M. (1984). Spectral sensitivity of a novel photoreceptive system mediating entrainment of mammalian circadian rhythms. *Nature*, **308**:186–8.

Thiele, G. and Meissl, H. (1987). Action spectra of the lateral eyes recorded from mammalian pineal glands. *Brain Research*, **424**:10–16.

Wehr, T.A., Skwerer, R.G., Jacobsen, F.M., Sack, D.A., and Rosenthal, N.E. (1987). Eye versus skin phototherapy of seasonal affective disorder. *American Journal of Psychiatry*, **144**:753–7.

Wolken, J.J. (1975). *Photoprocesses, photoreceptors, and evolution,* p. 45. Academic Press, New York.

Yamazaki, S., Goto, M., and Menaker, M. (1999). No evidence for extraocular photoreceptors in the circadian system of the Syrian hamster. *Journal of Biological Rhythms,* **14**:197–201.

Chapter 23

Personality and cognition

Murray W. Enns and Brian J. Cox

23.1 **Introduction**

The relationship between personality and depression is complex. Although it is commonly assumed that maladaptive personality traits act as vulnerability factors for depression, relatively few prospective studies have demonstrated that personality dysfunction increases risk for depression. Nevertheless, most investigators and clinicians would agree that personality has an important relationship with depressive illness in general. While many studies on the relationship of personality to depression have been reported, there are a limited number of studies that have examined the relationship between personality and SAD. The limited number of studies likely reflects, in part, the emphasis placed on biologically based theories involving the presumed role of light deprivation and exposure in the aetiology and treatment of SAD. There is, however, little reason to assume that light deprivation and exposure are devoid of psychological effects or that personality is a purely psychologically determined characteristic.

In this chapter we will review the studies that have examined the relationship between categorically or dimensionally assessed personality and SAD. As personality and cognitive style are closely related constructs, studies that have examined the relationship between cognitive variables such as dysfunctional attitudes, negative automatic thoughts, or attributional style and SAD will also be reviewed. Conceptually, several different relationships may exist between a personality variable and SAD. A personality factor may predispose an individual to the development of depression (vulnerability model), the occurrence of episodes of SAD may lead to changes in personality function (scar model), or an underlying process may contribute to both personality and SAD (continuity model). Personality may also influence the expression of SAD (pathoplasty model) and the depressed state may influence the measurement of personality (affective state dependency)(Akiskal *et al.* 1983; Enns and Cox 1997).

These models of the relationship between personality and depression are, of course, not mutually exclusive. Existing studies clearly demonstrate an association between a number of personality variables and SAD, but are not sufficient to accept or reject the vulnerability, scar, or continuity models. Several studies provide evidence that in SAD patients, personality trait assessment (for example, neuroticism) is significantly influenced by the depressed state. A number of studies also provide evidence that the presence of personality dysfunction (as observed while depressed) predicts poorer light-therapy response and/or poorer long-term outcome in SAD patients (pathoplasty model).

Because of the extensive psychiatric literature regarding the relationship between personality and depression in general, it is important to ask whether the personality factors implicated in SAD are the same as those in non-seasonal depression. It appears that both non-specific personality characteristics (related to both SAD and non-seasonal depression) and possibly specific traits (unique to SAD) may be involved. A hierarchical model of higher- and lower-order personality traits is useful to understand the relationship among various personality dimensions. The highest level of such a trait hierarchy consists of broad general dimensions of individual differences such as neuroticism and extroversion, while more specific traits such as self-criticism or hostility are at a lower level in the hierarchy (Watson *et al.* 1994). The five-factor model (for example, Costa and McCrae 1992), which describes higher-order dimensions of personality labelled neuroticism, extroversion, openness, agreeableness, and conscientiousness, provides a useful framework for understanding the personality factors associated with SAD.

A number of personality traits have been associated non-specifically with both SAD and non-seasonal depression. These include traits that reflect dysregulation of affect, preponderance of negative affects (including depressive, hostile, and anxious affects), and impulsivity. Examples include traits labelled as cluster B and cluster C personality disorders (DSM-III, DSM-III-R, DSM-IV), harm avoidance, 'oral' personality traits, and negative cognitive style. Each of these traits which are non-specifically associated with seasonal and non-seasonal depression can be broadly conceptualized as being related to the neuroticism construct.

In contrast, there has been little evidence of an association between openness to experience and non-seasonal depression, but there is preliminary evidence that SAD patients have higher levels of openness than both normals and non-seasonal depressed patients (Bagby *et al.* 1996; Jain *et al.* 1999). According to Costa and McCrae (1992), important elements of openness include attentiveness to inner feelings, divergent thinking, unconventionality, and willingness to question authority and entertain novel ideas. Highly open individuals may experience both positive and negative emotions more keenly than closed individuals. Accordingly, it may be that such individuals more keenly experience the negative affects associated with seasonal changes in biological rhythms. Furthermore, their enthusiastic open-mindedness and willingness to consider an unconventional treatment such as light therapy theoretically could enhance their responsiveness to light treatment.

Dimensionally assessed seasonality has also been associated with external locus of control of mood (LOCOM)(Murray *et al.* 1995) and moderately associated with openness (Jang *et al.* 1997). It is tempting to speculate that the higher-order construct of openness may bear a significant relationship to LOCOM and that highly 'open' individuals may generally experience their mood as something under control of their environment, including the seasonal environment. However, there are no empirical data yet available that address this issue.

In what follows we summarize the published literature on SAD and personality/cognition. We also attempt to integrate the observations and consider some directions for future research.

23.2 Comparisons of SAD patients with normal controls

Studies of the personality structure of patients with SAD have resulted in conflicting findings. An early report from Rosenthal's group (National Institute of Mental Health) indicated that patients with SAD were relatively free of personality disorders (Schulz *et al.* 1988). Schulz and colleagues (1988) conducted a comparison of patients with SAD (n = 28), normal controls (n = 29), and non-SAD depressed subjects (n = 12 in-patients). They reported that SAD patients and normal controls had a lower frequency of severe personality disorders than the non-SAD depressives (based on structured interviews). However, dimensional scores of SAD subjects on DSM-III-R cluster A, B, and C personality traits were all elevated in comparison with the normal controls. Their SAD patients were also reported to have Minnesota Multiphasic Personality Inventory (MMPI) (McKinley and Hathaway 1943) scores within normal limits, with the exception of a mild elevation of the psychopathic deviance scale. The authors considered the latter finding as a possible reflection of the presence of adaptive aspects of psychopathic features in the SAD subjects, for example, assertiveness and confidence (Ray and Ray 1982).

There are a number of methodological limitations with this report, however. The sample size was small, and both the non-SAD depressed comparison group and the SAD patient group likely were unrepresentative samples. The in-patient group had lengthy, disabling, treatment-resistant mood disorders (as reflected in their mean Global Assessmant of Functioning score of 45.6). The SAD group was recruited through media publicity, and as such, a selection bias could have resulted. Finally, the personality assessments were all conducted during active depressive illness, thus raising the possibility that some of the positive findings were due to the effect of the depressed state on the personality tests.

Several subsequent studies have compared the personality characteristics of SAD patients to normal control subjects (Berman *et al.* 1993; Hodges and Marks 1998; Pendse *et al.* 1999). Unfortunately each of these studies utilized a different measure of personality or cognition. Berman and colleagues (1993) conducted a three-way comparison of SAD patients (n = 30, assessed while depressed), bulimia nervosa patients (n = 30), and normal controls (n = 30). Since the main objective of the study was to examine the clinical overlap between bulimia and SAD, the subjects all completed the Eating Disorders Inventory (EDI) (Garner *et al.* 1983) which contains three subscales assessing personality dimensions, perfectionism, ineffectiveness, and interpersonal distrust. Patients with SAD scored higher than controls and lower than bulimic subjects on all three of these scales (though the results for perfectionism were significant only for the bulimia vs. control comparison).

Hodges and Marks (1998) compared small groups of patients with SAD (n = 10, assessed while depressed), non-seasonal depression (n = 11, assessed while depressed), and normal controls (n = 10) using two different measures of depressogenic cognitive style — the Automatic Thoughts Questionnaire (ATQ) (Hollon and Kendall 1980) and the Dysfunctional Attitudes Scale (DAS) (Weissman and Beck 1978). The ATQ measures negative automatic thoughts (including thoughts about personal maladjustment, negative self-concept, low self-esteem, and hopelessness) and the DAS measures maladaptive attitudes. The authors found that both SAD and non-SAD depressed subjects had higher (more pathological) scores than controls on each of these scales, but they found no significant difference between SAD and non-SAD depressed patients on any of the scales. Given the small sample size, however, this study only had statistical power to detect very large effect sizes.

Pendse and colleagues (1999) also conducted a three-way comparison of SAD patients (n = 23, assessed while depressed), non-SAD depressed patients (n = 23, all of whom had made suicide attempts and were depressed at assessment), and normal controls (n = 23) using the Karolinska Scales of Personality (KSP) (Schalling *et al.* 1987) and the Marke-Nyman Temperament questionnaire (MNT) (Sjöbring 1973). They observed that the SAD patients showed significantly higher scores on the somatic anxiety, muscular tension, psychasthenia, irritability, and suspicion scales and significantly lower (more pathological) scores on the validity and socialization scales compared to normal controls. Examination of the content of these scales suggests that those that were elevated in the SAD patients closely reflect symptoms and may correspond to the concept of neuroticism (the tendency to experience negative affects). The socialization and validity scales, in contrast, appear to be closely related to the construct of extroversion. Because the patients in the study were assessed during the acutely depressed phase of their illness, the observed pattern of results may be reflective of current distress rather than an accurate appraisal of pre-depressive personality. The authors also noted that the non-SAD depressed group had significantly greater scores than the SAD group on few scales (somatic and psychic anxiety and muscular tension), but these findings likely reflect the greater overall severity of a patient group selected for suicide attempts.

23.3 **Comparisons of SAD patients with non-seasonal depressed patients**

Several authors have reported comparisons of the personality of SAD patients with non-SAD depressed patients (Schuller *et al.* 1993; Reichborn–Kjennerud *et al.* 1994; Bagby *et al.* 1996; Levitan *et al.* 1998; Jain *et al.* 1999). Schuller and colleagues compared 24 SAD patients and 17 non-SAD depressed patients using the Depressive Experiences Questionnaire, which measures dependency and self-criticism (DEQ) (Blatt *et al.* 1976) and the Millon Clinical Multiaxial Inventory, which generates trait scores for each of the 11 DSM-III-R categories of personality disorder (MCMI) (Millon, 1983). They reported lower levels of dependency and self-criticism as well as lower levels of schizotypal and avoidant traits in the SAD patients. In contrast, the SAD patients reported higher levels of narcissistic traits than the non-SAD subjects. The authors attributed the latter observation to higher levels of adaptive aspects of narcissism including self-worth and self-confidence in the SAD group. The SAD patients and the non-SAD subjects were experiencing similar levels of depression symptoms at the time of assessment (an important strength of the study). However, the method of recruitment of the patients differed; SAD patients were recruited through the media, while the non-SAD patients were clinic referrals.

Reichborn–Kjennerud and colleagues (1994) evaluated 57 SAD patients in the summer (that is, while euthymic) using the Structured Interview for DSM-III-R Personality Disorders (SIDP) (Pfohl *et al.* 1989). The authors did not interview a comparison group of non-SAD patients, but they noted that the frequency and types of DSM-III-R personality disorders in their study group was similar to that reported previously for out-patients with non-seasonal major depression. Although satisfactory reliability of their diagnostic interviews was reported, the failure to use a comparison group is an important limitation in the interpretation of these results.

Levitan and colleagues (1998) compared the cognitive style of SAD (n = 26) and non-SAD depressed patients (n = 30) using the Attributional Style Questionnaire (ASQ) (Whitley 1991). They found no significant difference between groups in ASQ scores.

Two different groups have reported comparisons of SAD patients with depressed control subjects using the five-factor model of personality (Bagby *et al.* 1996; Jain *et al.* 1999). Bagby and colleagues compared clinically referred SAD (n = 43) and non-SAD depressed patients (n = 57) using the NEO Personality Inventory (NEO-PI-R) (Costa and McCrae 1992) and controlling for depression symptoms. Their main finding was a significantly higher score on the openness (O) dimension in SAD patients compared to non-seasonal depressives; SAD subjects scored more than one standard deviation higher on the O scale than a normative group. This elevation was explained predominantly by three facets of O — namely aesthetics, feelings, and ideas.

Jain and colleagues (1999) replicated the finding of elevated O scores in their comparison of 24 SAD patients with 13 bipolar depressed subjects. Importantly, this study included a longitudinal follow-up and personality reassessment of 20 of the SAD subjects. While the neuroticism and extroversion domains of the NEO-FFI (Costa and McCrae 1992) were found to change significantly when the SAD patients were reassessed in the summer (while euthymic), the elevation of O scores was unchanged. The finding of elevated O scores in SAD patients relative to both norms and two different depressed comparison groups, and the invariance of this finding between the depressed and euthymic state make this the most robust finding to date on the association between personality and SAD. In contrast, no consistent relationship between openness and non-seasonal depression has been observed (Bagby *et al.* 1997; Wolfstein and Trull 1997).

23.4 **The impact of personality on the outcome of SAD**

Whether or not personality/cognitive factors are important in the aetiology of SAD, it is possible that personality could have a significant influence on the outcome or clinical presentation of SAD (pathoplastic effect). A number of authors have observed that DSM-III/ DSM-III-R defined personality traits/disorders, particularly avoidant personality disorder, are associated with poorer response to light therapy and/or lower likelihood of summer remission of SAD symptoms (Lilie *et al.* 1990; Partonen and Lönnqvist 1995; Reichborn–Kjennerud and Lingjærde 1996).

Reichborn–Kjennerud and Lingjærde (1996) also evaluated the relationship between Tridimensional Personality Questionnaire (TPQ) (Cloninger *et al.* 1991) scores and response to light therapy in 33 patients with SAD. (The TPQ measures harm avoidance, reward dependence, and novelty seeking.) They observed a significant association between harm avoidance scores at baseline and outcome of 6 days of light therapy. This finding corroborates the observation that avoidant personality traits are associated with poorer outcome since the harm avoidance construct includes anticipatory worry, fear of uncertainty, shyness with strangers, and fatigability. It should also be noted that harm avoidance shows a strong relationship with neuroticism (Cloninger *et al.* 1994).

It may be that these forms of personality dysfunction interfere with interpersonal and behavioural changes that are associated with complete response to treatment for depression. This interpretation is in keeping with the results of a recent study of the impact of interpersonal processes on the outcome of light therapy (Geerts *et al.* 2000). Geerts and colleagues observed that interpersonal attunement and extroversion were associated with favourable outcome in 60 SAD patients treated with light therapy.

In contrast, Levitan and colleagues (1998) evaluated the relationship of ASQ scores to the outcome of light therapy in 26 SAD patients and the outcome of pharmacotherapy in 30 non-SAD depressed patients. While ASQ scores were associated with pharmacotherapy treatment outcome, they observed no relationship between attributional style and response to phototherapy.

23.5 **Affective state dependency of personality in SAD**

In the foregoing review of the relationship between personality/cognition and SAD, it was noted that assessment of personality was conducted with currently depressed patients in the majority of studies. It has, however, been well demonstrated in non-seasonal depression that the depressed state has an important impact on the assessment of many domains of personality (Enns and Cox 1997). A particularly salient example of this is the personality domain of neuroticism, which is a broad, general, and largely heritable personality trait, the core of which is a tendency to experience a variety of negative affective states (Costa and McCrae 1992). As such, the observation of an association between a personality or cognitive variable and SAD during acute depression needs to be replicated with euthymic patients before considering a possible aetiologic role of that factor in SAD.

Four published reports have already shown evidence of considerable affective state dependence of the personality traits associated with SAD (Lilie et al. 1990; Meesters 1992; Reichborn–Kjennerud et al. 1997; Jain et al. 1999). Lilie and colleagues (1990) studied 20 SAD patients in the winter and summer using the MMPI and the MCMI. They observed that 60 per cent of all subjects had some personality scale abnormality in the winter, while only 35 per cent scored in the abnormal range in the summer. They also commented that the most frequently elevated scales of both the MMPI and the MCMI appeared to be indirectly measuring depressive symptoms. Similar findings were observed with a Dutch version of the MMPI (Meesters 1992).

Reichborn–Kjennerud and colleagues (1997) examined dimensional scores on the Personality Disorders Questionnaire–Revised (PDQ-R) (Hyler et al. 1987) which measures DSM-III-R defined personality traits, in 45 SAD patients before and after treatment. They noted that the scores on several personality variables, including schizotypal, histrionic, narcissistic, and obsessivecompulsive traits were significantly lower after treatment. The personality dimensions of the five-factor model were assessed before and after treatment in 20 SAD patients in another recent study (Jain et al. 1999). Two of the five dimensions showed significant change; neuroticism scores decreased and extroversion scores increased with improvement in depression symptoms.

These findings suggest that much of the observed association between personality/ cognition and SAD could be attributable to state effects of depressed mood. The most robust and mood invariant association of personality with SAD is the O dimension of the five-factor model. However, there have been no longitudinal pre-morbid assessment studies that can confirm that elevated O antedates the onset of SAD.

23.6 **Seasonality and personality**

While SAD is a categorical diagnosis, an underlying dimensional construct of 'seasonality' (seasonal variability in mood, energy, appetite, sleep, and so on) which is presumed to be normally distributed in the general population has also been evaluated in relation to personality. An Australian group was the first to examine the relationship between personality and seasonality (Murray et al. 1995). The authors measured the correlations between the three dimensions of the Eysenck Personality Questionnaire (neuroticism, extroversion, and psychoticism) (Eysenck and Eysenck 1975) and the Global Seasonality Scale (GSS) of the Seasonal Pattern Assessment Questionnaire (SPAQ) (Rosenthal et al. 1984). They observed a moderate correlation between neuroticism and GSS ($r = 0.38$), as well as a correlation of $r = 0.44$ between GSS and a measure of external locus of control of moods. They interpreted this result as an indication that seasonality is indistinct from neurotic phenomena generally, and suggested that highly seasonal individuals may be very responsive to a range of stressors, including non-seasonal ones.

The observation of an association between GSS and neuroticism was replicated and extended by a Canadian group (Jang *et al.* 1997). Jang and colleagues observed significant correlations between both neuroticism and openness (from the NEO-FFI) and GSS in their study of 297 adults from a general population sample. They also reported that several dimensions of the Dimensional Assessment of Personality Pathology (DAPP) (Livesley *et al.* 1992) were significantly correlated with seasonality (affective lability, anxiousness, cognitive distortion, insecure attachment, identity problems, narcissism, submissiveness, and oppositionality). The content of several of these DAPP dimensions is fairly similar to the neuroticism dimension (Widiger 1998).

Nilsen and colleagues (1997) also examined the correlation between GSS seasonality and the personality dimensions of the Basic Character Inventory (BCI) (Torgersen 1980). Their main finding was a medium-sized correlation ($r = 0.29$) between oral (neurotic) traits and GSS. While these observations are consistent with the idea that seasonality is related to a more general tendency to experience negative affects, the magnitude of the observed correlations is such that a relatively small proportion of variance in seasonality (about 15 per cent) is explained by neuroticism or related traits.

Finally, Jang and colleagues (1998) used community twin data to examine the genetic correlation between GSS and personality factors. They reported that the observed correlations between GSS and several personality factors (neuroticism, cognitive dysregulation, affective lability, anxiousness, and stimulus seeking) were strongly attributable to genetic factors. For example, the genetic correlation between neuroticism and GSS was 0.52, indicating that about 27 per cent of the genetic influences affecting seasonality and neuroticism are the same.

A recent study failed to replicate the finding of an association between neuroticism and personality (Gordon *et al.* 1999). These authors found no significant correlation between a measure of neuroticism and GSS seasonality. In contrast to the three positive reports, this study was conducted amongst a group of 45 subjects diagnosed with SAD. The negative result likely relates to restricted variance of GSS and/or neuroticism scores in the patient sample.

The intriguing observations just summarized need to be considered in the light of some significant limitations of the GSS scale of the SPAQ. First, it has been noted that the GSS shows a skewed distribution in general population samples, with few subjects scoring over 18 (on the 24-point scale) and the large majority of subjects scoring between 0 and 8 (Kasper *et al.* 1989; Spoont *et al.* 1991). This unfavourable psychometric property may influence the magnitude of some observed correlations and limit the detection of others. More importantly, retrospective reports of the magnitude of seasonal variation in mood and other behaviours may be inflated in relation to prospectively measured seasonal change (Nayyar and Cochrane 1996). As such, part of the association between GSS and neuroticism may be related to the *tendency to report* seasonal variability rather than actual seasonal change in mood.

23.7 Cognitive sensitivity to light

Most investigations concerning the aetiology and treatment of SAD have given emphasis to presumed biological effects of bright-light exposure versus deprivation. One group of investigators has given further consideration to whether a cognitive or psychological sensitivity to light may play a role in the genesis of SAD (Richter *et al.* 1992; Bouhuys *et al.* 1994, 1995). Richter and colleagues (1992) conducted a comparison of morning light therapy (n = 7) and 'imagined light' treatment (while under hypnosis, n = 7) for SAD. They found an advantage for morning light on both self-reported and observer-rated depression symptoms. Thus the study did not support the hypothesis that response to phototherapy could be explained by non-specific cognitive reactions to the perception of light. However, the two treatment groups were small, and subjects were assigned to treatments non-randomly on the basis of hypnotizability.

Bouhuys and colleagues conducted a unique study of sensitivity to symbolic light in 29 remitted SAD patients and 29 non-depressed controls. Subjects were shown schematic drawings of ambiguous faces expressing different emotions, embedded in either light-coloured or dark-coloured backgrounds. The subjects were asked to rate the faces in regard to the degree of elation (vs. sadness), rejection (vs. invitation), and activation (vs. sleepiness). SAD patients perceived larger differences in activation between faces on light versus dark backgrounds than controls. Also, the larger the difference that SAD patients perceived in invitation between light and dark backgrounds, the earlier in the subsequent autumn/winter they became depressed. These results were interpreted as evidence of a possible cognitive bias that could contribute to negative interpersonal perceptions as the daylight hours decrease. That is, individuals with this cognitive bias would be relatively more exposed to faces which are interpreted as less active or inviting. However, since there was no non-SAD depression comparison group it is uncertain whether the findings are specific to patients with seasonal forms of depression. Furthermore, the study involved multiple comparisons and has not yet been replicated, so the possibility of a Type 1 error cannot be excluded.

23.8 Summary and conclusions

The literature reviewed in this chapter provides preliminary evidence of an important relationship between personality and SAD. A variety of different personality constructs have been evaluated in this literature, including many of the higher- and lower-order personality dimensions that have been associated with non-seasonal forms of depression. Although some reports have indicated that SAD patients have remarkably normal personality profiles, it is quite possible that a recruitment bias contributes to such observations.

The majority of reports indicate that personality dysfunction in SAD patients is quite similar in most respects to that in non-seasonal depression. Important exceptions to this general observation are the findings of an association between openness and SAD (Bagby et al. 1996; Jain et al. 1999), and the observation of 'cognitive sensitivity' to symbolic light in SAD patients (Bouhuys et al. 1994). Whether there is any interrelationship between openness and sensitivity to symbolic light has not been studied. However, the hypotheses that openness correlates with sensitivity to imagined light, that highly open individuals may be predisposed to develop SAD, and that openness and cognitive sensitivity to imagined light predict response to light treatment warrant investigation.

These hypotheses hold in common the idea that apart from biological effects, bright light may also have important psychological effects in individuals who are predisposed to SAD. That is, the seasonally changing light exposure acts as an important stressor in predisposed individuals (a stress-diathesis model). It is also possible that a combination of personality vulnerabilities that are not specific to SAD (for example, neuroticism) with specific vulnerabilities (for example, cognitive sensitivity to light) causes an even greater liability for seasonally recurring depression (another testable hypothesis).

As noted in the introduction of this chapter, studies reported to date do not allow us to draw definitive conclusions about the nature of the association between personality traits and SAD. There are limitations of many of the existing studies including possible recruitment biases, small sample sizes, failure to include both normal and non-SAD depressed comparison groups, the frequent practice of assessing personality during active depressive episodes, and the focus on a narrow range of personality variables. Many of the findings in the existing literature have not been replicated. Personality findings in SAD patients may reflect pre-existing vulnerability factors, 'scars' left by recurring depressions or common underlying processes. To provide clearer evidence, methodologically improved studies will be necessary.

Ideally, studies that simultaneously assess both higher- and lower-order personality factors, perform baseline assessments in euthymic patients, and include longitudinal follow-up should be conducted. Such studies are, of course, labour intensive and costly. Family studies examining the personality of never depressed, previously depressed, and currently depressed relatives of probands with SAD would also help sort out the nature of the SAD–personality relationship. Integration of studies of personality and SAD, with biological and treatment investigations, should also contribute to the generation of more unified hypotheses about the nature of SAD.

References

Akiskal, H.S., Hirshfeld, R.M., and Yerevanian, B.I. (1983). The relationship of personality to affective disorders. *Archives of General Psychiatry*, **40**:801–10.

Bagby, R.M., Schuller, D.R., Levitt, A.J., Joffe, R.T., and Harkness, K.L. (1996). Seasonal and non-seasonal depression and the five-factor model of personality. *Journal of Affective Disorders*, **38**:89–95.

Bagby, R.M., Bindseil, K.D., Schuller, D.R., Rector, N.A., Young, L.T., Cooke, R.G., *et al.* (1997). Relationship between the five factor model of personality and unipolar, bipolar and schizophrenic patients. *Psychiatry Research*, **70**:83–94.

Berman, K., Lam, R.W., and Goldner, E.M. (1993). Eating attitudes in seasonal affective disorder and bulimia nervosa. *Journal of Affective Disorders*, **29**:219–25.

Blatt, S.J., D'Affitti, J.P., and Quinlan, D.M. (1976). *Depressive experiences questionnaire* (unpublished manuscript). Department of Psychiatry, Yale University, New Haven, CT.

Bouhuys, A.L., Meesters, Y., Jansen, J.H., and Bloem, G.M. (1994). Relationship between cognitive sensitivity to (symbolic) light in remitted seasonal affective disorder patients and the onset time of a subsequent depressive episode. *Journal of Affective Disorders*, **31**:39–48.

Bouhuys, A.L., Meesters, Y., Jansen J.H., and Bloem G.M. (1995). Winterdepressie i: cognitieve gevoeligheid voor (symbolisch) licht voorspelt het begin van een nieuwe depressieve episode. *Tijdschrift voor Psychiatrie*, **37**:32–42.

Cloninger, C.R., Przybeck, T.R., and Svrakic D.M. (1991). The tridimensional personality questionnaire: US normative date. *Psychological Reports*, **69**:1047–57.

Cloninger, C.R., Przybeck, T.R., Svrakic, D.M., and Wetzel, R.D. (1994). *The Temperament and Character Inventory (TCI): a guide to its use and development*. Washington University, St. Louis, Missouri.

Costa, P.T. and McCrae, R.R. (1992). *Revised NEO Personality Inventory (NEO-PI-R) and NEO Five Factor Inventory (NEO-FFI): professional manual*. Psychological Assessment Resources, Odessa, FL.

Enns, M.W. and Cox, B.J. (1997). Personality dimensions and depression: review and commentary. *Canadian Journal of Psychiatry*, **42**:274–84.

Eysenck, H.J. and Eysenck, S.B. (1975). *Manual of the Eysenck personality questionnaire*. Hodder and Stroughton, London.

Garner, D.M., Olmsted, M.P., and Polivy, J. (1983). Development and validation of a multidimensional eating disorder inventory for anorexia nervosa and bulimia. *International Journal of Eating Disorders*, **2**:15–34.

Geerts, E., Kouwert, E., Bouhuys, N., Meesters, Y., and Jansen, J. (2000). Nonverbal interpersonal attunement and extravert personality predict outcome of light treatment in seasonal affective disorder. *Journal of Affective Disorders*, **59**:193–204.

Gordon, T., Keel, J., Hardin, T.A., and Rosenthal, N.E. (1999). Seasonal mood change and neuroticism: the same construct? *Comprehensive Psychiatry*, **40**:415–17.

Hodges, S. and Marks, M. (1998). Cognitive characteristics of seasonal affe ctive disorder: a preliminary investigation. *Journal of Affective Disorders*, **50**:59–64.

Hollon, S.D. and Kendall, P.C. (1980). Cognitive self-statements in depression: development of an automatic thoughts questionnaire. *Cognitive Therapy and Research*, **4**:383–95.

Hyler, S.E. and Rieder, R.O. (1987). *PDQ-R: Personality Diagnostic Questionnaire Revised*. New York State Psychiatric Institute, New York.

Jain, U., Blais, M.A., Otto, M.W., Hirshfeld, D.R., and Sachs, G.S. (1999). Five-factor personality traits in patients with seasonal depression: treatment effects and comparisons with bipolar patients. *Journal of Affective Disorders*, **55**:51–4.

Jang, K.L., Lam, R.W., Livesley, W.J., and Vernon P.A. (1997). The relationship between seasonal mood change and personality: more apparent than real? *Acta Psychiatrica Scandinavica*, **95**: 539–43.

Jang, K.L, Lam, R,W., Harris, J.A., Vernon, P.A., and Livesley, W.J. (1998). Seasonal mood change and personality: an investigation of genetic co-morbidity. *Psychiatry Research*, **78**:1–7.

Kasper, S., Wehr, T., Bartko, J., Gaist, P., and Rosenthal, N.E. (1989). Epidemiological findings of seasonal changes in mood and behavior. *Archives of General Psychiatry*, **46**:823–33.

Levitan, R.D., Rector, N.A., and Bagby, R.M. (1998). Negative attributional style in seasonal and nonseasonal depression. *American Journal of Psychiatry*, **155**:428–30.

Lilie, J.K., Lahmeyer, H.W., Watel, L.G., and Eastman, C.I. (1990). The relation of personality to clinical outcome in SAD. *Society for Light Treatment and Biological Rhythms Abstracts*, **2**:213.

Livesley, W.J., Jackson, D.N., and Schroeder, M.L. (1992). Factorial structure of traits delineating personality disorders in clinical and general population samples. *Journal of Abnormal Psychology*, **101**:432–40.

McKinley, J.C. and Hathaway, S.R. (1943). The identification and measurement of the psychoneuroses in medical practice: the Minnesota Multiphasic Personality Inventory. *Journal of the American Medical Association*, **122**:161–7.

Meesters, Y. (1992). Test-hertestbetrouwbaarheid van persoonlijkheidsvragenlijsten bij mensen met winterdepressieve klachten. *Nederlands Tijdschrift Voor De Psychologie*, **47**:143–7.

Millon, T. (1983). *Millon Clinical Multiaxial Inventory manual* (3rd edn). National Computer Systems, Minneapolis.

Murray, G.W., Hay, D.A., and Armstrong, S.M. (1995). Personality factors in seasonal affective disorder: is seasonality an aspect of neuroticism? *Personality and Individual Differences*, **19**:613–17.

Nayyar, K. and Cochrane, R. (1996). Seasonal changes in affective state measured prospectively and retrospectively. *British Journal of Psychiatry*, **168**:627–32.

Nilsen, K.B., Edvardsen, J., Richardsen, A., Konradsen, H., and Arne Holte, A. (1997). Årstidsavhengig affektvariasjon og personlighetstrekk blant unge voksne i Finnmark, Tromsø og Oslo. *Tidsskrift for Norsk Psykologforening*, **34**:595–603.

Partonen, T. and Lönnqvist, J. (1995). The influence of comorbid disorders and of continuation light treatment on remission and recurrence in winter depression. *Psychopathology*, **28**:256–62.

Pendse, B., Westrin, Å., and Engström, G. (1999). Temperament traits in seasonal affective disorder, suicide attempters with non-seasonal major depression and healthy controls. *Journal of Affective Disorders*, **54**:55–65.

Pfohl, B., Blum, N., Zimmerman, M., and Stangl, D. (1989). *Structured interview for DSM-III-R personality, SIDP-R*. Department of Psychiatry, University of Iowa, Iowa City.

Ray, J.J. and Ray, J.A.B. (1982). Some apparent advantages of subclinical psychopathy. *Journal of Social Psychology*, **117**:135–42.

Reichborn–Kjennerud, T., Lingjærde, O., and Dahl, A.A. (1994). Personality disorders in patients with winter depression. *Acta Psychiatrica Scandinavica*, **90**:413–19.

Reichborn–Kjennerud, T. and Lingjærde, O.(1996). Response to light therapy in seasonal affective disorder: personality disorders and temperament as predictors of outcome. *Journal of Affective Disorders*, **41**:10110.

Reichborn–Kjennerud, T., Lingjærde, O., and Dahl, A.A. (1997). DSM-III-R personality disorders in seasonal affective disorder: change associated with depression. *Comprehensive Psychiatry*, **38**:43–8.

Richter, P., Bouhuys, A.L., van den Hoofdakker, R.H., Beersma, D.G.M, Jansen, J.H., Lambers, P.A., *et al.* (1992). Imaginary versus real light for winter depression. *Biological Psychiatry*, **31**: 534–6.

Rosenthal, N.E., Sack, D., Gillin, J., Lewy, A.J, Goodwin, F.K., Davenport, Y., *et al.* (1984). Seasonal affective disorder: a description of the syndrome and preliminary findings with light therapy. *Archives of General Psychiatry*, **41**:72–80.

Schalling, D., Asberg, M., Edman, G., and Oreland, L. (1987). Markers for vulnerability to psychopathology: temperament traits associated with platelet MAO. *Acta Psychiatrica Scandinavica*, **76**:172–82.

Schuller, D.R., Bagby, R.M., Levitt, A.J., and Joffe, R.T. (1993). A comparison of personality characteristics of seasonal and nonseasonal major depression. *Comprehensive Psychiatry*, **34**:360–2.

Schulz, P.M., Goldberg, S., Wehr, T.A., Sack, D.A., Kasper, S., and Rosenthal N.E. (1998). Personality as a dimension of summer and winter depression. *Psychopharmacology Bulletin*, **24**:476–83.

Sjöbring, H.(1973). Personality structure and development, a model and its application. *Acta Psychiatrica Scandinavica*, **244**:113–57.

Spoont, M.R., Depue, R.A., and Krauss, S.S. (1991). Dimensional measurement of seasonal variation in mood and behavior. *Psychiatry Research*, **39**:269–84.

Torgersen, S. (1980). The oral, obsessive, and hysterical personality syndromes. *Archives of General Psychiatry*, **37**:1272–7.

Watson, D., Clark, L.A., and Harkness, A.R. (1994). Structures of personality and their relevance to psychopathology. *Journal of Abnormal Psychology*, **103**:18–31.

Weissman, A.N. and Beck, A.T. (1978). *Development and validation of the dysfunctional attitude scale: a preliminary investigation.* Paper presented at the American Educational Research Association meeting, Toronto, Canada.

Whitley, B. (1991), A short form of the expanded attributional style questionnaire. *Journal of Personality Assessment*, **56**:365–9.

Widiger, T.A. (1998). Four out of five ain't bad. *Archives of General Psychiatry*, **55**:865–6.

Wolfstein, M. and Trull, T.J. (1997). Depression and openness to experience. *Journal of Personality Assessment*, **69**:614–32.

Chapter 24

Neuroimaging

Russell G. Vasile and Janis L. Anderson

24.1 Introduction

This chapter reviews neuroimaging studies of patients with SAD in relation to similar studies of non-SAD patients. In general, the few SAD studies published thus far implicate brain areas where abnormalities have been found in non-SAD. The authors will examine the contribution of neuroimaging studies to hypotheses regarding the pathophysiology of seasonal and non-seasonal affective disorders. Potential clinical benefits from research in this field will be described.

24.2 Neuroimaging studies of SAD

The literature on neuroimaging of SAD includes two studies involving single photon emission computed tomography (SPECT), and two using positron emission computed tomography (PET). These physiologic techniques measure regional cerebral blood flow (rCBF) and localized regional glucose uptake respectively, and do not define structural anatomic features. (For technical information regarding these modalities see Prohovnik 1993; Van Heertum and Tikofsky 1995; Sackheim and Prohovnik 1993; Rauch and Renshaw 1995; Drevets and Raichle 1995; Kennedy *et al.* 1997; Rauch and Savage 1997; Alavi and Hirsch 1991.) An anatomical, not functional neuroimaging study utilized classic MRI to evaluate pituitary volume in SAD (Schwartz *et al.* 1997).

The studies cannot be compared precisely due to differences in sample selection, imaging techniques, and methods of data analysis. Indeed, one major issue that deserves greater attention is characterization of abnormalities potentially specific to subtypes of SAD, such as unipolar vs. bipolar SAD, or winter SAD vs. summer SAD — but larger sample sizes are essential to address this issue.

Following reports of decreased whole-cortex glucose metabolic rate (GMR) in non-SAD bipolar depressed patients compared with normal controls (Baxter *et al.* 1989; Martinot *et al.* 1990), Goyer contrasted cerebral glucose metabolism in 9 summer-SAD patients of whom 7 met DSM-III-R criteria for bipolar disorder, with 45 normal control subjects. In the summer-SAD group, Goyer found a decrease in cortical GMR compared with controls (Goyer *et al.* 1992). Comparisons of specific brain regions showed increased average, normalized GMR in the orbital frontal cortex (defined as anterior medial-, right-, and left-frontal plus right- and left-posterior frontal regions) of SAD patients as compared to normal control subjects. However, summer-SAD patients had a lower average, normalized GMR in the left inferior parietal lobule (consisting of the left parietal and parietal–occipital regions).

Goyer suggested that summer SAD had, in common with other major depressive disorders, a decrease in cortical GMR. However, whereas bipolar summer SAD was similar to bipolar non-SAD in global cortical GMR, it differed in the pattern of regional activity.

Other investigators have reported hypermetabolism in the orbital frontal and prefrontal cortex in obsessive–compulsive disorder (OCD) patients (Swedo et al. 1989; Baxter et al. 1987). Since none of his SAD patients had OCD, Goyer speculated that summer SAD and OCD have a common disturbance of metabolism in the left inferior parietal lobule and the orbital frontal cortex.

Cohen et al., in a PET investigation of 7 winter SAD patients (5 diagnosed as bipolar II) compared with 38 healthy controls, found globally lower GMR in SAD, whether the SAD patients were studied in an 'on-light' or 'off-light' condition (Cohen et al. 1992). The 'on-light' condition consisted of at least 10 days of 2.5 hours of 2500 lux of full spectrum light administered between 6.00 to 9.00 a.m. and then 6.00 to 9.00 p.m. Six of the seven SAD patients were studied sequentially in both the 'on-light' and the 'off-light' condition using a crossover design. The 'off-light' SAD patients were depressed and were found to have a 12.5 per cent lower overall or global grey-matter GMR as compared to normal controls (who were not exposed to light treatment). All SAD patients had an antidepressant response to light treatment. There was also a reduction in GMR in the superior subregion of the anterior medial frontal cortex and lower superior medial frontal cortical regions in SAD patients studied in the 'on-light' and 'off-lights' condition as compared to normal controls. Thus, these findings are consistent with those of Goyer reported in summer SAD. Cohen also found higher basal ganglia GMR in SAD patients than in controls.

Cohen et al. suggested that cerebral metabolism in SAD was characterized by hypoactivity in the superior prefrontal cortex and mid-prefrontal cortex, and hyperactivity in the medial orbito-frontal cortex. In addition, they reported that higher depression ratings, measured on the 21-item Hamilton Rating Scale and a supplementary atypical depression rating scale, were associated with lower metabolism in the superior medial prefrontal cortex. As is widely observed in winter SAD, atypical vegetative symptoms were common (Wehr et al. 1991) and the authors suggested a possible correlation with laterality of GMR.

Cohen et al. noted further findings in other regions. The 'off-light' patients with SAD as compared to normal controls had relatively higher GMR in right parietal and medial orbito-frontal cortex and lower GMR in the left parietal cortex. These abnormal prefrontal and parietal cortex regions appeared highly coupled (showing a positive correlation of GMR) in the SAD patients. Finally, Cohen reported that the SAD patients, following light treatment, exhibited increased cortical glucose utilization in the occipital region. It is not yet known if light treatment produces specific changes compared to other therapies, but a possible activation of the visual system in response to light is intuitively compelling.

Two groups have used SPECT techniques to study SAD. Murphy et al. (1993), utilizing the planar xenon SPECT method, reported a significant increase in global cerebral blood flow (CBF) in four winter-SAD patients compared to four age- and gender-matched normal controls following 2-hour exposure to 1500 lux of light. Unlike the Goyer and Cohen GMR data, untreated SAD patients did not differ from controls in global, regional, or hemispheric CBF. However, the SAD patients and control subjects did have a significantly different change in global CBF following light exposure. Whereas in the SAD group, the mean percentage change in CBF increased by 7.9 per cent, in the controls, global CBF decreased by 19 per cent. Murphy suggested that SAD patients had a physiologically distinct response to light as compared to control subjects. It is not clear whether pre-treatment differences between SAD patients and controls are easier to detect using GMR than CBF, nor whether the very small sample size did not allow a significant difference to be detected.

Our group observed differences in change in regional CBF between winter-SAD patients who responded as compared to those who did not respond to light treatment (Vasile *et al.* 1997). Ten depressed patients with winter SAD underwent SPECT functional brain imaging studies before and after light treatment (>2500 lux for 0.5–2 hours daily for approximately 1 week). Five patients had a therapeutic response to light treatment and five did not. There were four women and one man in each group. Relative increases in rCBF were observed in all brain regions compared to cerebellum in treatment responders, whereas non-responders showed no change or decreases in rCBF relative to cerebellum. Significant differences in mean percentage change in rCBF between responders and non-responders were detected in frontal and cingulate cortex and thalamus. Treatment responders exhibited a consistent trend toward increased rCBF in temporo-parietal, occipital, basal ganglia ROI, and in whole brain. These findings were consistent with the hypothesis that an increase in rCBF is associated with recovery from depression in SAD, as suggested by the Murphy *et al.* (1993) data.

The one neuroanatomic study in the literature on SAD found that neither winter depression nor change of season is associated with significant change in pituitary volume compared to normal controls, as measured by classic MRI (Schwartz *et al.* 1997). This finding, in a group of SAD patients with atypical depressive symptoms, suggests that the hypothalamic pituitary axis (HPA) is not overactive in seasonal depression and stands in contrast to a report of enlarged pituitary volume in non-seasonal major depression with melancholic features (Krishman *et al.* 1991). These studies are consistent with the hypothesis that the HPA in SAD is not overactive and underlie the potential importance of atypical as compared to classic endogenous depressive symptoms in understanding the pathophysiology of SAD.

Thus, the few published neuroimaging studies of SAD patients, limited by small sample size, suggest overall attenuated cortical activity during the depressed state, but leave open a number of questions regarding specific regional patterns and possible differences among diagnostic subgroups. The studies also highlight differences in rCBF and regional glucose utilization in response to light between SAD patients and control subjects, and between SAD responders and non-responders to light treatment. Questions regarding differences in specific anatomical sites between SAD patients and normal controls remain to be studied.

24.3 Neuroimaging studies of major depressive disorders

Several reviews have summarized the results of functional neuroimaging studies of depressive disorders. Most, but not all, published studies describe reductions in rCBF in anterior frontal, temporal, and parietal regions. The inferior orbital cortex and dorsolateral prefrontal cortex of the frontal lobe are frequently described as hypoperfused in the depressed state. To date, no imaging studies specifically compare patterns of rCBF in depressed patients with atypical depressive symptoms with those in patients with endogenous or non-atypical depressive symptoms. Several studies have included both unipolar and bipolar depressed patients, but no consistently reproducible pattern of rCBF has been reported between these subgroups of depressed patients (George *et al.* 1993; Bolwig 1993; Schwartz and Speed 1992; Dougherty and Rauch 1997; Yazici *et al.* 1992).

Diminished rCBF in the hippocampus and the caudate nucleus has been reported in late-life depression (Awata *et al.* 1998). Mayberg *et al.* (1994) have reported that depressed patients exhibit hypoperfusion in predominantly paralimbic regions. Amsterdam and Mozley (1992) reported asymmetry in temporal lobe perfusion in patients with major depression. The PET investigation of Bench *et al.* (1992), which found that depressed patients exhibited decreased rCBF in the left anterior cingulate and the left dorsolateral prefrontal cortex, lends further support to the hypothesis that prefrontal and limbic neuronal networks are functionally impaired in major depression.

A recent SPECT study described significant reductions in rCBF during the acutely depressed state in the left superior frontal, bilateral parietal, and right lateral temporal cortex in 16 patients with major depression. After successful antidepressant treatment, there were no significant differences in rCBF between the patients in remission and control subjects (Ogura *et al.* 1998). In another recent investigation, 22 depressed patients were studied with SPECT scans before and after two weeks of left prefrontal transcranial magnetic stimulation (TMS), using a parallel design, double-blind treatment paradigm (Teneback *et al.* 1999). At medication-free baseline, all subjects exhibited significantly diminished blood flow in the bilateral medial temporal lobes, left prefrontal cortex, and caudate that significantly declined with increased depression severity. Depressed adults who responded to TMS, compared with non-responders, showed increased inferior frontal lobe activity. Following treatment, there was an even greater difference in inferior frontal blood flow in responders compared with non-responders. TMS responders showed increased rCBF at treatment termination compared with baseline in limbic regions as a function of mood improvement. As yet, there is no consistent evidence linking specific pre- and post-treatment changes in rCBF or GMR to clinical response to a specific treatment modality.

SPECT studies of depressed patients have demonstrated the importance of identifying subgroups of depressed patients in assessing patterns of rCBF. Such subgroups have included psychotic or endogenously depressed patients, depressed patients with cognitive dysfunction, and elderly (as compared to younger) depressed patients (Dolan *et al.* 1993; Bench *et al.* 1993; Austin *et al.* 1992). Drevets *et al.* (1992) studied depressed subjects, all of whom met criteria for melancholia and recurrent depression. In this carefully defined subgroup of patients with familial depression, only the actively depressed group had an increase in rCBF in the left frontal cortex, suggesting that this abnormality reflects a state marker for depression. While both the depressed and remitted depressed patient groups had increased rCBF in the left amygdala, this difference achieved significance only in the depressed group. A similar finding of increased rCBF in left frontal lobes in acutely depressed unipolar depressives (but not depressed bipolar patients) has been reported by Tutus *et al.* (1998).

Recent speculations as to the pathophysiology of depressive disorders are increasingly based on dysfunction in two interrelated basal ganglia-thalamocortical circuits (Lafer *et al.* 1997):

1. a limbic neural circuit connecting the amygdala, anterior cingulate, and ventral striatum with medial and ventrolateral prefrontal cortex

2. a prefrontal neural circuit connecting the head of the caudate and thalamus with the dorsolateral prefrontal cortex.

Drevets has suggested imbalances within these circuits may contribute to depressive disorders. He speculates that dysfunction of modulatory systems within the prefrontal cortex, striatum, and brain stem may disinhibit affective responses generated through the amygdala and its projections (Drevets 1999).

Extensive dopaminergic, noradrenergic, serotonergic, and cholinergic projections mediate neurotransmission and neuroreceptor sensitivity in the neuromodulatory circuits just noted. Interactions among these neurotransmitters are linked to hypotheses explaining the therapeutic action of antidepressant medications. The antidepressant effect of enhanced serotonergic and dopaminergic activity may be based upon inhibitory modulation of basal ganglia-thalamocortical circuits. It is noteworthy that the SPECT and PET neuroimaging studies of SAD patients already described implicate basal ganglia-thalamocortical circuits, consistent with this explanation of affective dysregulation in depressive disorders.

24.4 Future directions in neuroimaging research on SAD

The described research strategies employed in neuroimaging studies of major depression provide insights into future directions in SAD research. Study designs with larger patient samples which identify bipolar and unipolar and elderly vs. younger patient subgroups will be required to further clarify neuroimaging changes in SAD. The limited SAD studies raise the possibility that studies comparing patients with 'atypical' vs. 'typical' vegetative depressive symptom patterns may yield regional differences in cerebral metabolic activity. Attention to issues of 'state' vs. 'trait' neuroimaging findings will be of importance, particularly as baseline markers predictive of treatment response.

SAD studies offer a potentially unique contribution since SAD patients are often euthymic and untreated in the summer. Recent developments in SPECT receptor imaging have enabled investigators to explore receptor activity in affective disorders. This promising methodology has also been employed to assess serotonin$_2$ receptor activity in a sample of 19 depressed patients compared to controls (D'haenen *et al.* 1992).

Studies integrating assessment of rCBF and regional glucose metabolic activity in relation to change in neurotransmitter and neuroreceptor activity involving limbic neuronal networks appears to be a promising research strategy. Studies of changes in neurotransmitter turnover in SAD could be linked to further neuroimaging investigations (Anderson *et al.* 1992). Further exploration of differences in rCBF and regional metabolic glucose utilization between responders and non-responders to light treatment in SAD and differences in neurotransmitter parameters await further studies. Of particular clinical relevance would be a specific baseline brain imaging finding predictive of response or non-response to light treatment. Studies of receptor sensitivity and density and relationship to treatment response now pursued in other fields have not yet been identified in SAD patients.

The correlation of physiologic and anatomic neuroimaging studies with recent research findings on G protein levels as a state marker for winter depression in patients with SAD (Avissar *et al.* 1999) represents another promising area for research. Functional MRI studies of affective disorders are now beginning to emerge, but none have specifically focused on SAD. The fact that SAD patients appear to share basal ganglia-thalamocortical abnormalities with non-SAD patients suggests that in addition to studies of circadian neuroanatomy and neurophysiology, a broader neuroanatomical focus will be essential for clarifying the pathophysiology of seasonal mood disorders. All of these areas present rich opportunities for further research.

References

Alavi, A. and Hirsch, L.J. (1991). Studies of central nervous system disorders with single photon computed tomography and positron emission tomography: evolution over the past two decades. *Seminars in Nuclear Medicine*, **XXI(1)**:58–91.

Amsterdam, J.D. and Mozley, D.P. (1992). Temporal lobe asymmetry with iofetamine (IMP) SPECT imaging in patients with major depression. *Journal of Affective Disorders*, **24**:43–53.

Anderson, J.L., Vasile, R.G., Mooney, J.J., Bloomingdale, K.L., Samson, J.A., and Schildkraut, J.J. (1992). Changes in norephinephrine output following light therapy for fall/winter seasonal depression. *Biological Psychiatry*, **32**:700–4.

Austin, M.P., Dougall, N., Ross, M., Murray, C., O'Carroll, R.E., Moffoot, A., *et al.* (1992). Single photon emission tomography with ^{99m}tc-exametazime in major depression and the pattern of brain activity underlying the psychotic/ neurotic continuum. *Journal of Affective Disorders*, **26**:31–44.

Avissar, S., Schreiber, G., Nechamkin, Y., Neuhaus, I., Lam, G.K., Schwartz, P., *et al.* (1999). The effects of seasons and light therapy on G protein levels in mononuclear leukocytes of patients with seasonal affective disorder. *Archives of General Psychiatry*, **56**:178–83.

Awata, S., Ito, H., Konno, M., Ono, S., Kawashima, R., Fukuda, H., *et al.* (1998). Regional cerebral blood flow abnormalities in late-life depression: relation to refractoriness and chronification. *Psychiatry and Clinical Nneuroscience*, **52**:97–105.

Baxter, L.R., Phelps, M.E., Mazziotta, J.C., Guze, B.H., Schwartz, J.M., and Selin, C.E. (1987). Local cerebral glucose metabolic rates in obsessive–compulsive disorder. *Archives of General Psychiatry*, **44**:211–18.

Baxter Jr, L.R., Schwartz, J.M., Phelps, M.E, Mazziotta, J.C., Guze, B.H., Selin, C.E., *et al.* (1989). Reduction of prefrontal cortex glucose metabolism common to three types of depression. *Archives of General Psychiatry*, **46**:243–50.

Bench, C.J., Friston, K.J., Brown, R.G., Scott, L., Frackowiak, R.S.J, and Dolan, R.J. (1992). The anatomy of melancholia. Abnormalities of regional cerebral blood flow in major depression, *Psychological Medicine*, **22**:607–15.

Bench, C.J., Friston, K.J., Brown, R.G., Frackowiak, R.S.J., and Dolan, R.J. (1993). Regional cerebral blood flow in depression measured by positron emission tomography: the relationship with clinical dimensions. *Psychological Medicine*, **23**:579–90.

Bolwig, T.G. (1993). Regional cerebral blood flow in affective disorder. *Acta Psychiatrica Scandinavia*, **371(Suppl)**:48–53.

Cohen, R.M., Gross, M., Nordahl, T.E., Semple, W.E., Oren, D.A., and Rosenthal, N.E. (1992). Preliminary data on the metabolic brain pattern of patients with seasonal affective disorder. *Archives of General Psychiatry*, **49**:545–52.

D'haenen, H., Bossuyt, A., Mertens, J., Bossuyt–Piron, C., Gijsemans, M., and Kaufman, L. (1992). SPECT imaging of serotonin$_2$ receptors in depression. *Psychiatry Research*, **45(4)**:227–37.

Dolan, R.J., Bench, C.J., Liddle, P.F., Fiston, K.J., Frith, C.D., Grasby, P.M., *et al.* (1993). Dorsolateral prefrontal cortex dysfunction in the major psychoses; symptom or disease specificity? *Journal of Neurology, Neurosurgery, and Psychiatry*, **56**:1290–4.

Dougherty, D. and Rauch, S.L. (1997). Neuroimaging and neurobiological models of depression. *Harvard Review of Psychiatry*, **5**:138–59.

Drevets, W.C. (1999). Prefrontal corticalamygdalar metabolism in major depression. *Annals of the New York Academy of Science*, **877**:614–37.

Drevets, W.C., Videen, T.O., Price, J.L., Preskorn, S.H., Carmichael, S.T., and Raichle, M.E. (1992). A functional anatomical study of unipolar depression. *Journal of Neuroscience*, **12(9)**:3628–41.

Drevets, W.C. and Raichle, M.E. (1995). *Positron emission tomographic imaging studies of human emotional disorders*. Massachusetts Institute of Technology Press, Cambridge, Massachusetts.

George, M.S., Ketter, T.A., and Post, R.M. (1993). SPECT and PET imaging in mood disorders. *Journal of Clinical Psychiatry*, **54**:6–13.

Goyer, P.F., Schultz, P.M. , Semple, W.E., Gross, M., Nordahl, T.E., King, C.A., *et al.* (1992). Cerebral glucose metabolism in patients with summer seasonal affective disorder. *Neuropsychopharmacology*, **7(3)**:233–40.

Kennedy, S.H., Javanmard, M., and Vaccarino, F.J. (1997). A review of functional neuroimaging in mood disorders: positron emision tomography and depression. *Canadian Journal of Psychiatry*, **42**:467–75.

Krishnan, K.R., Doraiswamy, P.M., Lurie, S.N., Figiel, G.S., Husain, M.M., Boyko, O.B., *et al.* (1991). Pituitary size in depression. *Journal of Clinical Endocrinology and Metabolism*, **72**:256–9.

Lafer, B., Renshaw, P.F., and Sachs, G.S. (1997). Major depression and the basal ganglia. *Psychiatric Clinics of North America*, **20(4)**:885–96.

Martinot, J.L., Hardy, P., Feline, A., Huret, J-D., Mazoyer, B., Attar–Levy, D., *et al.* (1990). Left prefrontal glucose hypometabolism in the depressed state: a confirmation. *American Journal of Psychiatry*, **147**:1313–17.

Mayberg, H.S, Lewis, P.J., Regenold, W., and Wagner Jr, H.N. (1994). Paralimbic hypoperfusion in unipolar depression. *Journal of Nuclear Medicine*, **35**:929–34.

Murphy, D.G.M., Murphy, D.M., Abbas, M., Palzidou, E., Binnie, C., Arendt, J., *et al.* (1993). Seasonal affective disorder: response to light as measured by electroencephalogram, melatonin suppression, and cerebral blood flow. *British Journal of Psychiatry*, **163**:327–31.

Ogura, A., Morinobu, S., Kawakatsu, S., Tosuka, S., and Komatani, A. (1998). Changes in regional brain activity in major depression after successful treatment with antidepressant drugs. *Acta Psychiatrica Scandinavian*, **98**:54–9.

Prohovnik, I.P. (1993). SPECT imaging of cerebral physiology. In *Review of psychiatry* (ed. J.M. Oldham, M.B. Riba, and A. Tasman). American Psychiatric Press, Washington, DC.

Rauch, S.L. and Renshaw, P.F. (1995). Clinical neuroimaging in psychiatry. *Harvard Review of Psychiatry*, **2**:297–312.

Rauch, S.L. and Savage, C.R. (1997). Neuroimaging and neuropsychology of the striatum. *Psychiatric Clinic of North America*, **20(4)**:741–68.

Sackeim, H.A. and Prohovnik, I. (1993). Brain imaging studies of depressive disorders, In *Biology of depressive disorders. Part A: a systems perspective* (ed. J.J. Mann and D.J. Kupfer), pp. 205–58. Plenum Press, New York and London.

Schwartz, J.A. and Speed, N.M. (1992). SPECT research in affective disorders. In *Biological psychiatry* (ed. G. Racagni), B.V. Vol. 1. Elsevier Science Publishers, London.

Schwartz, P.J., Loe, J.A., Bash, C.N., Bove, K., Turner, E.H., Frank, J.A., *et al.* (1997). Seasonality and pituitary volume. *Psychiatry Research: Neuroimaging Section*, **74**:151–7.

Swedo, S.E., Schapiro, M.B., Grady, C.L., Cheslow, D.L., Leonard, H.L., Kumar, A., *et al.* (1989). Cerebral glucose metabolism in childhood-onset obsessive–compulsive disorder. *Archives of General Psychiatry*, **46**:518–23.

Teneback, C.C., Nahas, Z., Speer, A.M., Molloy, M., Stallings, L.E., Spicer, S.M., *et al.* (1999). Changes in prefrontal cortex and paralimbic activity in depression following two weeks of daily left prefrontal TMS. *Journal of Neuropsychology and Clinical Neuroscience*, **11**:426–35.

Tutus, A., Simsek, A., Sofuoglu, S., Nardali, M., Kugu, N., Karaaslan, F., *et al.* (1998). Changes in regional cerebral blood flow demonstrated by single photon emission computed tomography in depressive disorders: comparison of unipolar vs. bipolar subtypes. *Psychiatry Research:Neuroimaging*, **83**:169–77.

Van Heertum, R.L. and Tikofsky, R.S. (ed.) (1995). *Cerebral SPECT imaging*. Raven Press, New York.

Vasile, R.G., Sachs, G., Anderson, J.L., Lafer, B., Matthews, E., and Hill, T. (1997). Changes in regional cerebral blood flow after light treatment for seasonal affective disorder: responders versus non-responders. *Biological Psychiatry* **42**:1000–5.

Wehr, T.A., Giesen, H.A., Schulz, P.M., Anderson, J.L., Joseph–Vanderpool, J.R., Kelly, K., *et al.* (1991). Contrasts between symptoms of summer depression and winter depression. *Journal of Affective Disorders*, **23**:173–83.

Yazici, K.M., Kapucu, O., Erbas, B., Varoglu, E., Gulec, C., and Bekdik, C.F. (1992). Assessments of changes in regional cerebral blood flow in patients with major depression using the ^{99m}Tc-HMPAO single photon emission tomography method. *European Journal of Nuclear Medicine*, **19**:1038–43.

Further reading

Brucke, T., Podreka, I., Angelberger, P., Wenger, S., Topitz, A., and Kufferle, B. (1991). Dopamine D$_2$ receptor imaging with SPECT: studies in different neuropsychiatric disorders. *Journal of Cerebral Blood Flow and Metabolism*, **11**:220–8.

Cummings, J.L. (1993). The neuroanatomy of depression. *Journal of Clinical Psychiatry*, **54(11)**:14–20.

Curran, S.M., Murray, C.M., Van Beck, M., Dougall, N., O'Carroll, R.E., Austin, M-P., et al. (1993). A single photon emission computerized topography study of regional brain function in elderly patients with major depression and with Alzheimer-type dementia. *British Journal of Psychiatry*, **163**:155–65.

D'haenen, H.A. and Bossuyt, A. (1994). Dopamine D-sub-2 receptors in depression measured with single photon emission computed tomography. *Biological Psychiatry*, **35(2)**:128–32.

Devous, M.D., Gullion, C.M., Grannemann, B.D., Trivedi, H., and Rush, A.J. (1993). Regional cerebral blood flow alterations in unipolar depression. *Psychiatry Research: Neuroimaging*, **50**:233–56.

Dolan, R.J., Bench, C.J., Brown, R.G., Scott, L.C., Friston, K.J., and Frackowiak, R.S.J. (1992). Regional cerebral blood flow abnormalities in depressed patients with cognitive impairment. *Journal of Neurology, Neurosurgery, and Psychiatry*, **55**:768–73.

Dolan, R.J., Bench, C.J., Liddle, P.F., Fiston, K.J., Frith, C.D., Grasby, P.M., et al. (1993). Dorsolateral prefrontal cortex dysfunction in the major psychoses; symptom or disease specificity? *Journal of Neurology, Neurosurgery, and Psychiatry*, **56**:1290–4.

Ebert, D., Feistel, H., and Barocka, A. (1991). Effects of sleep deprivation on the limbic system and the frontal lobes in affective disorders: a study with [Tc–99m] HMPAO SPECT. *Psychiatry Research: Neuroimaging*, **40**:247–51.

Ebert, D., Feistel, H., Barocka, A., and Kaschka, W. (1994). Increased limbic flow and total sleep deprivation in major depression with melancholia. *Psychiatry Research*, **5**:101–9.

Edmonstone, Y., Austin, M-P., Prentice, N., Dougall, N., Freeman, C.P.L., Ebmeier, K.P., et al. (1994). Uptake of [99m] Tc-exametazime shown by single photon emission computerized tomography in obsessive–compulsive diosorder compared with major depression and normal controls. *Acta Psychiatrica Scandinavia*, **90**:298–303.

Goodwin, G.M., Austin, M.P., Dougall, N., Ross, M., Murray, C., O'Carroll, R.E., et al. (1993). State changes in brain activity shown by the uptake of ^{99m}Tc-exametazime with single photon emission tomography in major depression before and after treatment. *Journal of Affective Disorders*, **29**:243–53.

Innis, R.B. (1992). Neuroreceptor imaging with SPECT. *Journal of Clinical Psychiatry*, **53(11)**:29–34.

Jezzard, P., Haxby, J., Sadato, N., Rueckert, L., and Mattay, V. (1995). Functional magnetic resonance imaging of the brain. *Annals of Internal Medicine*, **122**:296–303.

Lesser, I.M., Mena, I., Boone, K.B., Miller, B.L., Mehringer, C.M., and Wohl, M. (1994). Reduction of cerebral blood flow in older depressed patients. *Archives of General Psychiatry*, **51**: 677–86.

Maes, M., Dierckx, R., Meltzer, H.Y., Ingels, M., Schotte, C., Vandewoude, M., et al. (1993). Regional cerebral blood flow in unipolar depression measured with [Tc–99m]-HMPAO single photon emission computed topography: negative findings. *Psychiatry Research: Neuroimaging*, **50**:77–88.

Moretti, J.L., Caglar, M., and Weinmann, P. (1995). Cerebral perfusion imaging tracers for SPECT: which one to choose? *Journal of Nuclear Medicine*, **36**:359–63.

Nobler, M.S., Sackeim, H.A., Prohovnik, I., Moeller, J.R., Mukherjee, S., and Schnur, D.B. (1994). Regional cerebral blood flow in mood disorders. III: treatment and clinical response. *Archives of General Psychiatry*, **51**:884–97.

Philpot, M.P., Banerjee, S., Needham–Bennett, H., Costa, D., and Ell, P.J. (1993). ^{99m}Tc-HMPAO single photon emission tomography in late life depression: a pilot study of regional cerebral blood flow at rest and during a verbal fluency task. *Journal of Affective Disorders*, **28**:233–40.

Purl, B.K. and Lewis, S.W. (1992). Single photon emission computerized tomography (SPECT) in neuropsychiatry: a review. *Behavioral Neurology*, **5(3)**:139–47.

Reba, R.C. (1993). PET and SPECT: opportunities and challenges for psychiatry. *Journal of Clinical Psychiatry*, **54(Suppl)**:26–32.

Rezai, K., Andreasen, N.C., Alliger, R., Cohen, G., Swayze, V., and O'Leary, D.S. (1993). The neuropsychology of the prefrontal cortex. *Archives of Neurology*, **50**:636–42.

Rubin, E., Sackeim, H., Prohovnik, I., Moeller, J.R., Schnur, D.B., and Mukherjee, S. (1995). Regional cerebral blood flow in mood disorders. IV: comparison of mania and depression. *Psychiatry Research: Neuroimaging*, **61**:1–10.

Rubin, E., Sackeim, H.A., Nobler, M.S., and Moeller, J.R. (1994). Brain imaging studies of antidepressant treatments. *Psychiatric Annals*, **24(12)**:653–8.

Sackeim, H.A., Prohovnik, I., Moeller, J.R., Brown, J.R., Apter, S., Prudic, J., *et al.* (1990). Regional cerebral blood flow in mood disorders. I: comparisons of major depressives and normal controls at rest. *Archives of General Psychiatry*, **47**:60–70.

Scott, A.I., Dougall, N., Ross, M., O'Carroll, R.E., Riddle, W., Ebmeier, K.P., *et al.* (1994). Short-term effects of electroconvulsive treatment on the uptake of ^{99m}TC-Exametazime into brain in major depression shown with single photon emission tomography. *Journal of Affectivef Disorders*, **30**:27–34.

Silfverskiöld, P. and Risberg, J. (1989). Regional cerebral blood flow in depression and mania. *Archives of General Psychiatry*, **46**:253–9.

Thomas, P., Vaiva, G., Samaille, E., Maron, M., Alaix, C., Steinling, M., *et al.* (1993). Cerebral blood flow in major depression and dysthymia. *Journal of Affective Disorders*, **29**:235–42.

Chapter 25

Circadian clock

Diane B. Boivin

25.1 Introduction

Seasonal variations in mood and behaviour have been documented in epidemiological studies of the general population (Madden *et al.* 1996). Within the winter months, subjects frequently change their sleep habits, possess less energy, and experience variations in temperament. It has been proposed that human tolerance to changes in the lighting conditions, within seasons, varies according to a spectrum that includes at its end, clinical syndromes (for example, SAD) or subclinical syndromes (for example, sub-SAD) which have a genetic basis, at least for the winter forms (Madden *et al.* 1996).

Although physiological and behavioural changes have been reported in animals, it remains controversial whether humans are seasonal creatures. Several individuals, namely in the psychiatric community, would contend this view on an empirical basis. Psychiatric disorders such as bipolar affective disorders (Hunt *et al.* 1992), premenstrual dysphoric disorder (Parry *et al.* 1987), or even suicidal behaviours (Maes *et al.* 1993) frequently show increased rates of relapse around specific times of year. The condition coined in 1984 by Rosenthal and colleagues as SAD is a recurrent affective disorder tied with the changes of season (Rosenthal *et al.* 1984). Typically, patients diagnosed with SAD experience recurrent depressive episodes during either the autumn–winter months (winter form) or the spring–summer months (summer form), while recovering spontaneously outside of these seasons.

The winter form is the most frequent form of SAD. Atypical symptoms such as increased carbohydrate craving, increased weight gain, increased sleepiness, and reduced energy levels inspired several authors to draw some distant, yet interesting, comparisons with the seasonal changes of behaviour in hibernating species. Until now, most of the literature has dealt with the search for the pathogenesis of winter depression, which remains open, leaving the summer form for later inquiries. Predictably, the change in daylight exposure per day (the photoperiod) has been the first environmental factor blamed for the occurrence of winter depression.

The physiology of photoperiodism in seasonal species has guided the initial exploration of the pathological basis of winter SAD. It has been known for years that seasonal species adjust to their photoperiodic environment by adapting the temporal pattern of their diurnal rhythms, particularly those of hormones. It has been reported that melatonin, also called the 'hormone of darkness', was the messenger hormone responsible for conveying the duration of the dark period (scotoperiod) by adjusting the onset and offset of secretion in harmony with the subjective night. Similar observations have been made in human subjects studied under natural (Vondrašová–Jelínková *et al.* 1999) or artificial summer and winter photoperiods

(Wehr 1991). These healthy individuals adapted to their environment by patterning their hormonal rhythms to that of the imposed light–dark cycle. These results indicate that human subjects are at least capable of responding physiologically and behaviourally to the photoperiodic environment. Nevertheless, it remains unclear whether these observations have any practical implication or clinical relevance, since the modern-day addition of an auxiliary source of indoor lighting cancelled any effects of the photoperiodic environment (Wehr et al. 1995).

Until the later part of the twentieth century, human subjects were considered relatively insensitive to the light in their environment. In 1980, Lewy and colleagues disproved that assumption by reporting that bright-light exposure at night (> 2500 lux) was capable of inhibiting the nocturnal secretion of melatonin, presumably through its action on the endogenous circadian system (Lewy et al. 1980). In 1984, Rosenthal and colleagues hypothesized that the seasonal changes in light exposure, namely the reduction in the total daily light exposure, could significantly affect mood in humans and play a major role in the pathogenesis of winter SAD. Lewy and colleagues proposed that light therapy was effective mainly in the morning and induced its antidepressant effect by advancing the phase of the endogenous circadian system (Lewy et al. 1987). These results gave support to a putative role of the endogenous circadian pacemaker in the pathogenesis of winter SAD. So far, several circadian hypotheses, not mutually exclusive, have been proposed to explain the occurrence of SAD. This chapter will review the major circadian hypotheses of SAD, which comprise the photoperiod, the phase-delay, the melatonin, and the reduced amplitude hypotheses.

25.2 Effects of light on the endogenous circadian system

The first reported effect of light on the human circadian system was its capacity to inhibit nocturnal melatonin secretion. Initially, it was believed that light levels should exceed a minimal threshold of 2500 lux to exert a robust biological effect (Lewy et al. 1980). This was later refuted when it was discovered that much lower light intensities (100 lux) would be sufficient to significantly reduce melatonin secretion at night (Gaddy et al. 1993). The magnitude of melatonin suppression was shown to be dependent upon the illuminance levels of the light exposure and to be more pronounced with 2500 lux (Brainard et al. 1988).

Bright light was also found to exert a powerful resetting effect on the phase of the human circadian pacemaker according to its phase of initial administration (Czeisler et al. 1989; Honma and Honma 1988; Minors et al. 1991). In an experiment, prospectively designed to allow construction of a dose response curve to light in humans, we reported that even ordinary levels of indoor room light (about 180 lux) were able to advance the endogenous oscillation of core body temperature, plasma melatonin, and plasma cortisol in healthy young men (Boivin et al. 1996; Boivin and Czeisler 1998). These results have been reproduced by other teams (Waterhouse et al. 1998) and are consistent with the observation that photoperiod-responsive changes in human circadian rhythms may be suppressed by regular exposure to artificial room light (Wehr et al. 1995). These results also imply that changes in the timing of the sleep–wake cycle, as frequently occurs in depression, might change the timing of exposure to indoor room light and darkness, and may subsequently have a significant effect on the resultant rhythms.

In vertebrates and arthropods, the importance of circadian rhythms in photoperiodic time measurement has been known for a while (Pittendrigh et al. 1991). Studies in mammals also revealed that both day length and illuminance levels, which characterize the photoperiodic environment, can substantially modify light-induced phase shifts (Elliot 1994; Humlova and Illnerová 1992) or even the topology of the light-induced phase response curve (Elliot 1994). Recent evidence suggests that human subjects are sensitive to the photoperiodic environment, which can induce persistent changes in the intrinsic waveform of several circadian markers, as well as induce changes within sleep organization (Matthews *et al.* 1991; Wehr *et al.* 1993; Wehr 1991) or in the temporal relationship between several diurnal rhythms. For instance, the duration of the nocturnal secretion of plasma melatonin, high prolactin secretion, and rising levels of cortisol are significantly longer after humans have been exposed chronically to long nights rather than to short nights (Wehr 1991).

Light exposure often exerts another important effect on human circadian physiology, namely it can modify the amplitude of the circadian oscillation. It has been demonstrated that properly timed exposure to light and darkness can substantially reduce the amplitude of the circadian oscillation in humans, and drive the system to what has been called its singular region (Jewett *et al.* 1991). This observation, and the large (> 8 hours) phase shifts induced by 5-hour exposure to 10 000 lux daily for 3 days (Czeisler *et al.* 1989), were interpreted as evidence that the human circadian system is complex and capable of adapting its sensitivity to light by changes in amplitude and phase (Kronauer *et al.* 1993). Such changes of amplitude, and its indirect impact on the circadian phase, were hypothesized to play a role in the pathogenesis of SAD (Czeisler *et al.* 1987).

25.3 Diurnal variation of mood in healthy and winter-depressed subjects

A diurnal variation in subjective measures of mood in healthy volunteers has been reported (Monk *et al.* 1992), suggesting that there is an underlying circadian rhythm of mood. Given the deterioration of subjective mood rating following sleep deprivation in healthy subjects, an experimental protocol that bisects the relative influences of time elapsed since awakening and circadian phase ought to be employed to quantify this interaction.

In a recent collaborative research project (Boivin *et al.* 1997), 24 healthy, young subjects were enrolled in a 'forced desynchrony protocol'. Subjects spent between 19 to 33 days on a 28-hour or 30-hour sleep–wake schedule. Because entrainment of the endogenous circadian pacemaker to days much longer (or shorter) than 24 hours is not possible, these conditions induced desynchrony between the circadian timing system (which continues to oscillate according to its nearly 24-hour intrinsic period) and the imposed sleep–wake cycle. Subjective mood could then be assessed at a variety of circadian phases and times since waking. Under these settings, a significant variation of mood was observed with circadian phase. These results in healthy, young subjects indicated, for the first time, that subjective mood is influenced by a complex and non-additive interaction of circadian phase and duration of prior wakefulness. The nature of this interaction is such that moderate changes in the timing of the sleep–wake cycle may have significant effects on subsequent mood.

Despite the difference in affective states in healthy subjects and depressed patients, our results in healthy volunteers (Boivin *et al.* 1997) brings a circadian perspective to the well-known phenomenon of diurnal variation of mood in depression and the effects of sleep deprivation on patients with this condition. Very few studies have compared the diurnal variation of mood simultaneously in depressed and healthy controls. In one such study, seasonally depressed patients were enrolled in a 40-hour constant routine procedure (Graw *et al.* 1998). An improvement of mood levels was observed with sleep deprivation in 52 per cent of the patients versus 29 per cent of the controls. This rate of improvement falls within the range of that documented in non-seasonal depression (Wu and Bunney 1990). In non-seasonally depressed patients, a relationship has been observed between mood variability measures and the response to sleep deprivation (Gordijn *et al.* 1994). However, no such relationship has been observed for SAD patients. The reason for these differences are indeterminate and still today the relationship between the daily variation of mood, the endogenous circadian pacemaker, and depressive symptoms remains unclear.

In a recent original study (Koorengevel *et al.* 2000), a 54-year-old man with SAD was enrolled in a forced desynchrony experiment. He was scheduled on a program consisting of 20-hour days for a duration of 120 hours. He was studied during a depressive episode and following phototherapy. This study revealed the presence of a significant variation of mood levels as measured by the Adjective Mood Scale . During the depressive episode, the circadian variation of mood was shifted by about two hours earlier, compared to the recovery phase. The patient maintained a regular sleep schedule in the four days preceding his admission to the laboratory. These results suggest that the temporal relationship between the circadian rhythm of mood and the sleep–wake cycle might be disturbed during depressive episodes. Extension of this particular study should clarify whether the circadian variation of other behavioural parameters such as sleep organization, sleep propensity, and vigilance levels are atypical during winter depression.

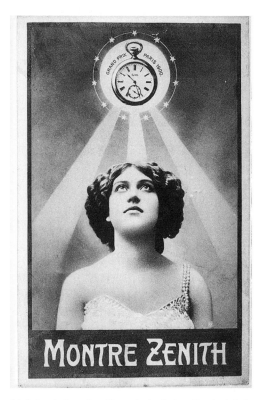

Fig. 25.1 Time-givers IV: light-dark cycles. The principal circadian lock is located in the suprachiasmatic nuclei of the brain, on which physical activity, knowledge of time, and state of health have a vital effect. Source: AWJ private collection.

25.4 Circadian hypotheses of winter depression

25.4.1 The phase-delay hypothesis

This hypothesis was proposed by Lewy and colleagues in 1987 to explain the antidepressant effects of light in winter depression (Lewy *et al.* 1987). The authors observed that morning exposure to bright light (for example, 10 000 lux from 6.00 to 8.00 a.m.) produced an advance in the time of onset of melatonin secretion. The authors concluded that the antidepressant effect of light therapy was attributed to its phase-advancing properties (for a review, see Lewy *et al.* 1988). They also observed that SAD patients tended to show a delay in the onset of plasma melatonin secretion compared to healthy controls during a depressive phase, and that respondents to morning bright light tended to exhibit a greater delay in their baseline values of melatonin onset.

The phase-delay hypothesis could be seen as a variant of the phase-advance hypothesis of endogenous depression. Lewy and colleagues simultaneously proposed that depressed patients should be 'phase type' according to the position of their endogenous circadian system (Lewy and Sack 1987). In contrast, the temporal distribution of REM (rapid eye movement) sleep earlier in the night in non-SAD depressed patients was interpreted as being the result of a phase advance of the endogenous circadian system. This hypothesis has been conceptualized into what has been called the 'internal coincidence model' (Wehr and Wirz–Justice 1981). According to this model, the endogenous circadian system is advanced relative to the sleep schedule such that sleep occurs at critical circadian phases at the end of the night. During these phases, sleep would exert a depressogenic effect in susceptible individuals. Therapeutic success has been reported in some patients by scheduling sleep episodes 5 to 6 hours earlier (Wehr *et al.* 1979).

There have been less sleep studies of SAD patients than of non-SAD depressed patients. In the initial description of the syndrome by Rosenthal and colleagues in 1984 (Rosenthal *et al.* 1984), sleep recordings during winter-depressive phases revealed a 17 per cent increase in total sleep time, an average increase of 23 per cent in sleep latency, and an average decrease of 46 per cent of slow wave sleep (SWS). However, the REM sleep latency and REM density were normal. Other polysomnographic recordings of seasonally depressed patients showed a decreased sleep efficiency, decreased SWS percentage, and increased REM density without modification of REM sleep latency (Anderson *et al.* 1994).

The absence of modifications of REM sleep variables have been confirmed by at least another group (Palchikov *et al.* 1997) and indicates that the sleep modifications of SAD patients is different from those observed in endogenous depression. In this study, SWS duration and percentage were significantly lower in respondents to phototherapy during winter months, when compared to non-respondents and controls. This difference disappeared after light therapy. No changes were observed after light therapy in sleep onset or REM sleep variable in SAD patients (Palchikov *et al.* 1997). These results would argue against a phase-shift hypothesis of winter depression because REM sleep is highly dependent on circadian phase (Dijk and Czeisler 1995). However, a significant phase advance of the diurnal rhythm of sleepiness was observed in this study and a prior one (Partonen *et al.* 1993).

The changes reported for SWS would rather support a role of homeostatic mechanisms in SAD and could be linked to impaired serotonin (5-HT) transmission (Palchikov *et al.* 1997). A recent study argued against this last possibility since the recuperative function of sleep was found to be normal in SAD patients after a 40-hour sleep deprivation constant routine procedure (Brunner *et al.* 1996). More studies are needed on the sleep changes of SAD patients and whether these changes would support a circadian and/or sleep–wake dependent hypothesis.

Overall, morning exposure to bright light was reported to be more effective than afternoon or evening exposure (Lewy *et al.* 1998*b*; Terman *et al.* 1998) in winter SAD, although it still remains a matter of debate (Wirz–Justice *et al.* 1993). This observation has served as the main argument for the phase-delay shift hypothesis for SAD. In 1987, Lewy and colleagues proposed that the endogenous circadian system was phase delayed relative to the sleep–wake cycle, and that morning phototherapy was effective by phase advancing the endogenous circadian rhythms of core body temperature and plasma melatonin (Lewy *et al.* 1987). This hypothesis was either supported (Avery *et al.* 1997; Dahl *et al.* 1993; Lewy *et al.* 1998*b*; Thompson *et al.* 1997) or challenged (Checkley *et al.* 1993; Eastman *et al.* 1993) experimentally by looking at the timing of various circadian markers.

If the phase-advance hypothesis was correct, patients would deteriorate following evening exposure to bright light due to a worsening of the phase-delay shift. On the contrary, evening phototherapy also produces an antidepressant effect without any reports of mood deterioration. Lewy and colleagues have argued that a direct energizing effect of light could explain the antidepressant effect of evening phototherapy despite the phase delay it induces (Lewy *et al.* 1988). Exogenous melatonin administered during the late afternoon or evening should also be therapeutic since it is known to induce a phase advance of the endogenous circadian system (Lewy *et al.* 1998*a*). So far, no convincing therapeutic effects were observed with exogenous melatonin (Wirz–Justice *et al.* 1990). The phase-shift hypothesis or its latest variants, the phase-instability or impaired entrainment hypotheses (Thompson *et al.* 1997), can neither be totally ruled out nor confirmed at this stage.

A serious limitation of most prior studies is the presence of masking effects induced by the rest–activity cycles on the observed rhythms. Few studies (Avery *et al.* 1997; Cajochen *et al.* 2000; Dahl *et al.* 1993; Graw *et al.* 1998) have used more sophisticated techniques, such as the constant routine procedure, to unravel the endogenous circadian phase of the core body temperature, plasma melatonin, and plasma cortisol rhythms. Even with the use of the constant routine procedure, care must be taken to control for the length of sleep episodes between the experimental conditions. For instance, Avery and colleagues (1997) reported a significant phase-advance shift of the circadian rhythm of plasma cortisol after a week of morning phototherapy compared to its baseline position and control subjects. However, SAD patients had a later rhythm at the start of the study compared to that of control subjects. Thus, an advance of the sleep schedule during the week of phototherapy might have contributed significantly to the differences between groups.

25.4.2 The photoperiod hypothesis

The cause of winter depression is still unknown, but the shortening of the photoperiodic environment during autumn/winter months has been incriminated as a triggering factor. Indeed, a therapeutic success has been reported by extending the duration of bright-light exposure each day (Rosenthal *et al.* 1984). It has subsequently been reported that the timing of the dawn and dusk light signals alone did not account for the therapeutic effect of phototherapy since a summer and winter 'skeleton photoperiod' (that is, no light administered between the dawn and dusk signals) were equally effective (Wehr *et al.* 1986). However, in this study, 5 of the 7 patients failed to return to their baseline mood levels before beginning their second treatment condition and a complex interaction was observed between the order and type of treatment. Therefore, the role of the photoperiodic environment in the pathogenesis of SAD cannot be totally excluded on the basis of this study. The question still remains whether in modern society SAD patients are exposing themselves to different levels of light across seasons, and whether the photoperiod hypothesis has any clinical relevance.

In modern society, urban dwellers are seldom exposed to light exceeding 1000 lux (Guillemette *et al.* 1998; Savides *et al.* 1986). Photoperiod-responsive changes in human circadian rhythms may be suppressed by regular exposure to artificial room light (Wehr *et al.* 1995), raising the question whether changes in outdoor lighting may have any effect on human circadian rhythms. Despite these concerns, human exposure to bright light varies with the seasons (Hébert *et al.* 1998). Whether it is the length of day, the total count of photons received, or exposure to critical illuminance levels, the photoperiodic environment appears important in the pathogenesis of SAD.

Guillemette and colleagues have shown, using objective measures of light exposure, that both healthy controls and subjects with sub-SAD are exposed to significantly varied amounts of bright light through the different seasons. The total exposure to light brighter than 1000 lux has been estimated at around 2.1 hours during the summer and 0.5 hour during the autumn/winter. In this study, no difference was noted between both groups, a result which suggests that subjective deterioration of mood cannot be explained by a reduction in the overall exposure to light. These results are consistent with those of a prior study conducted in winter (Oren *et al.* 1994) in which light-exposure profiles were comparable between SAD patients and healthy controls.

However, another study using subjective logs of exposure to sunlight (Eastman 1990) revealed that SAD patients exposed themselves to sunlight for about two hours more during summer days than control subjects. These results raise the possibility that seasonally depressed patients may have a greater need for bright light and may have an increased susceptibility to lower illuminance levels during the autumn and winter months. An interesting possibility is that the reduction of bright-light exposure during winter, combined with defective retinal adaptation (Remé *et al.* 1990), could worsen already impaired serotoninergic transmission (Schwartz *et al.* 1999). There is also evidence to support an exaggerated response of the human circadian system to changes in the photoperiod across seasons in SAD patients (Nathan *et al.* 1999). A complex interaction between retinal and environmental mechanisms remains possible and could play a major role in the pathogenesis of SAD.

25.4.3 The melatonin hypothesis

Another circadian hypothesis of SAD involves the photic regulation of melatonin secretion. It has been argued that melatonin is the messenger hormone responsible for transducing the duration of the scotoperiod by adjusting the onset and offset of its secretion in harmony with the subjective night. Recent studies support this view in relation to human subjects (Vondrašová–Jelínková *et al.* 1999; Wehr 1991). Therefore, melatonin was the first biological mechanism hypothesized to underlie the pathogenesis of SAD.

It is unclear, however, why a light treatment administered during the day, when melatonin levels are low or undetectable, could exert any antidepressant effect. Several studies have reported an absence of effect for phototherapy on the concentration of melatonin in the saliva (Partonen *et al.* 1996), and a normal circadian curve for plasma melatonin assayed over 24 hours in SAD patients (Checkley *et al.* 1993). At least one study reported an enhanced melatonin secretion in SAD patients compared to controls, with a reduction of melatonin levels after light therapy or during the summer (Danilenko *et al.* 1994). However, since the sleep schedule was not monitored during this study, it remains unclear whether these results are secondary to differences between groups in the timing of sleep or reflects an enhanced melatonin secretion regulated by the endogenous circadian pacemaker.

In its original formulation, the melatonin hypothesis was associated with the photoperiod hypothesis since it involved an increase in the duration of melatonin secretion associated with a short photoperiod (Rosenthal *et al.* 1986). A negative and direct effect of melatonin on mood and behaviour was also suggested. However, the administration of exogenous melatonin to SAD patients who responded to bright-light treatment did not induce a relapse into depression (Rosenthal *et al.* 1986). Moreover, the pharmacological manipulation of melatonin secretion by atenolol did not affect mood (Rosenthal *et al.* 1988). These results strongly argue against a direct effect of melatonin secretion on depressive symptoms.

Thus, a 'pure' melatonin hypothesis, without any relationship to a photoperiod hypothesis, is highly improbable in the pathogenesis of SAD. However, melatonin could potentially interact with 5-HT stimulation, but controversial findings have been reported on this issue (Childs *et al.* 1995; Partonen *et al.* 1996; Partonen and Lönnqvist 1998).

25.4.4 The reduced-amplitude hypothesis

The possibility that the circadian signal is weakened in SAD and that bright light exerts its antidepressant effect by enhancing circadian amplitude has been proposed (Czeisler *et al.* 1987). However, there is no convincing evidence to support this hypothesis (Checkley *et al.* 1993; Eastman *et al.* 1993; Levendosky *et al.* 1991). Furthermore, anecdotal reports of reduced amplitude in the diurnal curve of various hormones may well be explained by the masking effect of the rest-activity cycle (Glod *et al.* 1997).

25.5 Summary

At this stage, clear and simple connections cannot be drawn between the effects of light in SAD and the mechanisms involved in the photic resetting of the endogenous circadian pacemaker or the melatonin-suppressing effect of light. Despite this, the endogenous circadian system is most probably involved in the pathogenesis of winter depression. Namely, the interactions of the sleep–wake cycle and circadian system with neurotransmitter systems such as dopamine or 5-HT and with neurohormones remain potential avenues for future research.

Acknowledgements

Supported by the Canadian Psychiatric Research Foundation, the National Alliance for Research on Schizophrenia and Depression, the Levinschi Foundation, the Medical Research Council of Canada, and the 'Fonds de la Recherche en Santé du Québec'. The author is grateful to Leanne Ginsberg, Jason Singh, and Marie–Claude Charron for their editorial support.

References

Anderson, J.L., Rosen, L.N., Mendelson, W.B., Jacobsen, F.M., Skwerer, R.G., Joseph–Vanderpool, J.R., et al. (1994) Sleep in fall/winter seasonal affective disorder: effects of light and changing seasons. *Journal of Psychosomatic Research*, **38**:323–37.

Avery, D.H., Dahl, K., Savage, M.V., Brengelmann, G.L., Larsen, L.H., Kenny, M.A., et al. (1997) Circadian temperature and cortisol rhythms during a constant routine are phase-delayed in hypersomnic winter depression. *Biological Psychiatry*, **41**:1109–23.

Boivin, D.B., Duffy, J.F., Kronauer, R.E., and Czeisler, C.A. (1996) Dose-response relationships for resetting of human circadian clock by light. *Nature*, **379**:540–2.

Boivin, D.B., Czeisler, C.A., Dijk, D.J., Duffy, J.F., Folkard, S., Minors, D.S., et al. (1997) Complex interaction of the sleep–wake cycle and circadian phase modulates mood in healthy subjects. *Archives of General Psychiatry*, **54**:145–52.

Boivin, D.B. and Czeisler, C.A. (1998) Resetting of circadian melatonin and cortisol rhythms in humans by ordinary room light. *Neuroreport*, **9**:779–82.

Brainard, G.C., Lewy, A.J., Menaker, M., Fredrickson, R.H., Miller, L.S., Weleber, R.G., et al. (1988) Dose-response relationship between light irradiance and the suppression of plasma melatonin in human volunteers. *Brain Research*, **454**:212–18.

Brunner, D.P., Kräuchi, K., Dijk, D.J., Leonhardt, G., Haug, H.J., and Wirz–Justice, A. (1996) Sleep electroencephalogram in seasonal affective disorder and in control women: effects of midday light treatment and sleep deprivation. *Biological Psychiatry*, **40**:485–6.

Cajochen, C., Brunner, D.P., Kräuchi, K., Graw, P., and Wirz–Justice, A. (2000) EEG and subjective sleepiness during extended wakefulness in seasonal affective disorder: circadian and homeostatic influences. *Biolological Psychiatry*, **47**:610–17.

Checkley, S.A., Murphy, D.G., Abbas, M., Marks, M., Winton, F., Palazidou, E., et al. (1993) Melatonin rhythms in seasonal affective disorder. *British Journal of Psychiatry*, **163**:332–7.

Childs, P.A., Rodin, I., Martin, N.J., Allen, N.H.P., Plaskett, L., Smythe, P.J., et al. (1995) Effect of fluoxetine on melatonin in patients with seasonal affective disorder and matched controls. *British Journal of Psychiatry*, **166**:196–8.

Czeisler, C.A., Kronauer, R.E., Mooney, J.J., Anderson, J.L., and Allan, J.S. (1987) Biologic rhythm disorders, depression, and phototherapy: a new hypothesis. In *The psychiatric clinics of North America. Sleep disorders* (ed. M.K. Erman), pp. 687–709. W.B. Saunders Co., Philadelphia.

Czeisler, C.A., Kronauer, R.E., Allan, J.S., Duffy, J.F., Jewett, M.E., Brown, E.N., et al. (1989) Bright light induction of strong (Type 0) resetting of the human circadian pacemaker. *Science* **244**:1328–33.

Dahl, K., Avery, D.H., Lewy, A.J., Savage, M.V., Brengelmann, G.L., Larsen, L.H., et al. (1993) Dim light melatonin onset and circadian temperature during a constant routine in hypersomnic winter depression. *Acta Psychiatrica Scandinavica*, **88**:60–6.

Danilenko, K.V., Putilov, A.A., Russkikh, G.S., Duffy, L.K., and Ebbesson, S.O.E. (1994) Diurnal and seasonal variations of melatonin and serotonin in women with seasonal affective disorder. *Arctic Medical Research*, **53**:137–45.

Dijk, D.J. and Czeisler, C.A. (1995) Contribution of the circadian pacemaker and the sleep homeostat to sleep propensity, sleep structure, electroencephalographic slow waves, and sleep spindle activity in humans. *Journal of Neuroscience*, **15**:3526–38.

Eastman, C.I. (1990) Natural summer and winter sunlight exposure patterns in seasonal affective disorder. *Physiological Behavior*, **48**:611–16.

Eastman, C.I., Gallo, L.C., Lahmeyer, H.W., and Fogg, L.F. (1993) The circadian rhythm of temperature during light treatment for winter depression. *Biological Psychiatry*, **34**:210–20.

Elliot, J.A. (1994) Type 0 PRC in hamsters: influence of photoperiod and dim nocturnal illumination. *Society for Research on Biological Rhythms Abstracts*, 127.

Gaddy, J.R., Rollag, M.D., Ruberg, F.L., and Brainard, G.C. (1993) Light-induced melatonin suppression and pupil size. *Sleep Research*, **22**:406.

Glod, C.A., Teicher, M.H., Polcari, A., Mcgreenery, C.E., and Ito, Y. (1997) Circadian rest-activity disturbances in children with seasonal affective disorder. *Journal of the American Academy of Child and Adolescent Psychiatry*, **36**:188–95.

Gordijn, M.C., Beersma, D.G.M., Bouhuys, A.L., Reinink, E., and van den Hoofdakker, R.H. (1994) A longitudinal study of diurnal mood variation in depression; characteristics and significance. *Journal of Affective Disorders*, **31**:261–73.

Graw, P., Haug, H.J., Leonhardt, G., and Wirz-Justice, A. (1998) Sleep deprivation response in seasonal affective disorder during a 40-h constant routine. *Journal of Affective Disorder*, **48**:69–74.

Guillemette, J., Hébert, M., Paquet, J., and Dumont, M. (1998) Natural bright light exposure in the summer and winter in subjects with and without complaints of seasonal mood variation. *Biological Psychiatry*, **44**:622–8.

Hébert, M., Dumont, M., and Paquet, J. (1998) Seasonal and diurnal patterns of human illumination under natural conditions. *Chronobiology International*, **15**:59–70.

Honma, K. and Honma, S. (1988) A human phase response curve for bright light pulses. *Japanese Journal of Psychiatry and Neurobiology*, **42(1)**:167–8.

Humlova, M. and Illnerová, H. (1992) Resetting of the rat circadian clock after a shift in the light/dark cycle depends on the photoperiod. *Neuroscience Research*, **13**:147–53.

Hunt, N., Sayer, H., and Silverstone, T. (1992) Season and manic relapse. *Acta Psychiatrica Scandinavica*, **85**:123–6.

Jewett, M.E., Kronauer, R.E., and Czeisler, C.A. (1991) Light-induced suppression of endogenous circadian amplitude in humans. *Nature*, **350**:59–62.

Koorengevel, K.M., Beersma, D.G.M., Gordijn, M.C., Den Boer, J.A., and van den Hoofdakker, R.H. (2000) Body temperature and mood variations during forced desynchronization in winter depression: a preliminary report. *Biological Psychiatry*, **47**:355–8.

Kronauer, R.E., Jewett, M.E., and Czeisler, C.A. (1993) Commentary: the human circadian response to light — strong and weak resetting [comment]. *Journal of Biological Rhythms*, **8**:351–60.

Levendosky, A.A., Joseph–Vanderpool, J.R., Hardin, T., Sorek, E., and Rosenthal, N.E. (1991) Core body temperature in patients with seasonal affective disorder and normal controls in summer and winter. *Biological Psychiatry*, **29**:524–34.

Lewy, A.J., Wehr, T.A., Goodwin, F.K., Newsome, D.A., and Markey, S.P. (1980) Light suppresses melatonin secretion in humans. *Science*, **210**:1267–9.

Lewy, A.J. and Sack, R.L. (1987) Phase typing and bright light therapy of chronobiologic sleep and mood disorders. In *Chronobiology and psychiatric disorders* (ed. A. Halaris), pp. 181–206. Elsevier, New York.

Lewy, A.J., Sack, R.L., Miller, L.S., and Hoban, T.M. (1987) Antidepressant and circadian phase-shifting effects of light. *Science*, **235**:352–4.

Lewy, A.J., Sack, R.L., Singer, C.M., White, D.M., and Hoban, T.M. (1988) Winter depression and the phase-shift hypothesis for bright light's therapeutic effects: history, theory, and experimental evidence. *Journal of Biological Rhythms*, **3**:121–34.

Lewy, A.J., Bauer, V.K., Ahmed, S., Thomas, K.H., Cutler, N.L., Singer, C.M., *et al.* (1998*a*) The human phase response curve (PRC) to melatonin is about 12 hours out of phase with the PRC to light. *Chronobiology International*, **15**:71–83.

Lewy, A.J., Bauer, V.K., Cutler, N.L., Sack, R.L., Ahmed, S., Thomas, K.H., *et al.* (1998*b*) Morning vs evening light treatment of patients with winter depression. *Archives of General Psychiatry*, **55**:890–6.

Madden, P.A., Heath, A.C., Rosenthal, N.E., and Martin, N.G. (1996) Seasonal changes in mood and behavior. The role of genetic factors. *Archives of General Psychiatry*, **53**:47–55.

Maes, M., Meltzer, H.Y., Suy, E., and De Meyer, F. (1993) Seasonality in severity of depression: relationships to suicide and homicide occurrence. *Acta Psychiatrica Scandinavica* **88**:156–61.

Matthews, C.D., Guerin, M.V., and Wang, X. (1991) Human plasma melatonin and urinary 6-sulphatoxy melatonin: studies in natural annual photoperiod and in extended darkness. *Clinical Endocrinology*, **35**:21–7.

Minors, D.S., Waterhouse, J.M., and Wirz–Justice, A. (1991) A human phase-response curve to light. *Neuroscience Letters*, **133**:36–40.

Monk, T.H., Buysse, D.J., Reynolds III, C.F., Jarrett, D.B., and Kupfer, D.J. (1992) Rhythmic vs homeostatic influences on mood, activation, and performance in young and old men. *Journal of Gerontology*, 47:P221–7

Nathan, P.J., Burrows, G.D., and Norman, T.R. (1999) Melatonin sensitivity to dim white light in affective disorders. *Neuropsychopharmacology*, 21:408–13.

Oren, D.A., Moul, D.E., Schwartz, P.J., Brown, C., Yamada, E.M., and Rosenthal, N.E. (1994) Exposure to ambient light in patients with winter seasonal affective disorder. *American Journal of Psychiatry*, 151:591–3.

Palchikov, V.E., Zolotarev, D.Y., Danilenko, K.V., and Putilov, A.A. (1997) Effects of the seasons and of bright light administered at different times of day on sleep EEG and mood in patients with seasonal affective disorder. *Biological Rhythms Research*, 28:166–84.

Parry, B.L., Rosenthal, N.E., Tamarkin, L., and Wehr, T.A. (1987) Treatment of a patient with seasonal premenstrual syndrome. *American Journal of Psychiatry*, 144:762–6.

Partonen, T., Appelberg, B., and Partinen, M. (1993) Effects of light treatment on sleep structure in seasonal affective disorder. *European Archives of Psychiatry and Clinical Neuroscience*, 242:310–13.

Partonen, T., Vakkuri, O., Lamberg–Allardt, C., and Lönnqvist, J. (1996) Effects of bright light on sleepiness, melatonin, and 25-hydroxyvitamin D_3 in winter seasonal affective disorder. *Biological Psychiatry*, 39:865–72.

Partonen, T. and Lönnqvist, J. (1998) Seasonal affective disorder. *Lancet*, 352:1369–74.

Pittendrigh, C.S., Kyner, W.T., and Takamura, T. (1991) The amplitude of circadian oscillations: temperature dependence, latitudinal clines, and the photoperiodic time measurement. *Journal of Biological Rhythms*, 6:299–313 .

Remé, C., Terman, M., and Wirz–Justice, A. (1990) Are deficient retinal photoreceptor renewal mechanisms involved in the pathogenesis of winter depression? *Archives of General Psychiatry*, 47:878–9.

Rosenthal, N.E., Sack, D.A., Gillin, J.C., Lewy, A.J., Goodwin, F.K., Davenport, Y., *et al.* (1984) Seasonal affective disorder: a description of the syndrome and preliminary findings with light therapy. *Archives of General Psychiatry*, 41:72–80.

Rosenthal, N.E., Sack, D.A., Jacobsen, F.M., James, S.P., Parry, B.L., Arendt, J., *et al.* (1986) Melatonin in seasonal affective disorder and phototherapy. *Journal of Neural Transmission*, 21:257–67.

Rosenthal, N.E., Jacobsen, F.M., Sack, D.A., Arendt, J., James, S.P., Parry, B.L. *et al.* (1988) Atenolol in seasonal affective disorder: a test of the melatonin hypothesis. *American Journal of Psychiatry*, 145:52–6.

Savides, T.J., Messin, S., Senger, C., and Kripke, D.F. (1986) Natural light exposure of young adults. *Physiology and Behaviour* 38:571–4.

Schwartz, P.J., Turner, E.H., Garcia–Borreguero, D., Sedway, J., Vetticad, R.G., Wehr, T.A., *et al.* (1999) Serotonin hypothesis of winter depression: behavioral and neuroendocrine effects of the 5-HT1A receptor partial agonist ipsapirone in patients with seasonal affective disorder and healthy control subjects [Review]. *Psychiatry Research*, 86:9–28.

Terman, M., Terman, J.S., and Ross, D.C. (1998) A controlled trial of timed bright light and negative air ionization for treatment of winter depression. *Archives of General Psychiatry*, 55:875–82.

Thompson, C., Childs, P.A., Martin, N.J., Rodin, I., and Smythe, P.J. (1997) Effects of morning phototherapy on circadian markers in seasonal affective disorder. *British Journal of Psychiatry*, 170:431–5.

Vondrašová–Jelínková, D., Hájek, I., and Illnerová, H. (1999) Adjustment of the human melatonin and cortisol rhythms to shortening of the natural summer photoperiod. *Brain Research*, 816:249–53.

Waterhouse, J., Minors, D., Folkard, S., Owens, D., Atkinson, G., MacDonald, I., *et al.* (1998) Light of domestic intensity produces phase shifts of the circadian oscillator in humans. *Neuroscience Letters*, 245:97–100.

Wehr, T.A. (1991) The durations of human melatonin secretion and sleep respond to changes in daylength (photoperiod). *Journal of Clinical Endocrinology and Metabolism*, 73(6):1276–80.

Wehr, T.A., Wirz–Justice, A., Goodwin, F.K., Duncan, W., and Gillin, J.C. (1979) Phase advance of the circadian sleep–wake cycle as an antidepressant. *Science*, 206:710–13.

Wehr, T.A. and Wirz–Justice, A. (1981) Internal coincidence model for sleep deprivation and depression. In *Sleep '1980* (ed. W.P. Koella) pp. 26–33. Karger, Basel.

Wehr, T.A., Jacobsen, F.M., Sack, D.A., Arendt, J., Tamarkin, L., and Rosenthal, N.E. (1986) Phototherapy of seasonal affective disorder: time of day and suppression of melatonin are not critical for antidepressant effects. *Archives of General Psychiatry*, 43:870–5.

Wehr, T.A., Moul, D.E., Barbato, G., Giesen, H.A., Seidel, J.A., Barker, C., *et al.* (1993) Conservation of photoperiod-responsive mechanisms in humans. *American Journal of Physiology*, **265**:R846–57.

Wehr, T.A., Giesen, H.A., Moul, D.E., Turner, E.H., and Schwartz, P.J. (1995) Supression of men's responses to seasonal changes in day length by modern artificial lighting. *American Journal of Physiology*, **269**:R173–8.

Wirz–Justice, A., Graw, P., Kräuchi, K., Gisin, B., Arendt, J., Aldhous, M., *et al.* (1990) Morning or night-time melatonin is ineffective in seasonal affective disorder. *Journal of Psychiatry Research*, **24**:129–37.

Wirz–Justice, A., Graw, P., Kräuchi, K., Gisin, B., Jochum, A., Arendt, J., *et al.* (1993) Light therapy in seasonal affective disorder is independent of time of day or circadian phase. *Archives of General Psychiatry*, **50**:929–37.

Wu, J.C. and Bunney, W.E. (1990) The biological basis of an antidepressant response to sleep deprivation and relapse: review and hypothesis. *American Journal of Psychiatry* **147**:14–21.

Chapter 26

Genetic influences

Mary–Anne Enoch and David Goldman

26.1 Introduction

Winter SAD is characterized by the recurrent onset of major depression (MD) in the autumn or winter with remission in the spring/summer (Rosenthal *et al*. 1984). According to DSM-IV criteria, SAD is a subcategory of depression: the modifier 'with seasonal pattern' can be applied to recurrent MD disorder or MD episodes in bipolar I or II disorders (American Psychiatric Association 1994). There are six cardinal features of SAD: depressed mood, lack of energy, hypersomnia, craving for carbohydrates, overeating, and weight gain. Therefore SAD is one of the spectrum of disorders involving anxiety/ dysphoria but differs in showing a pattern of seasonal change (seasonality). Patients with SAD may also differ from those with non-seasonal depression by experiencing more hypersomnia, hyperphagia, and weight gain but less suicidal ideation and morning worsening of mood (Allen *et al*. 1993).

SAD may be induced in vulnerable individuals by diminished winter daylight (Rosenthal *et al*. 1984). With a lifetime prevalence of approximately 1 per cent (Partonen and Lönnqvist 1998), SAD may represent the pathological extreme of a spectrum of seasonal changes in mood and behaviour which have been estimated to occur in 27 per cent of normal individuals (Kasper *et al*. 1989). Is there any evidence for a genetic predisposition to SAD? If so, is SAD inherited as a distinct entity, or is there overlap between genes for seasonality and vulnerability to mood disorders, or are seasonality and depression inherited as separate traits? The aim of this chapter is to examine the evidence for a genetic component to SAD, seasonality, and depression, and also to evaluate the heritability of personality traits (for example, neuroticism) and other diagnoses (for example, bulimia nervosa (BN)) that are comorbid with SAD and which may therefore have shared genes. As SAD is a complex, spectrum disorder, many genes are probably involved and some of the important genetic variants could be commonly occurring but of only modest to moderate effect.

26.2 Familiality

Familiality of SAD

Several family studies which relied on family history data reported by SAD probands have found increased rates of mood disorders and alcoholism in first-degree relatives (Wirz–Justice *et al*. 1986; Rosenthal and Wehr 1987; Thompson and Isaacs 1988; Lam *et al*. 1989; White *et al*. 1990). The rates of seasonal depression in first-degree relatives of SAD patients is estimated as 13–17 per cent (Wirz–Justice *et al.* 1986; Rosenthal and Wehr 1987; Lam *et al.* 1989) compared to 1 per cent in the general population (Partonen and Lönnqvist 1998). In a more rigorously conducted family study of 68 patients, half with SAD and half with non-seasonal mood disorders, in which both proband and additional family informants provided family history, it was found that relatives of SAD probands had the same risk for other psychiatric disorders, except for increased alcoholism, as relatives of probands with non-seasonal depression (Allen *et al.* 1993). However, the authors did not include seasonal pattern in their study and therefore could not determine whether SAD was more common than MD in relatives of probands with SAD.

Familiality of MD

In the National Comorbidity Survey of 5877 respondents it was found that MD aggregated significantly in families: MD was twice as common in parents of probands with MD than in parents of those without MD, with an odds ratio of 2.74 (Kendler *et al.* 1997) — a similar odds ratio to that in other major family studies (Tsuang *et al.* 1980; Weissman *et al.* 1984; Gershon *et al.* 1982).

26.3 Heritability

Heritability of SAD

To date, there are no published studies on the heritability of SAD. However, twin studies provide extensive evidence for the heritability of MD and some evidence for the heritability of seasonality. In most studies of MD, a seasonal pattern specifier was not applied. Moreover, because of the relative abundance of non-seasonal depression compared with SAD, any study on MD will largely be of non-seasonal depression.

Heritability of seasonality

A univariate and multivariate analysis of 4639 twins from a community Australian twin registry found that genetic effects of seasonality, as assessed by the global seasonality score (GSS) (Rosenthal *et al.* 1987), account for at least 29 per cent of the variance in seasonality in men and women (Madden *et al.* 1996). However, in a study of 339 pairs of Canadian twins from higher latitudes, the heritability of the GSS was found to be 69 per cent in males and 45 per cent in females (Jang *et al.* 1997a). Changes in individual symptoms (except weight gain) were accounted for primarily by additive genetic effects in both sexes, and sex by genotype analyses suggested that genetic factors may be gender specific. These genetic differences may contribute to gender differences in the presentation of this disorder: SAD is more common, and seasonality tends to be more severe, in women (Kasper *et al.* 1989; Rosen and Rosenthal 1991), but men are usually more severely depressed (Blazer *et al.* 1998).

Heritability of MD

An Australian community study of 2662 pairs of twins found that the heritability of MD was 36–44 per cent in women and only 24 per cent in men (Bierut *et al.* 1999). In a study of 3790 US male and female pairs of twins from the population-based Virginia Twin Registry, MD was equally heritable in men and women (39 per cent) (Kendler and Prescott 1999). Although genetic factors may account for approximately the same proportion of the liability to MD in both sexes, the reduced correlation between opposite sex DZ pairs of twins indicates that some of the genes act differently in men and women (Kendler and Prescott 1999).

26.4 Comorbidity

Personality dimensions and seasonality

There appears to be a robust relationship between seasonality and personality traits, particularly neuroticism, and this relationship is replicable across clinical and general populations in both hemispheres, and using different instruments (Murray *et al.* 1995; Jang *et al.* 1997b). In a Canadian study of 297 pairs of twins from the general population, it was found that there were moderate genetic correlations (0.52 ranging down to 0.37) between seasonality and either neuroticism, cognitive dysregulation, affective lability, stimulus seeking, or anxiousness (Jang *et al.* 1998). A significant proportion of the genetic influences on seasonality and neuroticism are the same (0.27) (Jang *et al.* 1998). However, the impact of personality on seasonality may be more modest, accounting for perhaps 15 per cent of the total variance (Jang *et al.* 1997b).

Personality dimensions and depression

Family and twin studies have demonstrated that elevated neuroticism may be a vulnerability marker for MD (Kendler *et al.* 1993; Duggan *et al.* 1995). In a longitudinal study of 1733 female pairs of twins from the Virginia Twin Registry, it was estimated that 0.70 of the observed correlation between neuroticism and the liability to MD was due to shared genetic risk factors and approximately 0.55 of the genetic liability of MD appeared to be the same as of neuroticism (Kendler *et al.* 1993).

BN and SAD

There are several similarities between SAD and BN: female preponderance, carbohydrate craving, overeating, seasonal variation in symptoms, and increased rates of alcoholism in first-degree relatives. This overlap in clinical phenomenology raises the possibility that there may be genes in common.

BN and seasonality

Patients with BN have higher GSS scores and higher rates of SAD than controls (Brewerton *et al.* 1994). BN patients with high seasonality may represent a distinct subgroup with an earlier onset and more severe, unique course of illness compared to non-seasonal BN patients (Levitan *et al.* 1996). Patients with SAD not only have appetite and weight disturbances but also dysfunctional eating attitudes: SAD patients have higher scores on the Eating Disorders Inventory than controls (Berman *et al.* 1993).

BN and depression

An analysis of the co-occurrence of BN and MD in 1033 female pairs of twins from the Virginia Twin Registry found that additive genes accounted for a substantial proportion of variance of MD (43 per cent) and BN (50 per cent) (Walters *et al.* 1992). The genetic correlation of 0.46 between BN and MD suggests the presence of common genes (Walters *et al.* 1992). However, in a further analysis of MD, BN, and anxiety disorders, it was determined that genetic influences could be best explained by two factors loading on: (1) BN, phobia, and panic and (2) MD and generalized anxiety disorder (Kendler *et al.* 1995).

26.5 **Identifying the genetic origins of SAD**

Genetic analysis of complex diseases such as mood disorders is complicated by the fact that environmental as well as genetic factors are involved, and the impact of variation at any single gene is likely to be small. To detect subtle genetic effects large samples are needed. The four methods(Lander and Schork 1994) most widely used are:

1. linkage analysis: the inheritance pattern of phenotypes and genotypes are elucidated in pedigrees;

2. allele sharing methods: affected relatives are compared to detect excess genotype sharing;

3. association (case-control) studies: unrelated affected and unaffected individuals are compared;

4. analysis of inbred, transgenic, and gene-knockout animals (principally mice and rats).

Linkage analysis has been successfully employed in finding major genes (for example, in Huntington's Disease), but it has limited power to detect genes of modest effect (Risch and Merikangas 1996). Candidate gene association studies, including new approaches such as TDT (Transmission Disequilibrium Test) analysis (Ewens and Spielman 1995) and ethnic matching using markers (Pritchard and Rosenberg 1999), have far greater power for finding individual genes for complex diseases than linkage analysis (Risch and Merikangas 1996), and can avoid the problem of population stratification of cases and controls.

26.6 **Candidate gene analysis in SAD**

Several lines of evidence, reviewed in Chapter 21, suggest that serotonin dysfunction is of fundamental importance in the pathogenesis of SAD. Acute dietary depletion of tryptophan, the precursor of serotonin, has been found to reverse the beneficial effects of bright-light therapy in SAD patients (Neumeister *et al.* 1997), to precipitate temporary mood lowering or depression in healthy individuals at genetic risk for MD (Benkelfat *et al.* 1994), and to increase caloric intake and mood irritability in BN(Weltzin *et al.* 1995) whilst having no impact on controls.

Pharmacological responses in SAD patients also suggest possible dysfunction in serotonergic transmission: selective serotonin re-uptake inhibitors relieve the depressive symptoms of SAD patients (Lee *et al.* 1997; Lam *et al.* 1995) and meta-chlorophenylpiperazine (m-CPP), an agonist for several serotonin receptors (mainly 5-HT2C but also 5-HT2A and others), increases energy and euphoria in symptomatic SAD patients (Schwartz *et al.* 1997). These findings suggest that serotonin dysfunction in SAD may occur at or downstream of central serotonergic receptors.

An important starting point for understanding the vulnerability to SAD and seasonality may therefore be to evaluate the role of variation in the many genes involved in serotonin transmission, in particular those coding for receptors and the serotonin transporter (5-HTT). The most likely receptors are 5-HT1A, 5-HT2A, and 5-HT2C which appear to modulate mood, anxiety, and temperature. However, the 5-HT1A receptor seems to function normally in SAD (Schwartz *et al.* 1999).

There are few published studies of SAD patients who have been genotyped for serotonergic variants. Two studies implicate genetic variation in the 5-HTT and the 5-HT2A receptor in SAD. However, these case-control results should be viewed with caution until they are replicated. The shorter 's' allele of the 5-HTTLPR serotonin transporter promoter polymorphism drives transcription of the gene at a reduced rate, leading to diminished 5-HTT in human brain. This polymorphism has been associated with anxiety-related traits, particularly neuroticism and depression (Collier *et al.* 1996; Lesch *et al.* 1996; Mazzanti *et al.* 1998). The 's' allele has also been found to be more abundant in patients with SAD and to be associated with higher seasonality scores (Rosenthal *et al.* 1998). Hence the 's' allele may contribute to seasonality and to the risk of SAD. This proposition is supported by the recent finding that, as in patients with non-seasonal depression, symptomatic SAD patients have reduced 5-HTT availability in the thalamus/hypothalamus (Willeit *et al.* 2000).

A polymorphism, $-1438G/A$, in the promoter region of the gene for the 5-HT2A receptor has been associated with MD (Zhang *et al.* 1997), anorexia nervosa (Collier *et al.* 1997; Enoch *et al.* 1998), and obsessive–compulsive disorder (Enoch *et al.* 2001), but not with BN (Enoch 1998 *et al.*; Nacmias *et al.* 1999). Recently, this polymorphism was found to be more abundant in patients with SAD compared to controls (Enoch *et al.* 1999). However, there was no association with seasonality scores and there was no additive effect with 5-HTTLPR (Enoch *et al.* 1999). This fact, and the earlier finding of an association with MD but lack of association with BN (in which seasonality scores are also high), suggests that the 5-HT2A polymorphism may be associated with the dysphoria/anxiety element of SAD.

The few other studies on SAD and 5-HT genetic variation have been negative. In particular, no difference was found in SAD patients for two 5-HT2A amino-acid substitutions (Ala_{447}-Val_{447} and His_{452}-Tyr_{452}) (Ozaki *et al.* 1996) as well as for polymorphisms in tryptophan hydroxylase, the rate-limiting enzyme for serotonin synthesis (Han *et al.* 1999).

Although it is most likely that serotonergic dysfunction is of major importance in SAD, other neurotransmitter systems (catecholaminergic and dopaminergic) have been investigated. Catecholamine depletion, just like tryptophan depletion, has been shown to induce depressive symptoms in SAD patients, reversing the beneficial effects of light therapy (Neumeister *et al.* 1998). However, dopaminergic deficiency has not been shown to explain the pathology of SAD (Oren *et al.* 1994). A recent large study has shown that neither a functional polymorphism of catechol-O-methyltransferase (an enzyme involved in the metabolism of dopamine, noradrenaline, and adrenaline) nor dopamine DRD3 receptor polymorphisms are associated with neuroticism or depression (Henderson *et al.* 2000).

26.7 **Discussion**

Heritability studies provide substantial evidence for a genetic component in SAD. However, it is unclear whether SAD is inherited as a distinct entity from other conditions involving anxiety/dysphoria. In individuals from the community, heritability of seasonality and MD is moderate: approximately 30–45 per cent in both men and women. Although the quantitative role of genetic risk factors is approximately equal in both sexes, there is evidence, based on lower concordance of opposite sex pairs, for gender-specific action of genes. Predisposition to neuroticism may contribute to seasonality, with which 27 per cent of the genetic influences are shared, and to MD, with which 55 per cent of the genetic liability is shared. The lower transcribing 's' allele of the 5-HTTLPR transporter promoter polymorphism could explain a portion of the shared variance between neuroticism, seasonality, and MD since it has been associated with all three. Patients with SAD and BN have some symptoms in common, and the high seasonality scores in BN and lack of much genetic overlap between BN and MD suggest that SAD and BN may share some of the genes for seasonality.

The task of untangling the complexities of the genetic influences on SAD has only just begun. Large family datasets, including combinations of affected/unaffected sibling pairs and parent–child trios, need to be collected to do both TDT candidate gene association studies (particularly for the serotonin receptors) and also linkage analysis (to detect further candidate genes). Such efforts could delineate clinical subtypes and lead to the application of different and more specific treatment measures.

References

Allen, J.M., Lam, R.W., Remick, R.A., and Sadovnick, A.D. (1993) Depressive symptoms and family history in seasonal and nonseasonal mood disorders. *Am J Psychiatry* **150**(3):443–8.

American Psychiatric Association (1994) *Diagnostic and statistical manual of mental disorders* (4th edn). American Psychiatric Association, Washington DC.

Benkelfat, C., Ellenbogen, M.A., Dean, P., Palmour, R.M., and Young, S.N. (1994) Mood-lowering effect of tryptophan depletion. *Arch Gen Psychiatry* **51**:687–97.

Berman, K., Lam, R.W., and Goldner, E.M. (1993) Eating attitudes in seasonal affective disorder and bulimia nervosa. *J Affective Disord* **29**:219–25.

Bierut, L.J., Heath, A.C., Bucholz, K.K., Dinwiddie, S.H., Madden, P.A.F., Statham, D.J., *et al.* (1999) Major depressive disorder in a community-based twin sample. *Arch Gen Psychiatry* **56**:557–63.

Blazer, D.G., Kessler, R.C., and Swartz, M.S. (1998) Epidemiology of recurrent major and minor depression with a seasonal pattern: the National Comorbidity Survey. *Br J Psychiatry* **172**:164–7.

Brewerton, T.D., Krahn, D.D., Hardin, T.A., Wehr, T.A., and Rosenthal, N.E. (1994) Findings from the Seasonal Pattern Assessment Questionnaire in patients with eating disorders and control subjects: effects of diagnosis and location. *Psychiatry Res* **52**(1):71–84.

Collier, D.A., Stober, G., Li, T., Heils, A., Catalano, M., Bella, D. Di, *et al.* (1996) A novel functional polymorphism within the promoter of the serotonin transporter gene: a possible role in susceptibility to affective disorders. *Mol Psychiatry* **1**:453–60.

Collier, D.A., Arranz, M.J., Li, T., Mupita, D., Brown, N., and Treasure, J. (1997) Association between 5-HT2A gene promoter polymorphism and anorexia nervosa. *Lancet* **350**:412.

Duggan, C., Sham, P., Lee, A., Minne, C., and Murray, R. (1995) Neuroticism: a vulnerability marker for depression. Evidence from a family study. *J Affective Disord* **35**(3):139–43.

Enoch, M-A., Kaye, W., Rotondo, A., Greenberg, B., Murphy, D., and Goldman, D. (1998) 5-HT2A promoter polymorphism –1438G/A, anorexia nervosa, and obsessive–compulsive disorder. *Lancet* **351**:1785–6.

Enoch, M-A., Goldman, D., Barnett, R., Sher, L., Mazzanti, C.M., and Rosenthal, N.E. (1999) Association between seasonal affective disorder and the 5-HT2A promoter polymorphism, –1438G/A. *Mol Psychiatry* **4**:89–92.

Enoch, M-A., Greenberg, B.D., Murphy, D.L., and Goldman, D. (2001) Sexually dimorphic relationship of a 5-HT2A promoter polymorphism with obsessive–compulsive disorder.Biol Psychiatry **49**(4):385-8.

Ewens, W.J. and Spielman, R.S. (1995) The transmission/disequilibrium test: history, subdivision, and admixture. *Am J Hum Genet* **57**:455–64.

Gershon, E.S., Hamovit, J., Guroff, J.J., Dibble, E., Leckman, J.F., Sceery, W., *et al.* (1982) A family study of schizoaffective, bipolar I, bipolar II, unipolar and normal control probands. *Arch Gen Psychiatry* **39**:1157–67.

Han, L., Nielsen, D.A., Rosenthal, N.E., Jefferson, K., Kaye, W., Murphy, D., *et al.* (1999) No coding variant of the tryptophan hydroxylase gene detected in seasonal affective disorder, obsessive–compulsive disorder, anorexia nervosa, and alcoholism. *Biol Psychiatry* **45**(5):615–19.

Henderson, A.S., Korten, A.E., Jorm, A.F., Jacomb, P.A., Christensen, H., Rodgers, B., *et al.* (2000) COMT and DRD3 polymorphisms, environmental exposures, and personality traits related to common mental disorders. *Am J Med Genet* **96**(1):102–7.

Jang, K.L., Lam, R.W., Livesley, W.J., and Vernon, P.A. (1997a) Gender differences in the heritability of seasonal mood change. *Psychiatry Res* **70**:145–54.

Jang, K.L., Lam, R.W., Livesley, W.J., and Vernon, P.A. (1997b) The relationship between seasonal mood change and personality: more apparent than real? *Acta Psychiatr Scand* **95**:539–43.

Jang, K.L., Lam, R.W., Harris, J.A., Vernon, P.A., and Livesley, W.J. (1998) Seasonal mood change and personality: an investigation of genetic co-morbidity. *Psychiatry Res* **78**:1–7.

Kasper, S., Wehr, T.A., Bartko, J.J., Gaist, P.A., and Rosenthal, N.E. (1989) Epidemiological findings of seasonal changes in mood and behavior. *Arch Gen Psychiatry* **46**:823–33.

Kendler, K.S., Neale, M.C., Kessler, R.C., Heath, A.C., and Eaves, L.J. (1993) A longitudinal twin study of personality and major depression in women. *Arch Gen Psychiatry* **50(11)**:853–62.

Kendler, K.S., Walters, E.E., Neale, M.C., Kessler, R.C., Heath, A.C., and Eaves, L.J. (1995) The structure of the genetic and environmental risk factors for six major psychiatric disorders in women. *Arch Gen Psychiatry* **52**:374–83.

Kendler, K.S., Davis, C.G., and Kessler, R.C. (1997) The familial aggregation of common psychiatric and substance use disorders in the National Comorbidity Survey: a family history study. *Br J Psychiatry* **170**:541–8.

Kendler, K.S. and Prescott, C.A. (1999) A population-based twin study of lifetime major depression in men and women. *Arch Gen Psychiatry* **56**:39–44.

Lam, R.W., Buchanan, A., and Remick, R.A. (1989) Seasonal affective disorder — a Canadian sample. *Annals Clin Psychiatry* **1**:241–5.

Lam, R.W., Gorman, C.P., Michalon, M., Steiner, M., Levitt, A.J., Corral, M.R., *et al.* (1995) Multicenter, placebo-controlled study of fluoxetine in seasonal affective disorder. *Am J Psychiatry* **152**:1765–70.

Lander, E.S. and Schork, N.J. (1994) Genetic dissection of complex traits. *Science* **265**:2037–48.

Lee, T.M., Blashko, C.A., Janzen, H.L., Paterson, J.G., and Chan, C.C. (1997) Pathophysiological mechanism of seasonal affective disorder. *J Affective Disord* **46(1)**:25–38.

Lesch, K.P., Bengel, D., Heils, A., Sabol, S.Z., Greenberg, B.D., Petri, S., *et al.* (1996) Association of anxiety-related traits with a polymorphism in the serotonin transporter gene regulatory region. *Science* **274**:1527–31.

Levitan, R.D., Kaplan, A.S., and Rockert, W. (1996) Characterization of the 'seasonal' bulimic patient. *Int J Eat Disord* **19(2)**:187–92.

Madden, P.A.F., Heath, A.C., Rosenthal, N.E., and Martin, N.G. (1996) Seasonal changes in mood and behavior, the role of genetic factors. *Arch Gen Psychiatry* **53**:47–55.

Mazzanti, C.M., Lappalainen, J., Long, J.C., Bengel, D., Naukkarinen, H., Eggert, M., *et al.* (1998) Role of the serotonin transporter promoter polymorphism in anxiety-related traits. *Arch Gen Psychiatry* **55**:936–40.

Murray, G.W., Hay, D.W., and Armstrong, S.M. (1995) Personality factors in seasonal affective disorder: is seasonality an aspect of neuroticism? *Person Individ Diff* **19**:613–18.

Nacmias, B., Ricca, V., Tedde, A., Mezzani, B., Rotella, C.M., and Sorbi, S. (1999) 5-HT2A receptor gene polymorphisms in anorexia nervosa and bulimia nervosa. *Neurosci Lett* **277(2)**:134–6.

Neumeister, A., Praschak–Rieder, N., Heßelmann, B., Rao, M-L., Gluck, J., and Kasper, S. (1997) Effects of tryptophan depletion on drug-free patients with seasonal affective disorder during a stable response to bright light therapy. *Arch Gen Psychiatry* **54**:133–8.

Neumeister, A., Turner, E.H., Matthews, J.R., Postolache, T.T., Barnett, R.L., Rauh, M., *et al.* (1998) Effects of tryptophan depletion vs catecholamine depletion in patients with seasonal affective disorder in remission with light therapy. *Arch Gen Psychiatry* **55(6)**:524–30.

Oren, D.A., Moul, D.E., Schwartz, P.J., Wehr, T.A., and Rosenthal, N.E. (1994) A controlled trial of levodopa plus carbidopa in the treatment of winter seasonal affective disorder: a test of the dopamine hypothesis. *J Clin Psychopharmacol* **14(3)**:196–200.

Ozaki, N., Rosenthal, N.E., Pesonen, U., Lappalainen, J., Feldman–Naim, S., Schwartz, P.J., *et al.* (1996) Two naturally occurring amino acid substitutions of the 5-HT2A receptor: similar prevalence in patients with seasonal affective disorder and controls. *Biol Psychiatry* **40**:1267–72.

Partonen, T. and Lönnqvist, J. (1998) Seasonal affective disorder. *Lancet* **352(9137)**:1369–74.

Pritchard, J.K. and Rosenberg, N.A. (1999) Use of unlinked genetic markers to detect population stratification in association studies. *Am J Hum Genet* **65**:220–8.

Risch, N. and Merikangas, K. (1996) The future of genetic studies of complex human diseases. *Science* **273**:1516–17.

Rosen, L.N. and Rosenthal, N.E. (1991) Seasonal variations in mood and behavior in the general population: a factor analytic approach. *Psychiatry Res* **38**(3):271–83.

Rosenthal, N.E., Sack, D.A., Gillin, C., Lewy, A.J., Goodwin, F.K., Davenport, Y., *et al.* (1984) Seasonal affective disorder: a description of the syndrome and preliminary findings with light therapy. *Arch Gen Psychiatry* **41**:72–80.

Rosenthal, N.E. and Wehr, T.A. (1987) Seasonal affective disorders. *Psychiatr Annals* **17**:670–4.

Rosenthal, N.E., Brandt, G.H., and Wehr, T.A. (1987) *Seasonal Pattern Assessment Questionnaire.* National Institute of Mental Health, Bethesda, MD.

Rosenthal, N.E., Mazzanti, C.M., Barnett, R.L., Hardin, T.A., Turner, E.H., Lam, G.K., *et al.* (1998) Role of serotonin transporter promoter repeat length polymorphism (5-HTTLPR) in seasonality and seasonal affective disorder. *Mol Psychiatry* **3**:175–7.

Schwartz, P.J., Murphy, D.L., Wehr, T.A., Garcia–Borreguero, D., Oren, D.A., Moul, D.E., *et al.* (1997) Effects of meta-chlorophenylpiperazine infusions in patients with seasonal affective disorder and healthy control subjects. *Arch Gen Psychiatry* **54**:375–85.

Schwartz, P.J., Turner, E.H., Garcia–Borreguero, D., Sedway, J., Vetticad, R.G., Wehr, T.A., *et al.* (1999) Serotonin hypothesis of winter depression: behavioral and neuroendocrine effects of the 5-HT(1A) receptor partial agonist ipsapirone in patients with seasonal affective disorder and healthy control subjects. *Psychiatry Res* **86**(1):9–28.

Thompson, C. and Isaacs, G. (1988) Seasonal affective disorder — a British sample. *J Affective Disord* **14**:1–11.

Tsuang, M.T., Winokur, G., and Crowe, R.R. (1980) Morbidity risks of schizophrenia and affective disorders among first degree relatives of patients with schizophrenia, mania, depression and surgical conditions. *Br J Psychiatry* **137**:497–504.

Walters, E.E., Neale, M.C. , Eaves, L.J., Heath, A.C., Kessler, R.C., and Kendler, K.S. (1992) Bulimia nervosa and major depression: a study of common genetic and environmental factors. *Psychol Med* **22**(3):617–22.

Weissman, M.M., Gershon, E.S., Kidd, K.K., Prusoff, B.A., Leckman, J.F., Dibble, E., *et al.* (1984) Psychiatric disorders in the relatives of probands with affective disorders: the Yale University National Institute of Mental Health Collaborative Study. *Arch Gen Psychiatry* **41**:13–21.

Weltzin, T.E., Fernstrom, M.H., Fernstrom, J.D., Neuberger, S.K., and Kaye, W.H. (1995) Acute tryptophan depletion and increased food intake and irritability in bulimia nervosa. *Am J Psychiatry* **152**(11):1668–71.

White, D.M., Lewy, A.J., Sack, R.L., Blood, M.L., and Wesche, D.L. (1990) Is winter depression a bipolar disorder? *Compr Psychiatry* **31**:196–204.

Willeit, M., Praschak–Rieder, N., Neumeister, A., Pirker, W., Asenbaum, S., Vitouch, O., *et al.* (2000) [123I]-beta-CIT SPECT imaging shows reduced brain serotonin transporter availability in drug-free depressed patients with seasonal affective disorder. *Biol Psychiatry* **47**(6):482–9.

Wirz–Justice, A., Bucheli, C., Graw, P., Kielholz, P., Fisch, H.-U., and Woggon, B. (1986) Light treatment of seasonal affective disorder in Switzerland. *Acta Psychiatr Scand* **16**:733–7.

Zhang, H.Y., Ishigaki, T., Tani, K., Chen, K., Shih, J.C., Miyasato, K., *et al.* (1997) Serotonin2A receptor gene polymorphism in mood disorders. *Biol Psychiatry* **41**:768–73.

Perspectives

Chapter 27

Biological clock

Scott S. Campbell and Patricia J. Murphy

27.1 Introduction

The geophysical world provides a natural rhythmic structure to which humans and other animals need to adapt and respond. As a result, virtually all organisms have developed an internal timing system capable of not only reacting to the predictable nature of rhythmic environmental stimuli but also of anticipating these stimuli with a program of appropriately timed metabolic, physiologic, and behavioural events. The pervasive nature of such rhythmicity in physiology and behaviour suggests that this circadian (circa = about, dies = day) (Halberg 1959) temporal organization is vital to the overall well-being of the organism.

Among the numerous systems and functions mediated by the circadian timing system are hormonal output, body core temperature, rest and activity, sleep and wakefulness, and motor and cognitive performance. In all, literally hundreds of circadian rhythms in mammalian species have been identified (see for example, Aschoff and Wever 1981; Conroy and Mills 1970), and Aschoff (1965) has noted that 'there is apparently no organ and no function in the body which does not exhibit a similar daily rhythmicity'.

The physiological system governing the generation of these rhythms is an assemblage of neural structures, mediated by neurochemicals, which may be collectively called the biological clock. In this chapter we will examine how the human biological clock is influenced by light and melatonin, the two most widely-used and well-established chronobiotics. To provide a background for such an examination, we will begin this chapter with a brief description of some of the methodology and terms frequently employed in human chronobiological research, followed by a short historical perspective concerning the discovery of, and research into the human biological clock.

27.1.1 Measurement and terminology

A fundamental aspect of understanding the human biological timing system is becoming familiar with terms and measurement techniques used by investigators in the field of biological rhythms research. Figure 27.1 illustrates several of the most frequently used terms, as they apply to one of the most commonly measured circadian variables, body core temperature. Why body core temperature? As can be seen from Fig. 27.1, body temperature is characterized by a robust 24-hour variation. In addition, this is a variables for which it is relatively easy to obtain continuous, sensitive measurement across the 24-hour day. As such, the 24-hour variation in body temperature is considered by most researchers to reflect accurately the timing of the underlying biological clock.

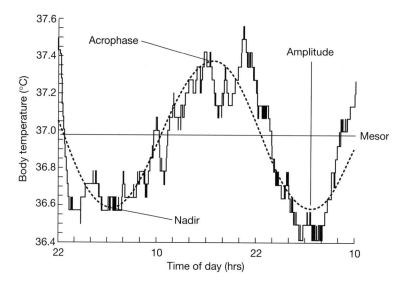

Fig. 27.1 Thirty-six-hour plot of body core temperature, showing smoothed cosine fit and parameters typically employed to describe salient features of the circadian oscillation. Nadir and acrophase are defined as the minimum and maximum points, respectively, of the fitted curve; mesor is the average value of the fitted curve; amplitude is defined as the value from peak to trough (or sometimes, peak to mesor) of the fitted curve.

Typically, the raw temperature curve obtained across a 24-hour (or longer) period is smoothed using some form of mathematical curve-fitting procedure. By convention, most investigators have used variations of least-squares cosine fitting technique (see for example, Brown and Czeisler 1992; Nelson *et al.* 1979) to obtain three measures that describe basic features of the circadian rhythms:

1. the *mesor*, or average value of the fitted curve;
2. the *amplitude*, defined as the value from peak to trough of the fitted curve;
3. the *nadir*, defined as the point on the fitted curve at which the minimum value occurs.

Instead of the nadir, some authors choose to report the *acrophase*, which is defined as the point on the fitted curve at which the maximum value occurs. When a simple cosine fit is employed, the nadir and the acrophase are, by definition, 12 hours apart.

The nadir is frequently used to designate the *phase* of the circadian rhythm under investigation, although any point in the variable's daily oscillation can be employed for this purpose. The phase of a rhythm describes its occurrence as a function of time, and designation of phase permits one to objectively describe temporal relationships, that is *phase relationships*, between two or more rhythmic processes, or between a circadian rhythm and the 24-hour day. Thus, a circadian rhythm is said to be *phase-advanced* when the nadir occurs at an earlier time, relative to a reference point, and is said to be *phase-delayed* when the nadir occurs at a later time. As we will see later, this is an important concept in biological rhythms research, since the phase of a rhythm, and its temporal relationship to other variables, can be altered by various stimuli and such manipulations often have a significant impact on physiology and behaviour.

More recently, an alternative marker of circadian phase has been employed by a growing number of research laboratories — the so-called dim light melatonin onset (DLMO) (see Lewy and Sack 1989). The production of melatonin by the pineal gland is rhythmic and is entrained by the light-dark cycle, and the daily onset of melatonin production is a relatively stable and clearly demarcated event. Thus, melatonin concentrations in blood or saliva, collected in dim, ambient light, at frequent intervals around the expected time of melatonin onset (typically between about 6.00 p.m. and midnight), can be measured, and circadian phase determined.

Phase position is typically defined as the point (time) at which melatonin concentrations exceed an absolute or relative threshold. DLMO has been considered by some investigators as providing a more reliable phase marker than body temperature, because it was thought to be relatively impervious to masking by environmental and behavioural factors, other than light. However, more recent evidence suggests that both body temperature and melatonin onset provide essentially the same accuracy and reliability as markers of the biological clock, both within a given individual across days and across a population, and both markers are considered to be valid reflections of the 'hands of the biological clock'.

In addition to the terms just discussed, a couple of additional ones that are employed primarily in studies utilizing the time-free environment (see following text) should be mentioned. Under these very special experimental conditions, in which subjects spend days, weeks, or even months in an apartment, with no cues to time of day, and only limited social contact, their subjective day-length is dictated by the biological clock. Under these conditions, subjects are said to free-run or to exhibit free-running rhythms. The frequency of the free-running rhythm (that is, the interval between successive temperature nadirs or some other circadian marker) is referred to as the free-running period or tau (τ).

27.1.2 Discovery of circadian principles

Because of their close link to the solar day, it was long believed that circadian rhythms were actually the product of such environmental cues. The proof that biological rhythms are regulated, instead, by factors inherent to the organism, could be derived only from studies of organisms living in the absence of external factors which may provide cues to time of day. The first published study to utilize such a methodology reported on the daily leaf movements in a plant, *Mimosa pudica* (de Mairan 1729; cited by Bünning 1960). Though the plant was kept in total darkness, its leaves continued to exhibit closure and unfolding at times roughly corresponding to dusk and dawn.

The further discovery, a century later, that such leaf movements showed a periodicity close to, but distinctly different from, the natural 24-hour cycle of light and darkness (de Candolle 1832; cited by Touitou and Haus 1992) provided perhaps the clearest indication that such rhythms were driven by endogenous mechanisms, rather than being the product of environmental stimuli. In the following decades, thousands of investigations established the existence of similar 'free-running' rhythms in species ranging from single-celled organisms to a wide variety of laboratory species. However, another 130 years would pass before the first attempts were made to study temporal components of human physiology and behaviour under analogous experimental conditions.

27.1.3 Human circadian rhythms

In the early 1960s, Aschoff and co-workers initiated a series of studies which, over the next 20 years, would lay the groundwork for much of what is known today about the human circadian system (for a comprehensive summary of much of this work, see Aschoff and Wever 1981; Wever 1979). All but a few pilot studies were conducted in an underground laboratory consisting of two studio apartments which were free of all environmental cues to time of day. The laboratory was heavily sound-dampened and the timing and intensity of illumination could be controlled from outside the apartments by the experimenters. In addition, the vast majority of subjects were studied in isolation in order to eliminate possible time cues provided by social contact.

The first experiments conducted in this unique environment (Aschoff 1965; Aschoff and Wever 1962) established that adult humans exhibit free-running rhythms of rest and activity averaging slightly longer than 25 hours. That is, a subject's average 'day' continued for about an hour longer than the natural day, though in some people the subjective day continued for a substantially longer period (up to 50 hours). Thus, subjects who thought that they had been in the time-free environment for, say, three weeks were often quite surprised to learn that a month or more had actually elapsed.

Several recent studies suggest that the human biological clock may, in fact, have an endogenous period of very close to 24, rather than 25 hours. Campbell and co-workers (Campbell *et al.* 1993) found that subjects who napped during their time in an otherwise traditional time-free protocol (the original studies specifically prohibited napping), exhibited free-running rhythms of rest-activity and temperature of 24.2 hours. Similar findings have since been reported using other experimental paradigms (for example, Czeisler *et al.* 1999).

27.2 **Effects of light on the biological clock**

The first hypothetical phase response curve (PRC) to light was proposed by Bünning (1936), based on his, and others', pioneering studies of diurnal oscillations in various plant species. These studies showed that such oscillations were not passively driven by the daily light-dark cycle but rather, were endogenously generated rhythms that were entrained by the daily alternation of light and darkness (Bünning and Stern 1930). Based on a relaxation oscillator model of the circadian clock, with a tension phase and a relaxation phase, Bünning proposed that such entrainment was achieved via a phase-dependent responsiveness to light. He summarized the hypothesis in 1960:

> If light (as example, a light break in the dark phase) ... is offered in the tension phase, this tension is made greater than it would otherwise have been. That is, the tension phase is extended by a given amount, for example, one to two hours. If the light treatment ... is repeated for several days, the adjustment process is also repeated until the light no longer falls in the tension phase. Thus, the phases ultimately occur several hours later than they did before this treatment. If, on the other hand, light is given in the relaxation phase, ... the relaxation process is brought to a halt one to two hours earlier than usual. The result is an advancing of the phase. (Bünning 1960; p. 6).

Such a hypothesis describing photic control of circadian rhythms was remarkable for the time, considering that the very existence of endogenous diurnal rhythmicity was still a matter of strenuous debate (Pittendrigh 1960). Subsequent research validated the phase-dependent nature of the endogenous clock's responsiveness to light, although the exact components of the PRC were shown to consist of a delay-sensitive phase in the early subjective night, an advance-sensitive phase in the late subjective night, and a non-responsive phase corresponding to an organism's subjective day. Such research also clarified the mechanism of entrainment by light and over the next three decades it was shown that the circadian systems of a wide variety of organisms responded in a similar manner to pulses of light (for reviews see, Gwinner 1975; Daan and Pittendrigh 1976; Pittendrigh 1981; Aschoff *et al.* 1982).

This included human circadian rhythms, which were shown to persist in the absence of external time cues, but at a period different from 24 hours (Aschoff and Wever 1962), indicating that synchronization of the human circadian clock was apparently in response to an external signal, or signals. Although the rigorous study of the human circadian system was still in its infancy, the importance of the natural light–dark (LD) cycle as a synchronizer of human circadian rhythms was generally acknowledged (see for example, Lobban 1958, 1960; Hellbrügge 1960; Sharp 1960).

The view that the LD cycle was an important Zeitgeber for the human circadian system was supported by studies of blind subjects. Most (see for example, Orth and Island 1969; Hollwich and Dieckhues 1971), but not all (Lund 1974, 1976), of these studies indicated that free-running rhythms of various functions failed to be entrained by social cues or established routines. Results of experiments in which normal subjects were exposed to forced living routines with periods ranging from 12 to 48 hours also supported the view. In those studies, in addition to reported entrainment of certain rhythms to the new period (usually sleep/ wake), other rhythms were reported to remain synchronized to a 24-hour periodicity, strongly suggesting entrainment by environmental factors, the most obvious being light.

Further support for the synchronizing capacity of light on the human circadian system was provided by Sharp (1960) who reported a phase delay in the plasma levels of leukocytes and in urine flow, in response to a 3-hour extension of darkness following normal wake time. A similar finding was reported several years later by Orth and Island (1969) who demonstrated that adrenocortical activity could be entrained to LD cycles which were dissociated from the timing of the subjects' sleep–wake cycles. Subsequent studies of human circadian rhythms, under more controlled experimental conditions, also seemed to confirm the role of the LD cycle as an effective synchronizer in humans. Artificial LD cycles were reported to effectively entrain subjects to non-24-hour periods (Aschoff 1969), and rapid re-entrainment of sleep– wake and temperature rhythms was accomplished by a single, 6-hour shift of the LD cycle (Aschoff 1967).

In these early studies, the LD cycle was temporally linked with periodic auditory tones, which signalled subjects to carry out various experimental procedures (for example, urine collection, performance test). On one occasion, however, shortly after the start of the study, the auditory signalling system failed. Despite the persisting LD cycle, subjects exhibited free-running rhythms (see Wever 1979, pp. 150–1 for a complete description). Subjects later confirmed that they perceived the auditory signals, but not the LD cycle, as a form of 'social contact' with the experimenters. Additional experiments designed to examine this chance finding more carefully (see for example, Wever 1970; Aschoff *et al.* 1971, 1975; Wever 1979; Aschoff and Wever 1981) led the investigators to question the strength (but not the existence) of the LD cycle as a synchronizer of human rhythms, relative to that of social cues. In one influential study (Aschoff *et al.* 1971), the authors concluded that a light–dark cycle was not necessary to entrain human circadian rhythms, 'at least for [the] 4 days' of the study.

Based on all subjects studied (n = 24), it was determined that the range of entrainment for a 'pure light–dark Zeitgeber' was smaller than + 1.0 hour, whereas the range of entrainment for the same light–dark cycle 'enriched' by social cues was about + 2.0 hours. The investigators concluded 'that the Zeitgeber effectiveness of light–dark cycles is small in comparison to that of social contacts' (Wever 1979, p. 191).

That light exposure could have a significant, direct impact on human physiological brain function was demonstrated unequivocally for the first time in a paper published by Lewy and co-workers in 1980. These investigators showed that light of substantially higher intensity than that used in the Andechs studies (2500 lux) was effective in suppressing night-time melatonin concentrations to daytime levels. Based on this finding, and on the intimate neuroanatomical links between the pineal gland and the endogenous circadian pacemaker located in the SCN, these investigators speculated that 'humans may require brighter light for the entrainment of circadian rhythms' than do other species (Lewy *et al.* 1980).

This paper marked a turning point in the study of the effects of light on the human circadian system, and over the next decade numerous investigators helped to further clarify and extend our knowledge in this area. Fifty years after the publication of Bünning's hypothetical PRC for plants, PRCs for humans were established, based on laboratory data (Honma and Honma 1988; Czeisler *et al.* 1989; Wever 1989; Minors *et al.* 1991), and more recent studies suggest that, under the proper circumstances, even moderately bright light may be sufficient to reset the biological clock (Boivin *et al.* 1996). Today, it is well accepted that ocular bright-light exposure can influence dramatically both the amplitude and phase of human circadian rhythms.

Recent studies also suggest that light can have an impact on the human biological clock even when administered to a non-ocular site. Based on a large body of literature demonstrating extraocular circadian phototransduction in a wide range of vertebrate species, we tested whether the biological clocks of a group of healthy, sighted adults between the ages of 18 and 62 years could be influenced by extraocular light exposure (Campbell and Murphy 1998). Using a fibre optic light source applied to the popliteal fossa of each leg (the area directly behind the kneecap), we administered light (approximately 13 000 lux) to subjects on one occasion, for a period of 3 hours. The circadian phase of body core temperature and melatonin onset were determined at baseline and following light exposure, and the degree of phase shifts was determined by comparing baseline and post-light measures.

We found that there was a systematic relationship between the timing of light exposure and the magnitude and direction of phase shifts, resulting in the generation of a PRC remarkably similar to that for ocular light exposure. In contrast, a sham light-exposure condition, in which the apparatus was attached to the legs but no light exposure occurred, resulted in no significant phase shifts. We have recently shown that the same type of light exposure can be used to reset the biological clock, even when subjects are sleeping (Campbell and Murphy 2000), and other investigators have used the procedure to successfully treat a circadian rhythm sleep disturbance in a totally blind woman (Erman *et al.* 1999).

27.3 **Effects of melatonin on the biological clock**

Acute administration of exogenous melatonin has been shown to phase shift the circadian rhythms of serum melatonin, body temperature, prolactin, and sleepiness (Mallo *et al.* 1988; McArthur *et al.* 1991; Zaidan *et al.* 1994). In addition, several groups have reported successful entrainment of sleep/wake, body core temperature, and endogenous melatonin rhythms with administration of both pharmacological and physiological levels of exogenous melatonin (Arendt *et al.* , 1985, 1986, 1988; Arendt and Marks 1983; Armstrong *et al.* 1986; Dahlitz *et al.* 1991; Folkard *et al.* 1990; Sack *et al.* 1991). The majority of these studies were conducted in otherwise healthy, blind individuals, in whom free-running circadian rhythms are often observed. It should be noted that, compared to sighted individuals, blind people may exhibit differential sensitivity to entraining stimuli. Therefore, one must use caution when generalizing these effects of exogenous melatonin to sighted populations.

The most comprehensive analyses of dose- and phase-dependent responses of exogenous melatonin have been conducted by Lewy and co-workers. These researchers have shown that a physiological dose of melatonin shifts the human circadian system according to a PRC (Lewy *et al.* 1992, 1998). In their first study, demonstrating a melatonin PRC in humans, sighted individuals were administered 0.5 mg melatonin in a split dose (that is, at two clock times separated by 2 hours) for 4 consecutive days (n = 27 trials in 9 subjects) following 1 week plus 2 days of placebo administration. In an additional three trials, conducted in three of the subjects, a single 0.5 mg dose was administered during the night-time hours (at 1.00 a.m., 3.00 a.m., or 5.00 a.m.) for 4 consecutive nights, and subjects were awakened briefly at the time of melatonin administration. The phase marker used to assess shifts was DLMO, which was measured after 1 week of placebo administration and after 4 consecutive days of melatonin administration. To assess its reliability as a marker of circadian phase, DLMO was also assessed in four trials prior to the week of placebo administration. The measure changed by a maximum of 21 minutes across the baseline week, indicating that it was a stable phase marker.

The shift in the time of DLMO following melatonin administration depended upon the circadian phase (relative to baseline DLMO) at which administration occurred, resulting in the first demonstration of a PRC to melatonin in humans. In general, phase advances occurred when melatonin was administered during the afternoon or early evening hours, and phase delays resulted from melatonin administration in the morning hours. The magnitude of phase advances was just over 1 hour, while phase delays of nearly 2 hours were reported. The experimental sessions in which phase advances were obtained far outnumbered phase delays, primarily because the times at which phase delays were most likely to be induced coincided with clock times at which subjects were typically asleep, and awakening them to administer melatonin introduced a potential confound in terms of differential exposure to ambient light.

A later replication of the human melatonin PRC (Lewy *et al.* 1998) utilized a slightly different experimental protocol. In that study, 6 individuals (ranging in age from 27 to 77 years) contributed 12 data points each to the PRC. DLMO was assessed in all subjects before and after a baseline week of placebo administration. Then, following 2 additional placebo days, a single, consolidated 0.5 mg dose was administered at the same clock time across the next 4 days and a post-melatonin DLMO was obtained. In this melatonin PRC, phase delays were more apparent, although the magnitude of neither advances nor delays was large; after 4 days of melatonin administration, the maximal phase shift was only 1.5 hours. Indeed, more than half of the phase shifts measured fell within one standard deviation (29 minutes) of the baseline variation in DLMO.

In addition to the question of robustness of melatonin-induced phase shifts, several other important issues remain to be addressed concerning the administration of melatonin in humans. For example, the inflection point of the PRC to melatonin in humans may not be the same as for light. Whereas phase delays typically occur when a light pulse precedes the nadir of the body temperature rhythm (Tmin), and phase advances occur when light is presented following Tmin, the same does not appear to be true for exogenous melatonin administration. Rather, when habitual wake time is termed circadian time 0 (CT0) and corresponds to a clock time of approximately 7.00 a.m. (Lewy *et al.* 1992, 1998) the crossover point from delays to advances occurs at approximately CT6 (which corresponds to about 1.00 p.m.), and from advances to delays, at approximately CT18 (which corresponds to about 1.00 a.m.).

In contrast, the PRC to light in humans has an inflection point at, or very near to, the daily minimum in body core temperature, which typically occurs earlier than habitual wake-time and earlier than 7.00 a.m., making the circadian time of the light PRC inflection point approximately CT22. Thus, although the melatonin PRC has been described as being approximately 12 hours out of phase with the light PRC (Lewy *et al.* 1998), the melatonin PRC's crossover points do not correspond as closely as implied to the inflection point of the light PRC.

There are other issues relating to melatonin administration that bear mentioning as well. The optimal dose for inducing phase shifts without producing side-effects (whether desirable or unwanted) remains unclear. Perhaps surprisingly, pharmacological doses have failed to induce phase shifts at times when physiological doses alter phase (for example, Wirz–Justice *et al.* 2000). The phase-dependent effects of a single dose (analogous to a single light pulse) on circadian phase requires further investigation. In this regard, several groups have studied the phase-resetting effects of single administrations of varying doses, and obtained extremely mixed results (Deacon and Arendt 1995; Wirz–Justice *et al.* 2000; Zaidan *et al.* 1994). There are considerable, age-related differences between individuals in the pharmacokinetics of melatonin — although age is not a complete explanation. The significance of the very large variations between individuals in endogenous levels of melatonin is not understood, and absolute melatonin levels or rhythm amplitude do not appear to be strongly related to any particular circadian rhythm dysfunction or other pathology.

In summary, it seems that individual differences in response to exogenous melatonin may be influenced in a complex manner by numerous factors including (but not limited to) the individual differences in pharmacokinetics, endogenous production levels, and perhaps internal circadian phase of the melatonin rhythm or circadian type. The circadian time of administration and ambient light exposure (both recent exposure and subsequent to melatonin intake) also influence the effects of exogenous melatonin on circadian phase.

The site of action of melatonin on the circadian timing system is also a matter of debate. The presence of high-affinity melatonin binding sites in the suprachiasmatic nucleus of rats and humans (Reppert *et al.* 1988) suggests that the synchronizing/stabilizing effects of melatonin may occur at the level of the primary pacemaker. However, direct resetting of the biological clock by melatonin in humans has not been demonstrated, although a study in rats did show immediate phase shifts in the SCN following melatonin injections (McArthur *et al.* 1991). There are, in addition, many acute, non-circadian effects of melatonin, including thermoregulatory and hypnotic effects, which could provide an indirect signal via feedback to the SCN which results in phase resetting of overt circadian rhythms.

Until investigation of the phase response to single or multiple administrations of melatonin at varying doses and under strictly controlled lighting conditions is more complete, and until there is some clarification regarding the optimal dose and time for melatonin administration, it will be very difficult to pin down the appropriate, effective regimen for application of melatonin for any clinical purpose.

Finally, an important concern that has yet to be systematically addressed is the safety of chronic melatonin administration in humans. It appears that to correct circadian rhythm abnormalities, melatonin, similar to timed bright-light exposure, would need to be used as a maintenance treatment, on a chronic basis. For this reason, the use of melatonin as a chronobiotic in the treatment of SAD or any circadian rhythm disorder should be undertaken with caution.

27.4 Implications for the aetiology and treatment of SAD

While a great deal more research is required to clarify a wide range of experimental and clinical questions, it is quite apparent that timed exposure to bright light and exogenous melatonin administration may have an important place in the treatment of various disorders involving circadian rhythms disturbance. To the extent that the biological clock may be implicated in the aetiology of SAD, the experimental examination of the nature of these chronobiotics clearly has important ramifications for improved diagnosis and treatment of this disorder.

Although light treatment was originally employed in the treatment of SAD based on the notion that patients could benefit simply from an increase in the duration of daily light exposure during the winter months (see, for example, Rosenthal *et al.* 1984), more recent evidence indicates that differential responses can be obtained depending on the time at which light is administered (Eastman *et al.* 1998; Terman *et al.* 1998; Wirz–Justice *et al.* 1998). For example, most clinicians report enhanced effectiveness of morning versus evening light, and at least one group has reported a significant correlation between clinical outcome and the degree to which the biological clock is advanced as a consequence of morning light exposure (Terman *et al.* 2001). Such findings clearly suggest that the biological timing system plays a critical role in the aetiology of SAD, or at least in the expression and resolution of the clinical picture of SAD.

In addition to a more complete understanding of the nature of chronobiotic effects on the biological clock and the mechanisms underlying their action, more pragmatic issues also require study. With respect to light treatment, patient compliance is a major problem. Many patients are unwilling or unable to commit the time required to achieve adequate, timely light exposure, on a daily basis, using current technology. Thus, a better understanding of dose-response issues, as well as the development of more user-friendly light administration devices, are likely to prove beneficial with more effective use of light treatment for SAD. As mentioned earlier, dose response is also an important issue with respect to exogenous melatonin administration. Furthermore, no study has examined the effects of chronic use of melatonin in terms of safety and effectiveness. It is quite likely that many such questions will be answered first, not in studies of patient populations, but rather in experimental studies of healthy subjects.

References

Arendt, J. and Marks, V. (1983). Can melatonin alleviate jet lag? [letter]. *British Medical Journal (Clinical Research),* **287**:638–9.

Arendt, J., Bojkowski, C., Folkard, S., Franey, C., Marks, V., Minors, D., *et al.* (1985). Some effects of melatonin and the control of its secretion in humans. In *Photoperiodism, melatonin, and the pineal* (ed. D. Evered and S. Clark), pp. 266–83. Pitman, London.

Arendt, J., Aldhous, M., and Marks, V. (1986). Alleviation of jet lag by melatonin: preliminary results of controlled double blind trial. *British Medical Journal (Clinical Research)*, **292**:652–9.

Arendt, J., Aldhous, M., and Wright, J. (1988). Synchronisation of a disturbed sleepwake cycle in a blind man by melatonin treatment [letter]. *Lancet*, **1**(8588):772–3.

Armstrong, S.M., Cassone, V.M., Chesworth, M.J., Redman, J.R., and Short, R.V. (1986). Synchronization of mammalian circadian rhythms by melatonin. *Journal of Neural Transmission*, **Suppl. 21**(1):375–94.

Aschoff, J. (1965). Circadian rhythms in man. *Science*, **148**:1427–32.

Aschoff, J. (1967). Human circadian rhythms in activity, body temperature and other functions. In *Life Sciences and Space Research V*, pp. 159–73. North Holland, Amsterdam.

Aschoff, J. (1969). Desynchronization and resynchronization of human circadian rhythms. *Aerospace Medicine*, **40(8)**:844–9.

Aschoff, J. and Wever R. (1962). Spontanperidik des menschen bei ausschluss aller Zeitgeber. *Naturwissenschaften*, **49**:337–42.

Aschoff, J., Fatranska, M., Giedke, H., Doerr, P., Stamm, D., and Wisser, H. (1971). Human circadian rhythms in continuous darkness: entrainment by social cues. *Science* **171**:213–15.

Aschoff, J., Hoffmann, K., Pohl, H., and Wever, R. (1975). Re-entrainment of circadian rhythms after phase-shifts of the Zeitgeber. *Nippon Seirigaku Zasshi*, **37(1)**:4–6.

Aschoff, J. and Wever, R. (1981). The circadian system of man. In *Handbook of Neurobiology* (ed. J. Aschoff). Plenum Press, New York.

Aschoff, J., Daan, S., and Groos, G.A. (ed.) (1982). *Vertebrate circadian systems: structure and physiology*. Springer–Verlag, Berlin.

Boivin, D., Duffy, J.F., Kronauer, R.E., and Czeisler, C.A. (1996). Dose-response relationships for resetting of the human circadian clock by light. *Nature*, **379(6565)**:540–2.

Brown, E.N. and Czeisler, C.A. (1992). The statistical analysis of circadian phase and amplitude in constant-routine core-temperature data. *Journal of Biological Rhythms*, **7(3)**:177–202.

Bünning, E. (1936). Die endogene tagesrhythmik als grundlage der photoperiodischen reaktion. *Berichte der Deutscen Botanischen Gesellschaft* **54**:590–607.

Bünning, E. (1960). Opening address: biological clocks. *Cold Spring Harbor Symposia on Quantitative Biology*, **25**:1–9.

Bünning, E. and K. Stern (1930). Über die tagesperiodischen bewegungen der primärblätter von phaseolus multiflorus II. Die bewegungen bei thermokonstanz. *Berichte der Deutschen Botanischen Gesellschaft* **48**:227–52.

Campbell S.S., Dawson, D., and Zulley, J. (1993). When the human circadian system is caught napping: evidence for endogenous rhythms close to 24 hours. *Sleep*, **16(7)**:638–40.

Campbell, S.S. and Murphy, P.J. (1998). Extraocular circadian phototransduction in humans. *Science*, **279**:396–9.

Campbell, S.S. and Murphy, P.J. (2000). Sleep alters human phase response to extraocular light. *Sleep*, **23(suppl. 2)**:A23.

Conroy, R.T. and Mills, J.N. (ed.) (1970). *Human circadian rhythms*. J. & A. Churchill, London.

Czeisler, C.A., Kronauer, R.E., Allan, J.S., Duffy, J.F., Jewett, M.E., Brown, E.N., *et al.* (1989). Bright light induction of strong (type 0) resetting of the human circadian pacemaker. *Science*, **244**:1328–33.

Czeisler, C.A., Duffy, J.F, Shanahan, T.L., Brown, E.N., Mitchell, J.F., Rimmer, D.W., *et al.* (1999). Stability, precision, and near-24-hour period of the human circadian pacemaker. *Science*, **284**:2177–81.

Daan, S. and Pittendrigh, C.S. (1976). A functional analysis of circadian pacemakers in nocturnal rodents. II: the variability of phase response curves. *Journal of Comparative Physiology*, **106**:253–66.

Dahlitz, M., Alvarez, B., Vignaum J., English, J., Arendt, J., and Parkes, J.D. (1991). Delayed sleep phase syndrome response to melatonin. *Lancet*, **337(8750)**:1121–4.

Deacon, S. and Arendt, J. (1995). Melatonin-induced temperature suppression and its acute phase-shifting effects in a dose-dependent manner in humans. *Brain Research* **688**:77–85.

Eastman, C.I., Young, M.A., Fogg, L.F., Liu, L., and Meaden, P.M. (1998) Bright light treatment of winter depression: a placebo-controlled trial. *Archives of General Psychiatry*, **55(10)**:883–9.

Erman, M.K., Parry, B.L., and Stahl, S.M. (1999). Successful treatment of disturbed sleep and circadian rhythms in a blind, enucleated individual with extraocular light therapy. *Sleep*, **22 (suppl. 1)**:B161.

Folkard, S., Arendt, J., Aldhous, M., and Kennett, H. (1990). Melatonin stabilises sleep onset time in a blind man without entrainment of cortisol or temperature rhythms. *Neuroscience Letters*, **113(2)**:193–8.

Gwinner, E. (1975). Circadian and circannual rhythms in birds. In *Avian biology*, (eds. D.S. Farner and J.R. King) Vol. 5, pp. 221–85. Academic Press, New York.

Halberg, F. (1959). Physiologic 24-hour periodicity: general and procedural considerations with reference to the adrenal cycle. *Zeitschrift fuer Vitamin-, Mormon- und Fermentforschung,* **10**:225–96.

Hellbrügge, T. (1960). The development of circadian rhythms in infants. *Cold Spring Harbor Symposia on Quantitative Biology,* **25**:311–23.

Hollwich, F. and Dieckhues, B. (1971). Circadian rhythms in the blind. *Journal of Interdisciplinary Cycle Research,* **2**:291–302.

Honma, K. and Honma, S. (1988). A human phase response curve for bright light pulses. *Japanese Journal of Psychiatry and Neurology,* **42**:167–8.

Kleinhoonte, A. (1929). Über die durch das licht regulierten autonomen bewegungen der Canavalia-Blätter. *Arch néerl Sci ex et nat,* **5**:1–110.

Lewy, A.J., Bauer, V.K., Cutler, N.L., Sack, R.L., Ahmed, S., Thomas, K.H., *et al.* (1998) Morning vs evening light treatment of patients with winter depression. *Archives of General Psychiatry,* **55(10)**:890–6.

Lewy, A.J., Wehr, T.A., Goodwin, F.K., Newsome, D.A., and Markey, S.P. (1980). Light suppresses melatonin secretion in humans. *Science,* **210**:1267–9.

Lewy, A.J. and Sack, R.L. (1989). The dim light melatonin onset (DLMO) as a marker for circadian phase position. *Chronobiology International,* **6**:93–102.

Lewy, A.J., Ahmed, S., Jackson, J.M.L., and Sack, R.L. (1992). Melatonin shifts circadian rhythms according to a phase response curve. *Chronobiology International,* **9**:380–92.

Lewy, A.J., Bauer, V.K., Ahmed, S., Thomas, K., Cutler, N., Singer, C., *et al.* (1998). The human phase response curve (PRC) to melatonin is about 12 hours out of phase with the PRC to light. *Chronobiology International,* **15(10)**:71–83.

Lobban, M.C. (1958). Excretory rhythms in indigenous arctic peoples. *Journal of Physiology,* **143**:69P.

Lobban, M.C. (1960). The entrainment of circadian rhythms in man. *Cold Spring Harbor Symposia on Quantitative Biology,* **25**:325–32.

Lund, R. (1974). Circadiane periodik physiologischer und psychologischer variablen bei 7 blinden versuchspersonen mit und ohne Zeitgeber [Doctoral thesis]. Technical University of Munich.

Lund, R. (1976). Circadiane rhythmen bei blinden. *30th Kongress der Deutschen Gesellschaft fuer Psychologie,* 391–2.

Mallo, C., Zaidan, R., Faure, A., Brun, J., Chazot, G., and Claustrat, B. (1988). Effects of a four-day nocturnal melatonin treatment on the 24 h plasma melatonin, cortisol, and prolactin profiles in humans. *Acta Endocrinology (Copenhagen),* **119**:474–80.

McArthur, A.J., Gillette, M.U., and Prosser, R.A. (1991). Melatonin directly resets the rat suprachiasmatic circadian clock in vitro. *Brain Research,* **565(1)**:158–61.

Minors, D.S., Waterhouse, J.M., and Wirz–Justice, A. (1991). A human phase-response curve to light. *Neuroscience Letters,* **133(1)**:36–40.

Nelson, W., Tong, Y.L., Lee, J.K., and Halberg, F. (1979). Methods for cosinor-rhythmometry. *Chronobiologia,* **6(4)**:305–23.

Orth, D.N. and Island, D.P. (1969). Light synchronization of the circadian rhythm in plasma cortisol (17-OHCS) concentration in man. *Journal of Clinical Endocrinology,* **29**:479–86.

Pittendrigh, C.S. (1960). Circadian rhythms and the circadian organization of living systems. *Cold Spring Harbor Symposia on Quantitative Biology,* **25**:159–84.

Pittendrigh, C.S. (1981). Circadian systems: entrainment. In *Handbook of behavioral neurobiology. Vol. 4: biological rhythms,* (ed. J. Aschoff) pp. 95–124. Plenum Press, New York.

Reppert, S., Weaver, D., Rivkees, S., and Stopa, E. (1988). Putative melatonin receptors are located in a human biological clock. *Science,* **242**:78–81.

Rosenthal, N.E., Sack D.A., Gillin, J.C., Lewy, A.J., Goodwin, F.K., Davenport, Y., *et al.* (1984). Seasonal affective disorder: A description of the syndrome and preliminary findings with light therapy. *Archives of General Psychiatry,* **41**:72–80.

Sack, R.L., Lewy, A.J., Blood, M.L., Stevenson, J., and Keith, D. (1991). Melatonin administration to blind people: phase advances and entrainment. *Journal of Biological Rhythms,* **6**:249–61.

Sharp, G.W.G. (1960). The effect of light on diurnal leukocyte variations. *Journal of Endocrinology*, 21:213–23.

Terman, M., Terman, J.S., and Ross, D.C. (1998) A controlled trial of timed bright light and negative air ionization for treatment of winter depression. *Archives of General Psychiatry*, 55(10):875–82.

Terman, J.S. , Terman, M., Lo, E.-S., and Cooper, T.B. (2001). Circadian time of mornig light administration and therapeutic response in winter depression. *Archives of General Psyciatry* 58:69–75.

Touitou, Y. and Haus, E. (1992). *Biological rhythms in clinical and laboratory medicine*. Springer–Verlag, New York.

Wever, R.A. (1970). Zur zeitgeber-strärke eines licht-dunkel-wechsels für die circadiane periodik des menschen. *Pflügers Archives*, 321:133–42.

Wever, R.A. (1979). *The circadian system of man: results of experiments under temporal isolation*. Springer–Verlag, New York.

Wever, R.A. (1989). Light effects on human circadian rhythms: a review of recent Andechs experiments. *Journal of Biological Rhythms*, 4:161–84.

Wirz–Justice, A. (1998). Beginning to see the light. *Archives of General Psychiatry*, 55(10):861–2.

Wirz–Justice, A., Kräuchi, K., Werth, E., Renz, C., Muller, S., Graw, P., et al. (2000). Does morning melatonin administration phase delay human circadian rhythms? *Seventh Meeting of the Society for Research on Biological Rhythms Abstracts*, p. 94.

Zaidan, R., Geoffriau, M., Brun, J., Taillard, J., Bureau, C., Chazot, G., et al. (1994). Melatonin is able to influence its secretion in humans: description of a phase response curve. *Neuroendocrinology*, 60:105–12.

Chapter 28

Clock organization

Martin R. Ralph

28.1 Introduction

The precision and accuracy of circadian rhythms, along with their existence in organisms throughout phylogeny, attest to the general importance of rhythmicity in nature. It is thought that the primary functions, or adaptive advantages, of endogenous rhythmicity are to provide a temporal organization for physiology and behaviour, and to optimize the timing of these processes with the cyclic environment. But although these assertions are credible, there is still little direct supporting evidence for an adaptive value. While this value is determined ultimately by the differential reproductive success of the genotype, the immediate advantages for the individual are manifest through greater fecundity, better health, optimal predator–prey relationships, and a longer life span. A potential adaptive value for the clock is demonstrated if experimental disruption of circadian rhythms leads to compromised health, reduced reproduction, and a decreased life expectancy.

In this chapter, we examine the relationship between the longevity of the organism and a loss of circadian rhythm integrity. This relationship is not simple, and the consequences of not having a biological clock, or of having a dysfunctional clock, are not well understood. Indeed, even where associations exist, it is usually not known whether disruptions of rhythmicity are the cause or consequence of compromised health or reproductive fitness. The intrinsic life span of a species is fixed within a given range by selection over evolutionary time, but the longevity of the individual is a product of its genetic background, environment, general health, ability to avoid predation, and random events. Rhythm disruption may contribute to a reduced longevity by affecting physiology and by impairing the organism's ability to deal with the exigencies of its cyclic environment.

28.2 Causes of rhythm dysfunction

A breakdown of rhythmic patterns occurs in various natural and artificial situations. Many organisms, including rodents, humans, and other primates, show fragmentation of activity rhythms or sleep–wake cycles as they reach a certain maturity (Peng *et al.* 1988; Brock 1991; Weitzman *et al.* 1991; Turek *et al.* 1996; Bliwise 1999). This condition, and especially a complete loss of rhythmicity, may be a reasonably accurate predictor of the animal's imminent demise (Wax and Goodrick 1978; Albers *et al.* 1981; Hurd and Ralph 1998). However, not all aged animals show the same degree of fragmentation, and some individuals retain robust rhythmicity up until their death. A population of aged animals, therefore, may be a highly heterogeneous group.

While ageing is a major factor contributing to rhythm breakdown, other important causes of rhythm dysfunction exist including injury, numerous neurological disorders (for review, see Zee and Grujic 1999), and nutritional state (Aguilar–Roblero *et al.* 1997; Langlais and Hall 1998; Bennett and Schwartz 1999). A prominent example of an association between circadian dysfunction and disease occurs in patients with Alzheimer's disease (Witting *et al.* 1990; Satlin *et al.* 1991; Van Someren *et al.* 1993). Here the disturbance to sleep and wakefulness is one of the hallmarks of the disease. Other medical conditions are also manifest as disruptions of circadian timekeeping, usually seen as a sleep disturbance in humans. Some sleep disorders such as delayed or advanced sleep phase syndrome (DSPS/ASPS) are, by definition, disturbances in circadian timekeeping. DSPS, or a loss of strong day–night distinction, is often presented following closed head injury and an 'internal desynchronization' has been suggested as a cause of various mood disorders, notably SAD and bipolar disorder (Buysse *et al.* 1999).

Social organization itself is a potential culprit for humans. For shift-workers, health and longevity may be at risk because circadian organization is compromised by the inappropriate timing of activity (Taylor and Pocock 1972; Folkard *et al.* 1985; Moore–Ede and Richardson 1985; Knutsson *et al.* 1986; Reinberg *et al.* 1989). Rapid transmeridian flight may also cause short-term rhythm disruption (Klein *et al.* 1972; Gander *et al.* 1993; Graeber 1994). Rigid adherence to work and school schedules often represents a temporal displacement of behaviour from more natural timing. Finally, institutionalized individuals, the elderly in particular, may be exposed to levels of illumination that are inadequate for normal entrainment.

However, the nature of the associations between rhythms, health, and longevity in both humans and other organisms is not clear-cut; there are different explanations for their existence. It can be argued, for example, that rhythm disruption is adaptive in some circumstances. During illness or injury, it may be advantageous to reduce the temporally gated drive to explore or to forage. Similarly, for seasonal breeders such as the golden hamster, it may be advantageous to reduce the influence of the clock at times when the temporal gating of locomotion underlying reproduction is not useful. In these examples, as in others, the peculiar circumstances might confer advantages for being able to disconnect the clock or to reduce its influence. (Interestingly, the importance of the clock is further substantiated by the need for such a mechanism.)

Nonetheless, a disruption of rhythmicity compromises what is considered to be a fundamental adaptive reason for having a clock — the temporal organization of physiology and behaviour. Such an occurrence would appear to negate the evolutionary significance of relying on a clock. Therefore, in situations where overt rhythms are fragmented or timing altered, it is reasonable to ask whether the breakdown of rhythmicity is the consequence or cause of other physical dysfunction or psychological impairment. For example, heart disease and poor sleep structure are often associated, and it is reasonable to assume that poor circulation compromises sleep. However, cardiac restructuring occurs at night during sleep (Sole 1986), so night-time wakefulness disrupts this important function. For psychiatric disorders such as depressive illnesses, many aspects of physiology are affected including sleep, immune function, gastrointestinal function, and temperature regulation. Are these effects ameliorated by an adaptive reduction in rhythm amplitude, or exacerbated by the loss of temporal organization?

In the laboratory, rhythm disruption has been induced by various means that may reflect natural situations. Fragmentation has been produced in rodents during repetitive shifts in the light–dark entraining cycle (Halberg and Cadotte 1975; Sakellaris *et al.* 1975; Nelson and Halberg 1986; Devan *et al.* forthcoming). This situation can be compared with the 'jet lag' experienced following successive transmeridian flights, or may mimic a pathological condition where rhythms no longer are able to be entrained to the external Zeitgeber. The propensity for fragmentation may also be laid down during gestation. Pups born to mothers who were given a calorie-restricted diet during gestation show low-amplitude, fragmented rhythms (Aguilar–Roblero *et al.* 1997). Similar disrupted patterns are exhibited by pups if their mothers are subjected to a mild stressor (such as handling) during the late stages of pregnancy (Cain *et al.* forthcoming). It is too early, however, to know whether these manipulations have any effect on the ultimate life expectancy of the organisms.

28.3 Mechanisms of rhythm dysfunction

Disturbances in the overt pattern of rhythmic behaviour and physiology could occur because either target systems have become disconnected from the central clock or the operation of the clock itself has been compromised. In both cases, the rhythmic influence of the central pacemaker would be reduced. This would result in either dampened, fragmented rhythms or a desynchrony among overt rhythms or both.

Because we usually observe only the overt influence of clock activity, it is difficult to determine whether fragmentation is due to a dysfunctional clock or to a reduced responsiveness to clock output. For age-related rhythm fragmentation, the source appears to be within the clock mechanism itself, and in older animals is likely to be a reflection of reduced cell–cell communication. Studies of the clock in the suprachiasmatic nucleus (SCN) of the hypothalamus *in vitro* demonstrate that the changes in overt patterns of behaviour during ageing are reflected in changes in the nucleus (Wise *et al.* 1988; Satinoff *et al.* 1993). Cellular electrical activity and the inducibility of c-*fos* expression within the nucleus are processes that show high-amplitude circadian rhythms in young adults, that become reduced in amplitude with age (Cai and Wise 1996; Cai *et al.* 1997).

Individual SCN pacemaker cells are capable of generating circadian oscillations *in vitro*, although periods range from about 18 hours to 30 hours (Welsh *et al.* 1995). The generation of overt, approximate 24-hour periodicity, appears to be a property of an ensemble of coupled pacemaker cells, therefore the dampening of circadian rhythms seen in aged animals may be due to a loss of cells or intercellular communication.

28.4 Rhythm dysfunction and reduced longevity

In the examples already presented, the same natural, accidental, or experimental situation that causes problems with circadian rhythms can also be shown to produce other health problems or risks via another route. It is difficult, therefore, to attribute unambiguously a decline in health or reduced life expectancy to disturbed rhythms. Nonetheless, a few recent studies have tackled this issue.

The most direct way of producing circadian disorganization is to remove the clock itself. Although there have been no reports of clock ablation affecting life span *per se*, SCN lesions have been shown to decrease survival in ground squirrels (Decoursey *et al.* 1997) and chipmunks (Decoursey *et al.* 2000) released back into the wild. The cause of the earlier demise appeared to be predation.

The value of having a clock that is tuned to the periodicity of the environment has been demonstrated in a number of species. In the lemur, *Microcebus murinus*, life span is shortened on accelerated photoperiodic cycles (Perret 1997). In insects (Pittendrigh and Minis 1972; Aschoff *et al.* 1979; Fleury *et al.* 2000), plants (Went 1960), and hamsters (Hurd and Ralph 1998), longevity has been shown to be maximal when the free-running period matches the period of the external cycle. However, the initial finding of this effect in *Drosophila* has not been verified in a subsequent study (Klarsfeld and Rouyer 1998). Similarly, when competing for limited resources, the survival of period-mutant strains of the cyanobacterium, *Synechococcus*, was favoured for organisms whose circadian periods matched that of their environment (Ouyang *et al.* 1998).

A general interpretation of these results is that a profound period difference between the endogenous rhythm and Zeitgeber leads to suboptimal phase relationships among processes within the organism or between organism and environment. However, it is debatable whether reduced longevity itself, or reproduction in the case of *Synechococcus*, demonstrates an adaptive advantage of a circadian clock. There may be a considerable cost that does not exist under natural conditions for relying on a mechanism that is chronically wrong for its environment. Hence, the adaptive value of the circadian clock in nature is not really tested.

In addition, the cause of the reduction in life span is not indicated in most of these experiments. In most studies, the physiology and behaviour of individuals is not monitored. Notable exceptions have been studies of the golden hamster. In cardiomyopathic (CM) hamsters, weekly 180° phase shifts of the light–dark cycle exacerbates the primary effect of the mutation on longevity (Penev *et al.* 1998), while exposure to constant light reduces the effect (Natelson *et al.* 1996).

For golden hamsters carrying the period mutation, *tau* (Ralph and Menaker 1988), longevity in a 24-hour light–dark cycle depends on whether the animals can entrain to the cycle (Hurd and Ralph 1998). This mutation, which is a reduced function allele of casein kinase-1-epsilon (*ck1e*) (Lowrey *et al.* 2000), causes the circadian period to be reduced to approximately 22 hours in the heterozygotes and to approximately 20 hours in the homozygous mutants. When raised on a 24-hour light cycle, the wild-type animals ($ck1e^{+/+}$) live the longest, followed by $ck1e^{tau/tau}$. However, the shortest-lived animals are the heterozygotes ($ck1e^{+/tau}$).

Examination of activity records shows that both homozygous groups had highly consolidated activity (although $ck1e^{tau/tau}$ animals were essentially oblivious to the light cycle). Heterozygotes, on the other hand, synchronized with the 24-hour cycle but had extremely early onsets of nocturnal behaviour, and the patterns were highly fragmented. The conclusion that was reached in this study was that the inability to synchronize properly with the environment resulted in an abnormal pattern of rhythmicity which led to the reduction in longevity.

28.5 Rhythm restoration and longevity

To determine whether life expectancy is actually influenced by the loss of rhythmic organization *per se*, it is necessary to demonstrate, in addition, that longevity is increased if the lost circadian organization is restored. The experiments with *Drosophila*, cyanobacteria, and hamsters already mentioned illustrate this indirectly. Essentially, a cure for the effects of abnormal entrainment in these period mutants is either a light–dark cycle that closely matches their circadian period or (for the hamster) no light cycle at all.

A reliable solution for the fragmentation that accompanies ageing (in hamsters) is to provide a new clock using transplantation techniques. Initially, SCN transplant studies were designed to test the hypothesis that this nucleus played the main role in generating and driving overt circadian rhythms. These experiments involved the restoration of rhythms to hosts that had been rendered arrhythmic with SCN lesions. Because the donor tissue was taken from a different circadian genotype, the source of the new rhythmicity was attributable to the implanted SCN (Ralph *et al.* 1990).

For aged animals whose locomotor patterns have deteriorated naturally, SCN implants have been shown to not only express a new, donor-specific periodicity, but also to raise the amplitude of the host's own SCN output (Hurd *et al.* 1995). In this way, the SCN graft, which has only limited access to brain targets, can influence the entire organism indirectly by affecting the host SCN. The result is the restoration of a more youthful pattern of locomotor behaviour, driven by the host clock, which has been associated with increased longevity: aged hosts with highly disorganized behaviour lived 20 per cent longer than expected following SCN grafting (Hurd and Ralph 1998).

Regardless of the underlying mechanism, the reduction of longevity when rhythms are disrupted, together with the increase that is produced when fragmented rhythms are reconsolidated, substantiates the claim that there is an adaptive significance to the organization that is provided by the circadian clock. Although it is not indicated by these experiments, it is likely that the premature demise of animals with fragmented rhythms is due to an overall reduction in health and well-being.

28.6 **Concluding remarks**

The breakdown of circadian rhythms in a variety of species, under natural and experimental conditions, is associated with a decrease in longevity. In no case though is there a suggestion that the circadian clock and the mechanism that defines the life span for the species are one and the same. It is important to remember that longevity and adaptive advantage are not equivalent. Increased longevity does not mean increased reproductive fitness.

However, the demonstration that rhythm restoration in aged hamsters is associated with an increase in life expectancy is a direct indication of the importance of maintaining robust rhythmicity. This is not a matter of manipulating the environment to eliminate the offending feature (for example, using period mutants on a T-cycle), but of repairing the animal's circadian system. This is a unique demonstration that the organization provided by the clock has a role that is perhaps more basic than synchronization with the cyclic environment.

It is more appropriate to view the SCN as one of the many organs and brain nuclei that have a specific role to play in maintaining the optimal, healthy functioning of the whole organism. When its function is compromised, so is the health and perhaps the life expectancy of the organism. In humans, it has been suggested that robust, 24-hour rest/activity rhythms might be useful in the prognosis of survival and tumour response in patients with colorectal cancer, as well as an indicator of quality of life (Mormont *et al.* 2000). It follows then that successful transplantation of the SCN, like any malfunctioning organ, presents the possibility of improving health and increasing the longevity of the individual. Of course, not all individuals gain from an SCN transplant. Young adults and aged animals with robust, high-amplitude rhythms do not improve.

This line of research raises three important general issues, especially if there is a clinical application to be considered. First, although the longevity of the individual may be increased, does this mean that health and well-being are also improved? It is generally taken as fact that improving health will promote a greater life expectancy, but in the case of circadian rhythmicity, this connection is still indirect. When the consolidation or amplitude of overt rhythms can be taken to indicate general health, then this question is partially answered.

Second, it is not known which restored rhythms (physiological or behavioural) are most critical to issues of physical and mental health. In SCN transplant studies, where the host SCN has been ablated, implanted tissues fail to restore many rhythms, particularly those that require neural connections with the SCN (Lehman *et al.* 1995). Transplantation into intact animals most likely gives a different pattern. The increased amplitude of the host's own locomotor rhythm suggests that restoration may be more inclusive.

Finally, the extent to which rhythmicity can be restored without invasive procedures such as brain tissue transplantation will determine the usefulness of this type of information to the general application of circadian biology to issues of human health and ageing.

References

Albers, H.E., Gerall, A.A., and Axelson, J.F. (1981) Circadian rhythm dissociation in the rat: effects of long-term constant illumination. *Neurosci Lett* **25**:89–94.

Aguilar–Roblero, R., Salazar–Juarez, A., Rojas–Castaneda, J., Escobar, C., and Cintra, L. (1997) Organization of circadian rhythmicity and suprachiasmatic nuclei in malnourished rats. *Am J Physiol* **273**:R1321–31.

Aschoff, J., Saint Paul, U.V., and Wever, R. (1971) The lifespan of flies under the influence of time shifts. *Naturwissenschaften* **58**:574.

Bennett, M.R. and Schwartz, W.J. (1999) Altered circadian rhythmicity is an early sign of murine dietary thiamine deficiency. *J Neurol Sci* **163**:6–10.

Bliwise, D.L. (1999) Sleep and circadian rhythm disorders in aging and dementia. In *Regulation of sleep and circadian rhythms* (ed. F.W. Turek and P.C. Zee), pp. 487–525. Marcel–Dekker, New York.

Brock, M.A. (1991) Chronobiology and aging. *J Am Geriatr Soc* **39**:74–91.

Buysse, D.J., Nofzinger, E.A., Keshavan, M.S., Reynolds III, C.F., and Kupfer, D.J. (1999) Psychiatric disorders associated with disturbed sleep and circadian rhythms. In *Regulation of sleep and circadian rhythms* (ed. F.W. Turek and P.C. Zee), pp. 597–641. Marcel–Dekker, New York.

Cai, A. and Wise, P.M. (1996) Age-related changes in jun-b and jun-d expression: effects of transplantation of fetal tissue containing the suprachiasmatic nucleus. *J Biol Rhythms* **11**:284–90.

Cai, A., Lehman, M.N., Lloyd, J.M., and Wise, P.M. (1997) Transplantation of fetal suprachiasmatic nuclei into middle-age rats restores diurnal Fos expression in host. *Am J Physiol* **272**:R422–8.

Decoursey, P.J., Krulas, J.R., Mele, G., and Holley, D.C. (1997) Circadian performance of suprachiasmatic nuclei (SCN)-lesioned antelope ground squirrels in a desert enclosure. *Physiol Behav* **62**:1099–108.

Decoursey, P.J., Walker, J.K., and Smith, S.A. (2000) A circadian pacemaker in free-living chipmunks: essential for survival? *J Comp Physiol* **A 186**:169–80.

Fleury, F., Allemand, R., Vavre, F., Fouillet, P., and Boulétreau, M. (2000) Adaptive significance of a circadian clock: temporal segregation of activities reduces intrinsic competitive inferiority in Drosophila parasitoids. *Proc R Soc Lond B* **267**:1005–10.

Folkard, S., Minors, D.S., and Waterhouse, J.M. (1985) Chronobiology and shift-work: current issues and trends. *Chronobiologia* **12**:31–54.

Gander, P.H., De Nguyen, B.E., Rosekind, M.R., and Connell, L.J. (1993) Age, circadian rhythms, and sleep loss in flight crews *Aviat Space Environ Med* **64**:185–9.

Graeber, R.C. (1994) Jet lag and sleep disruption. In *Principles and practice of sleep medicine* (ed. M.H. Kryger, T. Roth, and W.C. Dement), pp. 463–70. W.B. Saunders, Philadelphia.

Halberg, F. and Cadotte, I. (1975) Increased mortality in mice exposed to weekly 180 shifts of lighting regimen L.D. 12:12 beginning at 1 year of age. *Chronobiologia* **2(suppl. 1)**:26.

Hurd, M.W., Zimmer, K.A., Lehman, M.N., and Ralph, M.R. (1995) Circadian locomotor rhythms in aged hamsters following suprachiasmatic transplant. *Am J Physiol* **269**:R958–68.

Hurd, M.W. and Ralph, M.R. (1998) The significance of circadian organization for longevity in the golden hamster. *J Biol Rhythms* **13**:430–6.

Klarsfeld, A. and Rouyer, F. (1998) Effects of circadian mutations and LD periodicity on the life span of *Drosophila melanogaster*. *J Biol Rhythms* **13**:471–8.

Klein, K.E., Wegmann, H.M., and Hunt, B.I. (1972) Desynchronization of body temperature and performance circadian rhythms as a result of out-going and homegoing transmeridian flights. *Aerospace Med* **43**:119–32.

Knutsson, A., Akerstedt, T., and Orth–Gomer, K. (1986) Increased risk of ischaemic heart disease in shift workers. *Lancet* **2**:89–92.

Langlais, P.J. and Hall, T. (1998) Thiamine deficiency-induced disruptions in the diurnal rhythm and regulation of body temperature in the rat. *Metab Brain Dis* **13**:225–39.

Lehman, M.N., LeSauter, J., Kim, C., Berriman, S.J., Tresco, P.A., and Silver, R. (1995) How do fetal grafts of the suprachiasmatic nucleus communicate with the host brain? *Cell Transplant* **4**:75–81

Lowrey, P.L., Shimomura, K., Antoch, M.P., Yamazaki, S., Zemenides, P.D., Ralph, M.R., *et al.* (2000) Positional syntenic cloning and functional characterization of the mammalian circadian mutation, *tau*. *Science* **288**:483–91.

Moore–Ede, M.C. and Richardson, G.S. (1985) Medical implications of shift work. *Ann Rev Med* **36**:607–17.

Mormont, M.C., Waterhouse, J., Bleuzen, P., *et al.* (2000) Marked 24-h rest/activity rhythms are associated with better quality of life, better response, and longer survival in patients with colorectal cancer and good performance status. *Clin Cancer Res* **6**:3038–45.

Natelson, B.H., Ottenweller, J.E., Tapp, W.N., Bergen, M., and Soldan, S. (1996) Phototherapeutic effects in hamsters with heart disease. *Physiol Behav* **60**:463–8.

Nelson, W. and Halberg, F. (1986) Schedule-sh ift, circadian rhythms and lifespan of freely-feeding and meal-fed mice. *Physiol Behav* **38**:781–6.

Ouyang, Y., Andersson, C.R., Kondo, T., Golden, S.S., and Johnson, C.H. (1998) Resonating circadian clocks enhance fitness in cyanobacteria. *Proc Nat Acad Sci* **95**:8660–4.

Penev, P.D., Kolker, D.E., Zee, P.C., and Turek, F.W. (1998) Chronic circadian desynchronization decreases the survival of animals with cardiomyopathic heart disease. *Am J Physiol* **275**(***Heart, Circ Physiol 44***):H2334–7.

Peng, M.T., Jiang, M.J., and Hsu, H.K. (1980) Changes in running-wheel activity, eating and drinking and their day/night distributions thoughout the life span of the rat. *J Gerontol* **35**:339–47.

Perret, M. (1997) Change in photoperiodic cycle affects life span in a prosimian primate (*Microcebus murinus*). *J Biol Rhythms* **12**:136–45.

Pittendrigh, C.S. and Minis, D.H. (1972) Circadian systems: longevity as a function of circadian resonance in *Drosophila melanogaster*. *Proc Nat Acad Sci USA* **69**:1537–9.

Ralph, M.R. and Menaker, M. (1988) A mutation of the circadian system in golden hamsters. *Science* **241**:1225.

Ralph, M.R., Foster, R., Davis, F.C., and Menaker, M. (1990) Suprachiasmatic transplant determines circadian period. *Science* **247**:975–8.

Reinberg, A., Motohashi, Y., Bourdeleau, P., Touitou, Y., Nouguier, J., Levi, F., *et al.*(1989) Internal desynchronization of circadian rhythms and tolerance of shift work. *Chronobiologia* **16**:21–34.

Roosendaal, B., van Gool, W.A., and Swaab, D.F. (1987) Changes in vasopressin cells of the rat suprachiasmatic nucleus with aging. *Brain Res* **409**:259–66.

Sakellaris, P.C., Peterson, A., Goodwin, A., Winget, C.M., and Vernikos–Danellis, J. (1975) Response of mice to repeated photoperiod shifts: susceptibility to stress and barbiturates. *Proc Soc Exp Biol Med* **149**:677–80.

Satinoff, E., Li, H., Tcheng, T.K., Liu, C., McArthur, A.J. Medanic, M., *et al.* (1993) Do the suprachiasmatic nuclei oscillate in old rats as they do in young ones? *Am J Physiol* **265**:R1216–22.

Satlin, A., Teicher, M.N., Leiberman, H.R., Baldessarini R.J., Volicer, L., and Rheaume Y. (1991) Circadian locomotion activity rhythms in Alzheimer's disease. *Neuropsychopharmacology* **5**:115–26.

Sole, M. (1986) Hamster cardiomyopathy: understanding the pathogenesis of heart failure. *Hamster Info Serv* **8**:3–8.

Tapp, W.N. and Natelson, B.H. (1986) Life extension in heart disease: an animal model. *Lancet* **1**:238–40.

Taylor, P. and Pocock, S.J. (1972) Mortality of shift and day workers. *Brit J Int Med* **29**:201–7.

Turek, F.W. (1985) Circadian neural rhythms in mammals. *Ann Rev Physiol* **47**:49–64.

Turek, F.W. (1993) Aging, feedback and the circadian clock. *Brain Res* **18**:319.

Turek, F.W., Penev, P., Zhang, Y., Van Reeth, O., Takahashi, J.S., and Zee, P.C. (1996) Alterations in the circadian system in advanced age. In *Circadian clocks and their adjustment* (ed. D. Chadwick and K. Akrill), pp. 212–34. John Wiley, Chichester.

Van Someren, E.J.W., Hagebeuk, E.E.O., Swaab, D.F., *et al.* (1993) Circadian rest-activitiy disturbances in Alzheimer's disease. *Sleep Res* **22**:637.

Wax, T.M. and Goodrick, C.L. (1978) Nearness to death and wheel running behavior in mice. *Exp Gerontol* **13**:233–6.

Weitzman, E.D., Moline, M.L., Czeisler, C.A., and Zimmerman, J.C. (1991) Chronobiology of aging: temperature, sleepwake rhythms and entrainment. *Neurobiol Aging* **3**:299–309.

Welsh, D.K., Logothetis, D.E., Meister, M., and Reppert, S.M. (1995) Individual neurons dissociated from rat suprachiasmatic nucleus express independently phased circadian firing rhythms. *Neuron* **14**:697–706.

Went, F.W. (1960) Photo- and thermoperiodic effects in plant growth. *Cold Spring Harbor Symp Quant Biol* **25**:221–30.

Wise, P.M., Cohen, I.R., Weiland, N.G., and London, D.E. (1988) Aging alters the circadian rhythm of glucose utilization in the suprachiasmatic nucleus. *Proc Nat Acad Sci USA* **85**:5305–9.

Witting, W., Kwa, I.H., and Eikelenboom, P., *et al.* (1990) Alterations in the circadian restactivity rhythm in aging and Alzheimer's disease. *Biol Psychiatry* **27**:563–72.

Zee, P.C. and Grujic, M. (1999) Neurological disorders associated with disturbed sleep and circadian rhythms. In *Regulation of sleep and circadian rhythms* (ed. F.W. Turek and P.C. Zee), pp. 557–96. Marcel–Dekker, New York.

Chapter 29

Clock genes

Nicolas Cermakian and Paolo Sassone–Corsi

29.1 **Introduction**

Living organisms adapt to cyclic environmental conditions by using endogenous clocks that regulate a wide variety of physiological processes (Cermakian and Sassone–Corsi 2000; Pittendrigh 1993). Circadian rhythms are those that display a period close to 24 hours (the period being the duration of one cycle).

In animals, circadian rhythms are generated by specialized structures of the central nervous system (Hastings 1997; Moore and Silver 1998). The central clock structure in mammals is located within the suprachiasmatic nucleus (SCN) of the anterior hypothalamus. The SCN clock can function autonomously, without any external input, but it can be reset by environmental conditions (for example, day/night cycles). It has been known for some time that the circadian clocks rely on the function of specialized genes and on the interaction of their products (Dunlap 1999). However, the nature of these genes and a clearer picture of the molecular gears involved in circadian timekeeping have only recently been uncovered.

29.2 **Finding clock genes**

The first clock mutant ever identified was *period* (*per*) in the fruit fly *Drosophila melanogaster*, 30 years ago (Konopka and Benzer 1971). In recent years, many other genes have been identified, not only in the fly but also in cyanobacteria, fungi, and vertebrates, including fish, mice, and humans (Dunlap 1999). This was achieved mainly by genetic screening based on the identification of organisms for which the clock, and as a consequence circadian rhythms, present defects. For example, mutations in the *Drosophila per* gene can lead either to a shorter or longer period, or to complete loss of rhythmicity (Konopka and Benzer 1971). However, isolating clock mutants in mammals is a huge task that has been successful only in two cases up to now: the mouse *clock* gene (King *et al.* 1997) and the hamster gene for casein kinase Iε (Lowrey *et al.* 2000). Both were isolated through identification by positional cloning of the mutated gene in animals with abnormal rhythms. Fortunately, other clock genes were identified in the mouse, rat, and human based on their homology with genes first isolated in *Drosophila* and other organisms (Cermakian and Sassone–Corsi 2000; Dunlap 1999). For instance, mammals have three homologues of the fly *per* gene, called *per1, 2,* and *3* (Zylka *et al.* 1998), which appear to have acquired distinct roles within the clock of these organisms (Shearman *et al.* 2000).

A model for the functional interconnection between clock genes is presented in Fig. 29.1. Although these genes can be different in the various organisms studied, some key structural

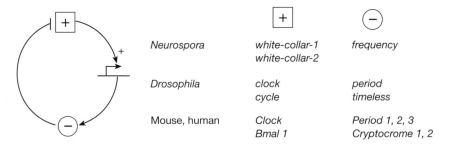

Fig. 29.1 Schematic representation of the negative feedback loop involved in most molecular circadian clocks. Positively acting factors (generally as heterodimers) (+) increase the transcription of other clock genes, which encode proteins (−) that feedback on their own expression by repressing the activity of the positive factors. On the right are given examples of genes encoding positive and negative factors of these loops from the fungi *Neurospora crassa*, the fruitfly *Drosophila melanogaster*, and mammals.

features are conserved. First, many clock genes encode protein with a PAS domain, a protein–protein interaction module first identified in the PER, AHR (arylhydrocarbon receptor), and SIM (singleminded) proteins (Huang *et al.* 1993). Second, many of these genes encode transcription factors or proteins that act in some way on gene regulation (Sassone–Corsi 1998). Indeed, as will be discussed in this chapter, the generation and modulation of rhythms rely mainly on activation and repression of gene expression. Third, the expression of many of these genes exhibit circadian rhythms (Dunlap 1999). Alternatively, even if the messenger RNA does not undergo fluctuations, oscillation in the abundance or the activity of the protein product can nevertheless be produced through post-transcriptional or post-translational regulation (Dunlap 1999).

29.3 **Feedback loops**

Despite the differences in the genes and proteins involved in the circadian clocks of various model organisms, the molecular device in which they are organized is the same: all circadian clocks studied rely primarily on regulatory feedback loops, usually at the level of transcription (Cermakian and Sassone–Corsi 2000; Dunlap 1999). This is schematized in Fig. 29.1 — positively acting factors increase the transcription of other clock genes, which encode proteins that feedback on their own expression by repressing the activity of the positive factors. For example, in *Drosophila*, the product of the *clock* and *cycle* genes are transcription factors that activate in concert to express *period* (*per*) and *timeless* (*tim*) genes (Darlington *et al.* 1998). The PERIOD and TIMELESS proteins then accumulate in the cytoplasm of cells and, when they reach a sufficient level, they dimerize, enter the nucleus (Gekakis *et al.* 1995), and inhibit the binding of the CLOCK-CYCLE dimer to DNA (Lee *et al.* 1999). This leads to a down-regulation of *per* and *tim* messenger RNA back to initial levels: the circadian loop is closed.

Recent data about the clock in *Neurospora* (Lee *et al.* 2000), *Drosophila* (Glossop *et al.* 1999), and the mouse (Shearman *et al.* 2000), however, indicate that the reality is more complex. Rather than a single feedback loop, the circadian clock is probably composed of a network of interlocked loops. In *Drosophila*, PER and TIM, in addition to repressing the activity of the CLOCK-CYCLE on their own promoters, also in some way promote activation of the *clock* gene (Glossop *et al.* 1999). In mammals, one of the PER proteins, PER2, positively gives feedback in an analogous way on the *Bmal1* gene (the homologue of *Drosophila cycle*) (Shearman *et al.* 2000).

Other clock genes encode regulators of the circadian feedback loops (Cermakian and Sassone–Corsi 2000). A typical example is the *double-time* (*dbt*) gene in *Drosophila* (Price *et al.* 1998). This gene encodes a kinase (that is, an enzyme adding phosphate groups on other proteins). The DBT protein phosphorylates PER, inducing in this way the degradation of this clock protein. The decrease in the amount of PER delays the entry of PER and TIM in the nucleus and their repressive action on transcription. Indeed, flies with mutations of the *dbt* gene exhibit a short period of circadian rhythms (Price *et al.* 1998). Hamsters with a mutated casein kinase Iε (the homologue of fly DBT) also present activity–rest rhythms with a period of only 20 hours (Lowrey *et al.* 2000).

29.4 **Input and output pathways**

Two other classes of clock genes mediate the input to and the output from the clock (see Fig. 29.2 and Cermakian and Sassone–Corsi 2000). The input pathways allow the clock to be entrained or reset by various stimuli, either environmental signals or physiological cues. The major environmental signal is the alternation of day and night (Pittendrigh 1993). People experiencing jet lag after a trip through time zones recover from it after several days; the new light–dark cycle affects their clock and entrains it to the right phase. Animals use the length of the photoperiod (duration of light during the day) to evaluate changes in seasons and adapt to circannual rhythms (period of about a year).

In mammals, light is perceived by the retina and the information is relayed to the SCN via the retinohypothalamic tract (RHT). Glutamate is released from the RHT and activates receptor on SCN neurons, initiating signalling cascades leading ultimately to phase shifting of the clock (Ding *et al.* 1994). Light induces the expression of immediate early genes (IEG), for example, c-*fos* (Kornhauser *et al.* 1990) and of clock genes, for example, *mPer1* and *mPer2* (Albrecht *et al.* 1997; Shearman *et al.* 1997) in the SCN. The transcriptional induction of these genes seems to be an important event for phase shifting of the clock. It is not completely clear which intracellular pathways lead to the up-regulation of these genes, but MAPKs (mitogen-activated protein kinases; see Obrietan *et al.* 1998) and CREB (cAMP-response element binding protein; see Ginty *et al.* 1993) are known to be involved. Moreover,

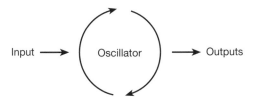

Fig. 29.2 The circadian clock is composed of three components: an oscillator or pacemaker, which generates and sustains rhythms, even in constant conditions; input pathways, regulating oscillator response to various stimuli (for example, light–dark cycles in the environment); and output pathways, which convey rhythmic information from the pacemaker to other physiological systems.

clock phase shifting and induction of IEG in the SCN have recently been shown to be associated with remodelling of chromatin (Crosio *et al.* 2000).

Although the role of IEG in clock phase shifting is unknown, it is thought that a change in the amount of *Per* gene protein products can lead to a delay or an advance by impeding or promoting nuclear translocation of negative factors of the circadian feedback loop (Maywood *et al.* 1999). In addition to the RHT and its neurotransmitter glutamate, other neural pathways affect the clock, using other neurotransmitters, for example, neuropeptide Y (Card and Moore 1989) and serotonin (Pickard and Rea 1997). Melatonin has also been shown to have a phase-shifting action on the clock (Liu *et al.* 1997). In *Drosophila*, light is received in clock cells by a protein called CRYPTOCHROME (Emery *et al.* 1998) and triggers degradation of TIM protein (Ceriani *et al.* 1999). The consequence is an advance or a delay of the phase of the clock, depending on the actual state of the feedback loop.

The SCN exerts its effects on physiology by neuronal or humoral signals (Cermakian and Sassone–Corsi 2000). A well-characterized output pathway links the SCN to the pineal gland (Foulkes *et al.* 1997). This structure synthesizes melatonin in a rhythmic fashion, but is not itself a clock structure and needs rhythmic signals from the SCN.

How is the regulation of the output achieved at the molecular level? Several recent studies provide examples of clock-controlled genes whose expression is activated by the CLOCK-BMAL1 (or CYCLE) dimer binding to an E-box in their promoters: this is, for instance, the case of *vrille* in *Drosophila* (Blau and Young 1999) and *dbp* in the mouse (Ripperger *et al.* 2000). Since the activity of the dimer varies in a circadian manner, as a consequence of the feedback loops already described, the expression of these output genes oscillates. Output genes typically encode peptides (Jin *et al.* 1999; Renn *et al.* 1999) that then convey the message to other tissues, or transcription factors (Blau and Young 1999; Ripperger *et al.* 2000) which themselves control the rhythmic expression of downstream effector genes.

29.5 Clock genes in humans

Homologues of the clock genes isolated in rodents have been found in humans (Katzenberg *et al.* 1998), and the molecular devices underlying circadian rhythms will probably prove to be very similar, if not identical, in these different mammals. The genetic basis of circadian clocks in humans strongly suggests a link between clock gene mutations and diseases or disorders. Given the organization of the circadian system (input–pacemaker–output; see Fig. 29.2), such mutations could in theory lead to abnormalities in entrainment, pacemaker functions, or coupling of pacemaker to effector systems (Moore 1997).

Various syndromes affecting the circadian system have been identified (Moore 1997). In a few cases, a genetic origin could be demonstrated. Patients affected with the Smith–Magenis syndrome (SMS) present various symptoms, including mental retardation, behavioural abnormalities, and congenital anomalies, as well as sleep disturbances and abnormal melatonin production (Potocki *et al.* 2000). SMS is caused by a large hemizygous deletion of chromosome 17, band p11.2 (Chen *et al.* 1997). However, the specific gene whose deletion is responsible for the circadian troubles has yet to be identified.

A familial advanced sleep-phase syndrome (FASPS) has been observed in three families (Jones *et al.* 1999). The individuals affected by FASPS have a clock with a period that is constantly shorter than normal, as well as profound phase advance in sleep–wake, temperature, and melatonin rhythms. These phenotypes are strikingly similar to those observed in hamsters with a mutated gene for the casein kinase Iε (Lowrey *et al.* 2000) which suggests that FASPS is caused by a mutation in a gene important for the regulation of the clock.

A last example of the link between clock genes and circadian behaviour is provided by a single nucleotide polymorphism in the human *Clock* gene, which is associated with diurnal preference (that is, morningness–eveningness preference; see Katzenberg *et al.* 1998).

Although the genetic cause of SAD is not known yet, melatonin regulation appears to be unaffected in SAD patients. The defect might rather be at the level of clock regulation by afferent pathways involving NPY and serotonin (Partonen and Lönnqvist 1998). Understanding SAD and designing efficient treatments will undoubtedly benefit from studies on the genes and molecular mechanisms involved in the circadian clock.

Acknowledgements

We thank all the members of the Sassone–Corsi laboratory for helpful discussions. N.C. was supported by a Canadian Institutes of Health Research post-doctoral fellowship. Work in our laboratory is supported by grants from CNRS, INSERM, CHUR, Human Frontier Science Program, Organon Akzo/Nobel, Fondation pour la Recherche Médicale, and Association pour la Recherche sur le Cancer.

References

Albrecht, U., Sun, Z.S., Eichele, G., and Lee, C.C. (1997). A differential response of two putative mammalian circadian regulators, *mper1* and *mper2*, to light. *Cell* **91**:1055–64.

Blau, J. and Young, M.W. (1999). Cycling *vrille* expression is required for a functional Drosophila clock. *Cell* **99**:661–71.

Card, J.P. and Moore, R.Y. (1989). Organization of lateral geniculate-hypothalamic connections in the rat. *Journal of Comparative Neurology* **284**:135–47.

Ceriani, M.F., Darlington, T.K., Staknis, D., Mas, P., Petti, A.A., Weitz, C.J., *et al.* (1999). Light-dependent sequestration of TIMELESS by CRYPTOCHROME. *Science* **285**:553–6.

Cermakian, N. and Sassone–Corsi, P. (2000). Multilevel regulation of the circadian clock. *Nature Reviews Molecular Cell Biology* **1**:59–67.

Chen, K.S., Manian, P., Koeuth, T., Potocki, L., Zhao, Q., Chinault, A.C., *et al.* (1997). Homologous recombination of a flanking repeat gene cluster is a mechanism for a common contiguous gene deletion syndrome. *Nature Genetics* **17**:154–63.

Crosio, C., Cermakian, N., Allis, C.D., and Sassone–Corsi, P. (2000). Light induces chromatin modification in cells of the mammalian circadian clock. *Nature Neuroscience* **3**:1247-47.

Darlington, T.K., Wager–Smith, K., Ceriani, M.F., Staknis, D., Gekakis, N., Steeves, T.D.L., *et al.* (1998). Closing the circadian loop: CLOCK-induced transcription of its own inhibitors *per* and *tim*. *Science* **280**:1599–603.

Ding, J.M., Chen, D., Weber, E.T., Faiman, L.E., Rea, M.A., and Gillette, M.U. (1994). Resetting the biological clock: mediation of nocturnal circadian shifts by glutamate and NO. *Science* **266**:1713–17.

Dunlap, J.C. (1999). Molecular bases for circadian clocks. *Cell* **96**:271–90.

Emery, P., So, W.V., Kaneko, M., Hall, J.C., and Rosbash, M. (1998). CRY, a *Drosophila* clock and light-regulated cryptochrome, is a major contributor to circadian rhythm resetting and photosensitivity. *Cell* **95**:669–79.

Foulkes, N.S., Borjigin, J., Snyder, S.H., and Sassone–Corsi, P. (1997). Rhythmic transcription: the molecular basis of circadian melatonin synthesis. *Trends in Neurosciences* **20**:487–92.

Gekakis, N., Saez, L., Delahaye–Brown, A.M., Myers, M.P., Sehgal, A., Young, M.W., *et al.* (1995). Isolation of *timeless* by PER protein interaction: defective interaction between timeless protein and long-period mutant. *Science* **270**:811–15.

Ginty, D.D., Kornhauser, J.M., Thompson, M.A., Bading, H., Mayo, K.E., Takahashi, J.S., *et al.* (1993). Regulation of CREB phosphorylation in the suprachiasmatic nucleus by light and a circadian clock. *Science* **260**:238–41.

Glossop, N.R., Lyons, L.C., and Hardin, P.E. (1999). Interlocked feedback loops within the *Drosophila* circadian oscillator. *Science* **286**:766–8.

Hastings, M.H. (1997). Central clocking. *Trends in Neurosciences* **20**:459–64.

Huang, Z.J., Edery, I., and Rosbash, M. (1993). PAS is a dimerization domain common to Drosophila period and several transcription factors. *Nature* **364**:259–62.

Jin, X., Shearman, L.P., Weaver, D.R., Zylka, M.J., de Vries, G.J., and Reppert, S.M. (1999). A molecular mechanism regulating rhythmic output from the suprachiasmatic circadian clock. *Cell* **96**:57–68.

Jones, C.R., Campbell, S.S., Zone, S.E., Cooper, F., DeSano, A., Murphy, P.J., *et al.* (1999). Familial advanced sleep-phase syndrome: a short-period circadian rhythm variant in humans. *Nature Medicine* **5**:1062–5.

Katzenberg, D., Young, T., Finn, L., Lin, L., King, D.P., Takahashi, J.S., *et al.* (1998). A CLOCK polymorphism associated with human diurnal preference. *Sleep* **21**:569–76.

King, D.P., Zhao, Y., Sangoram, A.M., Wilsbacher, L.D., Tanaka, M., Antoch, M.P., *et al.* (1997). Positional cloning of the mouse circadian *Clock* gene. *Cell* **89**:641–53.

Konopka, R.J. and Benzer, S. (1971). Clock mutants of Drosophila melanogaster. *Proceedings of the National Academy of Sciences of the USA* **68**:2112–16.

Kornhauser, J.M., Nelson, D.E., Mayo, K.E., and Takahashi, J.S. (1990). Photic and circadian regulation of c-*fos* gene expression in the hamster suprachiasmatic nucleus. *Neuron* **5**:127–34.

Lee, C., Bae, K., and Edery, I. (1999). PER and TIM inhibit the DNA binding activity of a Drosophila CLOCK-CYC/dBMAL1 heterodimer without disrupting formation of the heterodimer: a basis for circadian transcription. *Molecular and Cellular Biology* **19**:5316–25.

Lee, K., Loros, J.J., and Dunlap, J.C. (2000). Interconnected feedback loops in the *Neurospora* circadian system. *Science* **289**:107–10.

Liu, C., Weaver, D.R., Jin, X., Shearman, L.P., Pieschl, R.L., Gribkoff, V.K., *et al.* (1997). Molecular dissection of two distinct actions of melatonin on the suprachiasmatic circadian clock. *Neuron* **19**:91–102.

Lowrey, P.L., Shimomura, K., Antoch, M.P., Yamazaki, S., Zemenides, P.D., Ralph, M.R., *et al.* (2000). Positional syntenic cloning and functional characterization of the mammalian circadian mutation tau. *Science* **288**:483–92.

Maywood, E.S., Mrosovsky, N., Field, M.D., and Hastings, M.H. (1999). Rapid down-regulation of mammalian period genes during behavioral resetting of the circadian clock. *Proceedings of the National Academy of Sciences of the USA* **96**:15211–16.

Moore, R.Y. (1997). Circadian rhythms: basic neurobiology and clinical applications. *Annual Review of Medicine* **48**:253–66.

Moore, R.Y. and Silver, R. (1998). Suprachiasmatic nucleus organization. *Chronobiology International* **15**:475–87.

Obrietan, K., Impey, S., and Storm, D.R. (1998). Light and circadian rhythmicity regulate MAP kinase activation in the suprachiasmatic nuclei. *Nature Neuroscience* **1**:693–700.

Partonen, T. and Lönnqvist, J. (1998). Seasonal affective disorder. *Lancet* **352**:1369–74.

Pickard, G.E. and Rea, M.A. (1997). Serotonergic innervation of the hypothalamic suprachiasmatic nucleus and photic regulation of circadian rhythms. *Biology of the Cell* **89**:513–23.

Pittendrigh, C.S. (1993). Temporal organization: reflections of a Darwinian clock-watcher. *Annual Review of Physiology* **55**:16–54.

Potocki, L., Glaze, D., Tan, D.X., Park, S.S., Kashork, C.D., Shaffer, L.G., *et al.* (2000). Circadian rhythm abnormalities of melatonin in Smith–Magenis syndrome. *Journal of Medical Genetics* **37**:428–33.

Price, J.L., Blau, J., Rothenfluh, A., Abodeely, M., Kloss, B., and Young, M.W. (1998). *double-time* is a novel Drosophila clock gene that regulates PERIOD protein accumulation. *Cell* **94**:83–95.

Renn, S.C., Park, J.H., Rosbash, M., Hall, J.C., and Taghert, P.H. (1999). A *pdf* neuropeptide gene mutation and ablation of PDF neurons each cause severe abnormalities of behavioral circadian rhythms in Drosophila. *Cell* **99**:791–802.

Ripperger, J.A., Shearman, L.P., Reppert, S.M., and Schibler, U. (2000). CLOCK, an essential pacemaker component, controls expression of the circadian transcription factor DBP. *Genes and Development* **14**:679–89.

Sassone–Corsi, P. (1998). Molecular clocks: mastering time by gene regulation. *Nature* **392**:871–4.

Shearman, L.P., Zylka, M.J., Weaver, D.R., Kolakowski Jr, L.F., and Reppert, S.M. (1997). Two *period* homologs: circadian expression and photic regulation in the suprachiasmatic nuclei. *Neuron* **19**:1261–9.

Shearman, L.P., Sriram, S., Weaver, D.R., Maywood, E.S., Chaves, I., Zheng, B., *et al.* (2000). Interacting molecular loops in the mammalian circadian clock. *Science* **288**:1013–19.

Zylka, M.J., Shearman, L.P., Weaver, D.R., and Reppert, S.M. (1998). Three *period* homologs in mammals: differential light responses in the suprachiasmatic circadian clock and oscillating transcripts outside of brain. *Neuron* **20**:1103–10.

Chapter 30

Future directions

Timo Partonen

30.1 Tasks

Since the first systematic description of winter SAD (Rosenthal *et al.* 1984), substantial research has been devoted to investigating the clinical picture and treating patients. However, there are still areas in which novel studies would be of great benefit. First, the ICD-10 diagnostic criteria for SAD remain provisional and need further validation as well as reference with the DSM-IV criteria. Studies of community-based samples will help estimate prevalence rates in different age ranges and latitudes of residence. Second, the aetiology of winter SAD seems far more complex than initially thought. Basic science is now providing important insights into the nature of SAD and valuable methods by which its genetic basis and pathogenesis can be addressed in more detail. These methods include physiological assessment such as examination of the properties of singularities, brain imaging techniques, and applications of molecular biology and genetics into medicine. Third, the mechanisms and sites of action of bright-light exposure await clarification in order for highly specific therapies and the optimal strategies for clinical management to be developed.

30.2 Singularities

Biological rhythms in body functions and behaviour allow living individuals to anticipate environmental changes. These rhythms are generated by inherited timekeeping mechanisms known as clocks (see the chapter by Campbell and Murphy). They are driven by signals from the individual's natural habitat in order to match the solar day and to reset their current phase relative to local time. They do not only measure the length of day but also generate the daily variation in activity. Their accuracy depends on individual response characteristics of these clocks, on which knowledge of time, physical activity, and state of health have a vital influence. Not only internal or social stimuli but also physical time givers can to a great extent modify complex behaviours such as eating, drinking, and sleeping in animals. These may have a marked effect on daily behaviour patterns in humans. In fact, throughout all our brief history of time, cycles of day and night have provided the basis for assessment of time of day and the length of day has yielded information about season.

It has been suggested that during evolution not only animals but also humans have developed an ability to detect and respond to changes in the photoperiod (Wehr *et al.* 1993). Based on analysis of responses to a range of experimental light–dark schedules, a variety of models have been formulated for the clocks measuring the length of the photoperiod. More experimental data on the response of the human circadian system are still needed for validation of models allowing the prediction of phase shifts to photic stimuli of any temporal pattern and any light intensity (Kronauer *et al.* 1999).

It is known that extensive phase shifts, advances, or delays, can be induced by exposing individuals to light near the time for body core temperature minimum. Exposure to bright light has also been shown to induce a physiological singularity, stopping the circadian clock (Jewett *et al.* 1991). The ability of a circadian system, such as the body clock, to reach a point of singularity seems to be a fundamental property of the circadian rhythms (Pedersen and Johnsson 1994). The phase singularity in biological systems may represent a cessation of individual oscillators or, alternatively, reflect a desynchronization of all the oscillators, bringing the biological system to a standstill.

The induction of a singularity in the circadian clock may also become a useful option for treatment. Exposing individuals with a phase singularity to a timed pulse of light has a potential to result in a phase shift of a great magnitude. By this means, extensive phase shifts could be achieved in a notably short period of time and used effectively in the treatment of chronobiological disorders, including winter SAD, for cases in which there are disabling advances or delays of the phase of circadian rhythms.

30.3 **Fractals**

Functional changes in brain activity can be visualized with quantitative electroencephalogram (qEEG), magnetoencephalography (MEG), functional magnetic resonance imaging and spectroscopy (fMRI and MRS), and tomography using serial X-ray computations, positron emission, or single-photon emission (cine CT, PET, or SPET). Research on winter SAD has also benefited from this universal development of brain imaging (see the chapter by Vasile and Anderson).

It is well known that healthy biological systems show spatial and temporal heterogeneity. The establishment that anatomical structures at different spatial scales or physiological processes at different time scales are related to one another reflects a fractal property (Kuikka and Tiihonen 1998). It makes the subject more capable of meeting the unpredictable environment of daily life and gives hence an adaptive advantage. The lack of sufficient heterogeneity and adaptation has been observed in many brain disorders but may also be found in mental disorders.

Nuclear medicine, with its evolving techniques, will soon be used for a variety of diagnostic purposes, as well as for targeting treatments in clinical practice. The method of fractal analysis may be of substantial help with the interpretation of complex data consisting of numerous observations on spatial and temporal changes such as brain images and circadian rhythm data. It provides us with tools to describe, quantify, and suggest mechanisms that reduce the spatial and temporal variability in biological systems.

30.4 **Molecules**

Research using the methods of molecular biology and genetics has been developing fast and is about to step into the post-genomic era with the near completion of the mapping of the human genome. Additional studies will discover whether the present polymorphisms of the known genes or some other genetic contributions explain differences in the phenotype of winter SAD and are clinically important (see the chapter by Enoch and Goldman). Studies on the function of single or a group of genes are likely to contribute to a better understanding of the basis of winter SAD from physiological to molecular levels. Of key significance may well be the unique response to light exposure among these patients.

In the course of evolution, selection for or against the unique response to light exposure may have resulted in differences in the circadian clock function. It may have affected the temporal organization of circadian rhythms and made the body clock more or less flexible to stimuli. However, the extent of individual responses to light exposure seems to be controlled by a processor separate from the principal circadian oscillator. This phenotypic difference is partly genetically determined and there is a significant degree of heritability, as shown in some animal species. The linkage of the phenotypes of winter SAD to the corresponding genotypes would benefit from the assessment of valid endophenotypes and would require the best available instruments to fulfil the task.

References

Jewett, M.E., Kronauer, R.E., and Czeisler, C.A. (1991) Light-induced suppression of endogenous circadian amplitude in humans. *Nature* **350**:59–62.

Kronauer, R.E., Forger, D.B., and Jewett, M.E. (1999) Quantifying human circadian pacemaker response to brief, extended, and repeated light stimuli over the phototopic range. *J Biol Rhythms* **14**:500–15.

Kuikka, J. and Tiihonen, J. (1998) Fractal analysis — a new approach in brain receptor imaging. *Ann Med* **30**:242–8.

Pedersen, M. and Johnsson, A. (1994) A study of the singularities in a mathematical model for circadian rhythms. *Biosystems* **33**:193–201.

Rosenthal, N.E., Sack, D.A., Gillin, J.C., Lewy, A.J., Goodwin, F.K., Davenport, Y., *et al.* (1984) Seasonal affective disorder: a description of the syndrome and preliminary findings with light therapy. *Arch Gen Psychiatry* **41**:72–80.

Wehr, T.A., Moul, D.E., Barbato, G., Giesen, H.A., Seidel, J.A., Barker, C., *et al.* (1993) Conservation of photoperiod-responsive mechanisms in humans. *Am J Physiol* **265**:R846–57.

Appendix

Useful information can be found at the following web sites:

- the home page of SADAssociation, a support organization for SAD, at *http://www.sada.org.uk/*

- the home page of the National Electronic Library for Mental Health at *http://www.nelmh.org/*

- a summary of the report of the Canadian Consensus Group on SAD at *http://www.fhs.mc-master.ca/direct/depress/sad2.html*

- The Cochrane Library, an electronic publication, at *http://www.update-software.com/cochrane/cochrane-frame.html*

- the home page of the Society for Light Treatment and Biological Rhythms at *http://www.sltbr.org/*

- professional instruments for the assessment of SAD at *http://www.cet.org/professional_-assessment_instrume.htm*

- the home page of the Centre for Evidence-Based Mental Health at *http://www.cebmh.com/*

Index